Medications and Sleep

Guest Editor

TIMOTHY ROEHRS, PhD

SLEEP MEDICINE CLINICS

www.sleep.theclinics.com

December 2010 • Volume 5 • Number 4

SAUNDERS an imprint of ELSEVIER, Inc.

W.B. SAUNDERS COMPANY
A Division of Elsevier Inc.

1600 John F. Kennedy Boulevard • Suite 1800 • Philadelphia, PA 19103-2899

http://www.sleep.theclinics.com

SLEEP MEDICINE CLINICS Volume 5, Number 4
December 2010, ISSN 1556-407X, ISBN-13: 978-1-4377-2496-7

Editor: Sarah E. Barth
Developmental Editor: Donald Mumford

Sleep Medicine Clinics (ISSN 1556-407X) is published quarterly by Elsevier Inc., 360 Park Avenue South, New York, NY 10010-1710. Months of issue are March, June, September and December. Business and Editorial Offices: 1600 John F. Kennedy Blvd., Ste. 1800, Philadelphia, PA 19103-2899. Customer Service Office: 3251 Riverport Lane, Maryland Heights, MO 63043. Periodicals postage paid at New York, NY and additional mailing offices. Subscription prices are $161.00 per year (US individuals), $80.00 (US residents), $346.00 (US institutions), $198.00 (foreign individuals), $111.00 (foreign residents), and $381.00 (foreign institutions). Foreign air speed delivery is included in all *Clinics* subscription prices. All prices are subject to change without notice. **POSTMASTER:** Send change of address to *Sleep Medicine Clinics*, Elsevier Health Sciences Division, Subscription Customer Service, 3251 Riverport Lane, Maryland Heights, MO 63043 Customer Service, (orders, claims, online, change of address): **Elsevier Health Sciences Division, Subscription Customer Service, 3251 Riverport Lane, Maryland Heights, MO 63043. Tel: 1-800-654-2452 (U.S. and Canada); 314-447-8871 (outside U.S. and Canada). Fax: 314-447-8029. E-mail: journals customerservice-usa@elsevier.com (for print support); journalsonlinesupport-usa@elsevier.com (for online support).**

Reprints. For copies of 100 or more of articles in this publication, please contact the Commercial Reprints Department, Elsevier Inc., 360 Park Avenue South, New York, NY 10010-1710. Tel.: 212-633-3812; Fax: 212-462-1935; E-mail: reprints@elsevier.com.

Printed and bound in the United Kingdom
Transferred to Digital Print 2011

GOAL STATEMENT

The goal of *Sleep Clinics of North America* is to keep practicing physicians up to date with current clinical practice by providing timely articles reviewing the state of the art in patient care.

ACCREDITATION

The *Sleep Clinics of North America* is planned and implemented in accordance with the Essential Areas and Policies of the Accreditation Council for Continuing Medical Education (ACCME) through the joint sponsorship of the University of Virginia School of Medicine and Elsevier. The University of Virginia School of Medicine is accredited by the ACCME to provide continuing medical education for physicians.

The University of Virginia School of Medicine designates this educational activity for a maximum of 15 *AMA PRA Category 1 Credits*™ for each issue, 60 credits per year. Physicians should only claim credit commensurate with the extent of their participation in the activity.

The American Medical Association has determined that physicians not licensed in the US who participate in this CME activity are eligible for a maximum of 15 *AMA PRA Category 1 Credits*™ for each issue, 60 credits per year.

Credit can be earned by reading the text material, taking the CME examination online at http://www.theclinics.com/home/cme, and completing the evaluation. After taking the test, you will be required to review any and all incorrect answers. Following completion of the test and evaluation, your credit will be awarded and you may print your certificate.

FACULTY DISCLOSURE/CONFLICT OF INTEREST

The University of Virginia School of Medicine, as an ACCME accredited provider, endorses and strives to comply with the Accreditation Council for Continuing Medical Education (ACCME) Standards of Commercial Support, Commonwealth of Virginia statutes, University of Virginia policies and procedures, and associated federal and private regulations and guidelines on the need for disclosure and monitoring of proprietary and financial interests that may affect the scientific integrity and balance of content delivered in continuing medical education activities under our auspices.

The University of Virginia School of Medicine requires that all CME activities accredited through this institution be developed independently and be scientifically rigorous, balanced and objective in the presentation/discussion of its content, theories and practices.

All authors/editors participating in an accredited CME activity are expected to disclose to the readers relevant financial relationships with commercial entities occurring within the past 12 months (such as grants or research support, employee, consultant, stock holder, member of speakers bureau, etc.). The University of Virginia School of Medicine will employ appropriate mechanisms to resolve potential conflicts of interest to maintain the standards of fair and balanced education to the reader. Questions about specific strategies can be directed to the Office of Continuing Medical Education, University of Virginia School of Medicine, Charlottesville, Virginia.

The faculty and staff of the University of Virginia Office of Continuing Medical Education have no financial affiliations to disclose.

The authors/editors listed below have identified no professional or financial affiliations for themselves or their spouse/partner:
Sarah Barth (Acquisitions Editor); Helen A. Baghodoyan, PhD; Cynthia Brown, MD (Test Author); Sachiko Chikahisa, PhD; Maryann C. Deak, MD; Ehren R. Dodson, PhD; Ralph Lydic, PhD; Mark W. Mahowald, MD; Hashir Majid, MD; William H. Moorcroft, PhD; Seiji Nishino, MD, PhD; Francoise J. Roux, MD, PhD; Noriaki Sakai, DVM, PhD; Carlos H. Schenck, MD; and Christopher J. Watson, PhD.

The authors/editors listed below identified the following professional or financial affiliations for themselves or their spouse/partner:
D. Troy Curry, MD is a researcher for Pfizer, Merck & Co., Somaxon, Evotec, Actelion, Vanda, Neurogen, Sanofi-Aventis, Ventus, Respironics, Jazz Pharmaceuticals; has received honoraria from and is on the speakers bureau for Glaxo-Smith Kline.
Robert N. Glidewell, PsyD is employed by Lynn Institute for Healthcare Research and LLC, Aspen Pointe; and owns stock in Behavioral Sleep Medicine.
Janine M. Hall-Porter, PhD is an industry funded research/investigator for Pfizer, Merck & Co., Somaxon, Evotec, Actelion, Vanda, Neurogen, Sanofi-Aventis, Ventus, Respironics, and Jazz Pharmaceuticals.
Max Hirshkowitz, PhD, D ABSM is an industry funded research/investigator, is a consultant, and serves on the Speakers' Bureau for Sanofi-Aventis, Takeda, and Cephalon.
Meir H. Kryger, MD is a consultant for Merck and Purdue, and is an industry funded research/investigator for Respironics and Resmed.
Andrew D. Krystal, MD, MS receives grant/research support from NIH, Sanofi-Aventis, Cephalon, GlaxoSmithKline, Merck, Neurocrine, Pfizer, Sepracor, Somaxon, Takeda, Transcept, Respironics, Neurogen, Evotec, Astellas, Abbott, and Neuronetics; and is a consultant for Abbott, Actelion, Arena, Astellas, Axiom, AstraZeneca, BMS, Cephalon, Eli Lilly, GlaxoSmithKline, Jazz, Johnson and Johnson, King, Merck, Neurocrine, Neurogen, Neuronetics, Novartis, Organon, Ortho-McNeil-Janssen, Pfizer, Respironics, Roche, Sanofi-Aventis, Sepracor, Somaxon, Takeda, Transcept, Kingsdown Inc., and CHDI.
Teofilo Lee-Chiong, Jr, MD (Consulting Editor) is on the Advisory Board/Committee for the American College of Chest Physicians and the American Academy of Sleep Medicine.
Timothy Roehrs, PhD (Guest Editor) is a consultant for Sanofi, Takada, and Evotec.
Thomas Roth, PhD receives grant support and is a consultant and speaker for Cephalon, Sanofi, and Sepracor; receives grant support and is a consultant for Aventis, GSK, Merck, Neurocrine, Pfizer, SchoeringPlough, Somaxon, Somnus, Syrex, Takeda, TransOral/Granscept, Ventus, Wyeth, and Xenoport; and is a consultant for Abbott, Accadia, Acogolix, Acorda, Actelion, Addrenex, Alchemers, Alza, Ancel, Arena, AstraZenca, AVER, Bayer, BMS, BTG, Cypress, Dove, Eisai, Elan, Eli Lilly, Evotec, Forest, Hypnion, Impax, Intec, Intra-Cellular, Jazz, J&J, King, Lundbeck, McNeil, MediciNova, Neurim, Neurogen, Novartis, Ocera, Orexo, Organon, Otsuka, Prestwick, Proctor and Gamble, Purdue, Resteva, Roche, Servier, Shire, Steady Sleep Rx, Vanda, Vivometrics, and Yamanuchi.
Paula K. Schweitzer, PhD is an industry funded research/investigator for Pfizer, Merck, Actelion, Vanda, Neurogen, Somaxon, and Ventus.
James K. Walsh, PhD is an industry funded research/investigator for Pfizer, Merck & Co., Somaxon, Evotec, Actelion, Vanda, Neurogen, Sanofi-Aventis, Ventus, Respironics, and Jazz Pharmaceuticals, and has provided consulting services to Pfizer, Sanofi-Aventis, Cephalon, Schering-Plough/Organon, Neurocrine, Takeda America, Actelion, Sepracor, Jazz, Respironics, Transcept, Neurogen, GlaxoSmithKline, Somaxon, Eli Lilly, Evotec, Merck, Kingsdown, Vanda, Ventus, and Somnus.
John W. Winkelman, MD, PhD is a consultant for Covance, GSK, Impax Laboratories, Luitpold Pharmaceuticals, Neurogen, Pfizer, and Zeo Inc.; is an industry funded research/investigator for GSK and Sepracor; and is on the Speakers' Bureau for Sanofi-Aventis and Sepracor.
Phyllis C. Zee, MD, PhD is a consultant for Philips/Respironics and Sanofi-Aventis, is on the Advisory Committee/Board for Merck, and is an industry funded research/investigator for Takeda.

Disclosure of Discussion of Non-FDA Approved Uses for Pharmaceutical Products and/or Medical Devices

The University of Virginia School of Medicine, as an ACCME provider, requires that all faculty presenters identify and disclose any off-label uses for pharmaceutical and medical device products. The University of Virginia School of Medicine recommends that each physician fully review all the available data on new products or procedures prior to clinical use.

TO ENROLL

To enroll in the Sleep Clinics of North America Continuing Medical Education program, call customer service at 1-800-654-2452 or visit us online at www.theclinics.com/home/cme. The CME program is available to subscribers for an additional fee of $114.00.

Sleep Medicine Clinics

RELATED INTEREST

Medical Clinics of North America, May 2010 (Vol. 94, No. 3)
Sleep Medicine
Christian Guilleminault, MD, DBiol, *Guest Editor*

THE CLINICS ARE NOW AVAILABLE ONLINE!

Access your subscription at:
www.theclinics.com

Contributors

CONSULTING EDITOR

TEOFILO LEE-CHIONG Jr, MD
Professor of Medicine and Chief, Division
of Sleep Medicine, National Jewish Health;
Associate Professor of Medicine, University
of Colorado Denver School of Medicine,
Denver, Colorado

GUEST EDITOR

TIMOTHY ROEHRS, PhD
Director of Research, Department of Internal
Medicine, Sleep Disorders and Research
Center, Henry Ford Hospital, Henry Ford
Health System; Professor, Department
of Psychiatry and Behavioral Neuroscience,
Wayne State University, School of Medicine,
Detroit, Michigan

AUTHORS

HELEN A. BAGHDOYAN, PhD
Professor, Department of Anesthesiology,
University of Michigan, Ann Arbor, Michigan

SACHIKO CHIKAHISA, PhD
Visiting Assistant Professor, Sleep and
Circadian Neurobiology Laboratory,
Stanford University School of Medicine,
Palo Alto; Assistant Professor, Department
of Integrative Physiology, Institute of Health
Biosciences, The University of Tokushima
Graduate School, Tokushima, Japan

D. TROY CURRY, MD
Sleep Medicine Associate, Sleep Medicine
and Research Center, St Luke's Hospital,
Chesterfield, Missouri

MARYANN C. DEAK, MD
Clinical Instructor in Medicine, Division
of Sleep Medicine, Department of Medicine,
Harvard School of Medicine, Boston,
Massachusetts

EHREN R. DODSON, PhD
Department of Neurology, Circadian Rhythms
and Sleep Center, Northwestern University,
Chicago, Illinois

ROBERT N. GLIDEWELL, PsyD
Director, Sleep Medicine and Research
Program, Lynn Institute for Healthcare
Research, Colorado Springs,
Colorado

JANINE M. HALL-PORTER, PhD
Research Associate, Sleep Medicine
and Research Center, St Luke's Hospital,
Chesterfield, Missouri

MAX HIRSHKOWITZ, PhD, D ABSM
Tenured Associate Professor, Baylor College
of Medicine, Department of Medicine and
Menninger Department of Psychiatry;
Director, MED VAMC Sleep Disorders and
Research Center, Houston, Texas

ANDREW D. KRYSTAL, MD, MS
Director, Insomnia and Sleep Research Program; Professor of Psychiatry and Behavioral Sciences, Duke University School of Medicine, Duke University Medical Center, Durham, North Carolina

MEIR H. KRYGER, MD
Clinical Professor, Department of Medicine, University of Connecticut School of Medicine, Farmington; Director of Research and Education, Gaylord Sleep Medicine, Wallingford, Connecticut

TEOFILO LEE-CHIONG Jr, MD
Professor of Medicine and Chief, Division of Sleep Medicine, National Jewish Health; Associate Professor of Medicine, University of Colorado Denver School of Medicine, Denver, Colorado

RALPH LYDIC, PhD
Professor, Department of Anesthesiology, University of Michigan, Ann Arbor, Michigan

MARK W. MAHOWALD, MD
Professor, Department of Neurology, Minnesota Regional Sleep Disorders Center, Hennepin County Medical Center; Department of Psychiatry (CHS) and Neurology (MWM), University of Minnesota Medical School, Minneapolis, Minnesota

HASHIR MAJID, MD
Assistant Professor of Medicine, Section of Pulmonary, Critical Care and Sleep Medicine, Department of Medicine, Baylor College of Medicine, Houston, Texas

WILLIAM H. MOORCROFT, PhD
Founder and Chief Consultant, Northern Colorado Sleep Consultants, Fort Collins, Colorado

SEIJI NISHINO, MD, PhD
Professor, Sleep and Circadian Neurobiology Laboratory, Stanford University School of Medicine, Palo Alto, California

TIMOTHY ROEHRS, PhD
Director of Research, Department of Internal Medicine, Sleep Disorders and Research Center, Henry Ford Hospital, Henry Ford Health System; Professor, Department of Psychiatry and Behavioral Neuroscience, Wayne State University, School of Medicine, Detroit, Michigan

THOMAS ROTH, PhD
Director, Department of Internal Medicine, Sleep Disorders and Research Center, Henry Ford Hospital, Henry Ford Health System; Professor, Department of Psychiatry and Behavioral Neuroscience, Wayne State University School of Medicine, Detroit, Michigan

FRANCOISE J. ROUX, MD, PhD
Assistant Professor of Medicine, Section of Pulmonary and Critical Care Medicine, Yale Center for Sleep Medicine, Yale University School of Medicine, New Haven, Connecticut

NORIAKI SAKAI, DVM, PhD
Postdoctoral Fellow, Sleep and Circadian Neurobiology Laboratory, Stanford University School of Medicine, Palo Alto, California

CARLOS H. SCHENCK, MD
Professor, Department of Psychiatry, Minnesota Regional Sleep Disorders Center, Hennepin County Medical Center; Department of Psychiatry (CHS) and Neurology (MWM), University of Minnesota Medical School, Minneapolis, Minnesota

PAULA K. SCHWEITZER, PhD
Sleep Medicine and Research Center, St Luke's Hospital, Chesterfield, Missouri

JAMES K. WALSH, PhD
Executive Director and Senior Scientist, Sleep Medicine and Research Center, St Luke's Hospital, Chesterfield; Adjunct Professor, Department of Psychology, Saint Louis University, St Louis, Missouri

CHRISTOPHER J. WATSON, PhD
Research Investigator, Department of Anesthesiology, University of Michigan, Ann Arbor, Michigan

JOHN W. WINKELMAN, MD, PhD
Associate Professor in Psychiatry, Brigham and Women's Hospital, Harvard School of Medicine, Boston, Massachusetts

PHYLLIS C. ZEE, MD, PhD
Department of Neurology, Circadian Rhythms and Sleep Center, Northwestern University, Chicago, Illinois

Contents

primary sleep disorders, no other functional or clinical significance is found with these changes. Selective slow wave sleep deprivation does not produce specific impairment and insomniacs do not show consistent deficiencies in slow wave sleep. Given the observation of these normal reductions in slow wave sleep with age, the absence of functional impairment associated with specific slow wave sleep deprivation, and no consistent sleep stage changes reported in insomnia, the functional and clinical significance of drug-related changes in stage 3 and 4 sleep, either reduction or enhancement, remains to be shown.

Comorbid insomnia has a pervasive role in the course of general medical and psychiatric illness. This article reviews the literature on the reciprocal interactions between insomnia and medical and psychiatric illness and on pharmacotherapy approaches for comorbid insomnia. The focus is on several of the comorbidities that are most common or relevant for the sleep clinician, including major depressive disorder, chronic pain, obstructive sleep apnea, chronic obstructive pulmonary disease, end-stage renal failure, dementia, alcohol use disorders, and comorbid insomnia during terminal illness.

Therapeutics for Sleep-disordered Breathing   647

Francoise J. Roux and Meir H. Kryger

Obstructive sleep apnea (OSA) is a common disorder, and obesity is a known risk factor for its development. Continuous positive airway pressure (CPAP) therapy is the standard treatment in OSA but is not always well accepted by the patients, partly because of its pressure-related side effects. Daytime hypersomnia is not always present in patients with OSA, and this subgroup of patients is even less likely to accept CPAP therapy. As a result, the long-term compliance with CPAP can vary between individuals. In addition, CPAP may not completely alleviate the symptoms associated with OSA, such as daytime hypersomnia. This article reviews the established evidence supporting medical therapy as an alternative to CPAP for OSA. Despite multiple trials with various medications, the current data do not support any particular pharmacologic treatment that could be significantly beneficial, suggesting that the pathophysiology underlying OSA is multifactorial and requires a better understanding to develop an effective medication.

Therapeutics of Narcolepsy   659

Hashir Majid and Max Hirshkowitz

Narcolepsy, an uncommon neurologic disorder, afflicts approximately 1 in 2000 individuals in the United States. Although management has improved significantly, especially with use of modafinil and sodium oxybate, impairment of function and quality of life persists in a considerable number of patients. Current therapeutic approaches are based on symptomatic relief and are often associated with undesirable side effects. This article describes the monoaminergic, cholinergic, and GABAergic systems and describes narcolepsy medications that work through these systems. The recently discovered orexin/hypocretin system is also described. The authors conclude that potential hypocretin-based therapy seems to hold promise for the future.

The Pharmacologic Management of Restless Legs Syndrome and Periodic Leg Movement Disorder   675

Maryann C. Deak and John W. Winkelman

Several essential principles should be considered in determining appropriate treatment of restless legs syndrome (RLS), such as potential secondary causes of RLS, timing and frequency of RLS symptoms, and impact of activity level. Different classes of medication have been used in the treatment of RLS, including both dopaminergic and non-dopaminergic agents. Periodic limb movements of sleep (PLMS) are a polysomnographic finding of stereotyped repetitive movements of the legs during sleep, which are present in more than 80% of RLS patients. Periodic limb movement disorder (PLMD) is defined as the presence of PLMS in patients with otherwise unexplained hypersomnia or insomnia. The diagnosis of PLMS can only be made after other sleep disorders have been excluded. Pharmacologic therapy of primary RLS, secondary RLS, and PLMD are discussed in this article.

Foreword

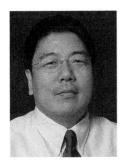

Teofilo Lee-Chiong Jr, MD
Consulting Editor

The internet is a tremendous source of instant information (and disinformation). Anyone who desires to learn about medications and their effects on sleep, including the drug therapy of insomnia, can easily, by a few simple keystrokes, move freely among an almost countless number of web portals. Admittedly, many of the data are unverified and many claims are unsupported by evidence. Nonetheless, what follows is a snapshot of the Internet taken on the morning of September 23, 2010 at 09:52-10:23 Mountain Time. Anyone who had access to the www. at that time would have read that:

0 Botanical compounds demonstrated to be consistently effective for treating insomnia

1 Serotonin antagonist and reuptake inhibitor drugs approved for use in insomnia

2 Melatonin receptor subtypes present in humans and other mammals

5 Percentage of clinical cases of chronic insomnia diagnosed as paradoxical insomnia

7 Hours of sleep an adult gets each night

8 Benzodiazepine receptor agonists specifically approved by the FDA for treatment of insomnia

10 FDA-approved agents for the treatment of insomnia

11 Longest recorded time a human had stayed awake (in days)

15 Percentage of adults developing acute adjustment insomnia during a 1-year period

25 Years an average adult sleeps during a lifetime

30 Percentage of adults suffering from chronic insomnia

90 Normal sleep efficiency (percentage)

484 Results on pubmed.gov on search term "cognitive behavioral therapy for insomnia"

1395 Results on pubmed.gov on search term "medications for insomnia"

263,000 Internet hits on "cognitive behavioral therapy for insomnia"

523,000 Internet hits on "melatonin for insomnia"

2,720,000 Internet hits on "medications for insomnia"

101,000,000 Search results for "insomnia" found on Google.com.

Needless to say, the greatest challenge of the next decade and for the next generation of soon-to-be-adults is discriminating between established, emerging, and fabricated science; distinguishing fact from fallacy; and recognizing helpful advice from deceitful deception. Unfortunately, the Internet, where everyone claims to be an authority, guru, expert, master, or specialist, and where opinion without reflection flows unfettered by accountability is *not* the place to start learning how to do so.

Teofilo Lee-Chiong Jr, MD
Division of Sleep Medicine
National Jewish Health
University of Colorado Denver School of Medicine
1400 Jackson Street, Room J221
Denver, CO 60206, USA

E-mail address:
Lee-ChiongT@njc.org

doi:10.1016/j.jsmc.2010.09.004

sleep.theclinics.com

Sleep Med Clin 5 (2010) xi
doi:10.1016/j.jsmc.2010.09.001
1556-407X/10/$ — see front matter © 2010 Elsevier Inc. All rights reserved.

Preface
Medications and Sleep

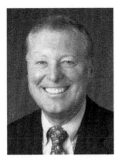

Timothy Roehrs, PhD
Guest Editor

Welcome to this issue of *Sleep Medicine Clinics* on the topic of Medications and Sleep. Any medication that crosses the blood-brain barrier carries the potential to alter sleep. Effects on sleep, either disruptive or therapeutic, may include alterations in the speed of sleep onset, the continuity of sleep, or the duration of sleep. Effects on sleep stages, often referred to as sleep architecture, may include changes in the normal age-related amounts of various sleep stages, or the ultradian rhythm of sleep, that is, the 90- to 120-min cycling through non-REM and REM sleep. Drug-induced changes in sleep and/or sleep stage architecture do not necessarily imply a disturbance of sleep. In some cases, the changes may be therapeutic, while in other cases, they may be benign or, at the least, not well understood. As clearly indicated in the first article by Watson et al, the complexity and range of neurobiologic mechanisms identified as controlling or influencing sleep and wake are the basis on which the many drugs discussed in this issue, with varying therapeutic targets and biological mechanisms, can affect sleep and wake.

The articles of the first half of this issue focus on the pharmacology of drug classes, their effects on sleep wake processes and theoretical discussions regarding how to assess hypnotic efficacy and safety, and the functional significance of sleep stage alterations. In Part 2, pharmacologic therapeutics for the major sleep disorders are described. These articles detail the major features of the various sleep disorders and then present various drugs used to treat the disorders. It is our hope that this issue will be informative and useful for both the relatively new sleep disorders practitioner and the more experienced practitioner, as well as for the clinical researcher.

Timothy Roehrs, PhD
Department of Internal Medicine
Sleep Disorders and Research Center
Henry Ford Hospital
Henry Ford Health System
2799 West Grand Boulevard, CFP-3
Detroit, MI 48202, USA

Department of Psychiatry and Behavioral Neuroscience
Wayne State University, School of Medicine
2751 East Jefferson
Detroit, MI 48207, USA

E-mail address:
Troehrs1@hfhs.org

Sleep Med Clin 5 (2010) xiii
doi:10.1016/j.jsmc.2010.09.003
1556-407X/10/$ — see front matter © 2010 Elsevier Inc. All rights reserved.

Neuropharmacology of Sleep and Wakefulness

Christopher J. Watson, PhD, Helen A. Baghdoyan, PhD, Ralph Lydic, PhD*

KEYWORDS

- Neurotransmitters • Receptors • Translational research
- Drug development

Sleep states are comprised of a constellation of physiologic and behavioral traits, and the mechanisms by which sedative-hypnotic medications alter these traits remain unclear. Drugs that enhance states of sleep also alter autonomic physiology, behavior, cognition, and affect. The complexities of brain neurochemistry and the extensive neural circuits regulating levels of behavioral arousal contribute to the present inability to understand exactly how sedative-hypnotics promote sleep. An additional complexity is that many sedative-hypnotic drugs have behavioral state-specific actions. For example, some sedative-hypnotic drugs promote the non-rapid eye movement (NREM) phase of sleep at the expense of decreasing the rapid eye movement (REM) phase of sleep. In spite of the foregoing limitations, there has been progress in developing sleep medications that maximize desired actions such as rapid sleep onset, minimal next day effect, low or no abuse potential, and creation of a drug-induced state that is indistinguishable from physiologic sleep. To date, however, no sedative-hypnotic produces all of these desired effects.

Rational drug design is an approach that has been successful in the development of antibiotic medications. Rational drug development of sedative-hypnotic medications is an approach based on understanding the receptor-binding properties of a molecule and how a molecule alters ligand binding, neurotransmitter synthesis, release, reuptake, and degradation. All of the foregoing cellular mechanisms can then be interpreted in the context of the overall drug effect. For sedative-hypnotic medications the desired action is, of course, promoting a safe and restorative sleep-like state. This article and **Fig. 1** provide an overview of neurotransmitters and brain regions currently known to modulate states of sleep and wakefulness. This overview of sleep neuropharmacology can be read as a précis of a recent book chapter[1] and interested readers are referred elsewhere for detailed reviews on sleep.[2–8]

γ-AMINOBUTYRIC ACID

The major inhibitory neurotransmitter in the brain is γ-aminobutyric acid (GABA), and activation of $GABA_A$ receptors causes neuronal inhibition by increasing chloride ion conductance. Because of their powerful inhibitory effects, $GABA_A$ receptors are the targets of most sedative-hypnotic and general anesthetic drugs. $GABA_A$ receptors exist as multiple subtypes[9] and these subtypes are differentially located throughout the brain.[10] The differences in clinical effects caused by various benzodiazepine (eg, diazepam) and nonbenzodiazepine (eg, eszopiclone) sedative-hypnotics are attributed to the relative selectivity of these drugs

Disclosure Statement: This work supported by National Institutes of Health grants: HL40881, HL65272, HL57120, MH45361, and the Department of Anesthesiology. This work was not an industry-supported study and the authors have no financial conflicts of interest.
Department of Anesthesiology, University of Michigan, 7433 Medical Sciences Building I, 1150 West Medical Center Drive, Ann Arbor, MI 48109-5615, USA
* Corresponding author.
E-mail address: rlydic@umich.edu

Sleep Med Clin 5 (2010) 513–528
doi:10.1016/j.jsmc.2010.08.003

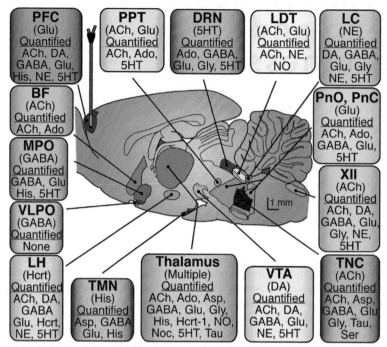

Fig. 1. Brain regions modulating sleep and wakefulness. The rat brain (sagittal view; *Modified from* Paxinos G, Watson C. The rat brain in stereotaxic coordinates. 6th edition. New York: Academic Press, 2007.) schematizes the location, shape, and size of some brain regions that regulate sleep and wakefulness. The microdialysis probe is drawn to scale and is shown sampling from the prefrontal cortex. **Key:** brain region name-bold print; major neurotransmitters used for signaling to other brain regions-in parentheses; neurochemical analytes relevant for arousal-state control that have been measured in that brain region-listed under the header "Quantified". ACh, acetylcholine; Ado, adenosine; Asp, aspartate; BF, basal forebrain; DA, dopamine; DRN, dorsal raphé nucleus; GABA, g-aminobutyric acid; Glu, glutamate; Gly, glycine; His, histamine; Hcrt, hypocretin; 5HT, serotonin; LC, locus coeruleus; LDT, laterodorsal tegmental nucleus; LH, lateral hypothalamus; MPO, medial preoptic area; NE, norepinephrine; NO, nitric oxide; Noc, nociceptin; PFC, prefrontal cortex; PPT, pedunculopontine tegmental nucleus; PnC, pontine reticular formation, caudal part; PnO, pontine reticular formation, oral part; Ser, serine; TMN, tuberomamillary nucleus; TNC, trigeminal nucleus complex; Tau, taurine; VLPO, ventrolateral preoptic area; VTA, ventral tegmental area; XII, hypoglossal nucleus. (*From* Watson CJ, Baghdoyan HA, Lydic R. A neurochemical perspective on states of consciousness. In: Suppressing the Mind: Anesthetic Modulation of Memory and Consciousness: Edited by A.G. Hudetz and R.A. Pearce, Springer/Humana Press; 2010. p. 33–80; with permission.)

for different GABA$_A$ receptor subtypes.[10] The complexity imparted by the numerous GABA$_A$ receptor subtypes is humbling. Although there is detailed knowledge about the many subunit isoforms that comprise GABA$_A$ receptor subtypes,[9] information is lacking about which of the many possible subtypes actually are expressed in specific brain regions,[11–13] and which subtypes are localized synaptically verses extrasynaptically.[14] Extrasynaptically localized GABA$_A$ receptors possess a delta subunit and have particular relevance for sleep medicine.[15,16]

A better understanding of the in vivo characteristics and anatomic localization of GABA$_A$ receptor subtypes will contribute to rational drug development. The preclinical studies described in this section illustrate the complexity of the problem and provide examples of how the effects of

GABAergic drugs on behavior vary as a function of brain region. For example, although systemic administration of GABAmimetic drugs promotes sleep, sedation, or general anesthesia, enhancing GABAergic transmission within the pontine reticular formation actually increases wakefulness and decreases sleep. The pontine reticular formation is part of the ascending reticular activating system and contributes to the generation of REM sleep. Direct administration into the pontine reticular formation of drugs that increase GABAergic transmission increases wakefulness and inhibits sleep.[17–20] Similarly, pharmacologically increasing the concentration of endogenous GABA within the pontine reticular formation increases the time required for isoflurane to induce general anesthesia.[21] Consistent with this finding are data showing that endogenous GABA levels in the pontine reticular formation are greater during wakefulness than during REM sleep[22] or during the loss of wakefulness caused by isoflurane (**Fig. 2**).[21] Inhibiting GABAergic signaling at $GABA_A$ receptors within the pontine reticular formation causes an increase in REM sleep and a decrease in wakefulness.[18,19,23,24] Likewise, decreasing extracellular GABA levels in the pontine reticular formation of rat decreases wakefulness and increases sleep,[20] and shortens the time required for isoflurane to induce loss of consciousness.[21] Furthermore, blocking $GABA_A$ receptors in the pontine reticular formation increases time needed to regain wakefulness after isoflurane anesthesia.[18] Considered together, these data demonstrate a wakefulness-promoting role for GABA in the pontine reticular formation.

In brain regions containing neurons that promote wakefulness, GABAergic inhibition has been shown to cause an increase in sleep.[25] These brain regions include the dorsal raphé nucleus (see **Fig. 1**), tuberomammillary nucleus of the posterior hypothalamus (see **Fig. 1**), medial preoptic area (see **Fig. 1**), and ventrolateral periaqueductal gray.[7,25–27]

ACETYLCHOLINE

Acetylcholine is distinguished as being the first identified neurotransmitter. Although the first neurochemical theory of sleep[28] correctly posited that acetylcholine plays a primary role in generating the brain-activated states of wakefulness and REM sleep, cholinergic drugs are not part of the standard pharmacologic armamentarium of sleep disorders medicine. Nonetheless, understanding the mechanisms by which cholinergic neurotransmission generates and maintains REM sleep is crucial, because acetylcholine interacts with other transmitter systems that are targets of sleep pharmacotherapy (eg, GABAergic and

monoaminergic). Much of the research on the regulation of sleep by acetylcholine has focused on transmission mediated by muscarinic cholinergic receptors. Five subtypes (M_1-M_5) of the muscarinic receptor have been identified,[29] and the M2 subtype plays a key role in the generation of REM sleep.[30]

Cholinergic signaling originating from the laterodorsal tegmental (LDT) and pedunculopontine tegmental (PPT) nuclei and the basal forebrain (see **Fig. 1**) promotes the cortically activated states of wakefulness and REM sleep.[31] LDT/PPT neurons can be divided into two populations based on discharge pattern. One population discharges maximally during wakefulness and REM sleep (referred to as Wake-On/REM-On) and another population fires only during wakefulness (Wake-On/REM-Off).[2] This finding helps explain how acetylcholine can promote both wakefulness and REM sleep. LDT/PPT neurons project to numerous wakefulness-promoting brain regions.[2] Cholinergic terminals in the pontine reticular formation arise from the LDT/PPT,[2] and muscarinic receptors are present in the pontine reticular formation.[30,32,33] Many studies have administered cholinomimetics to the pontine reticular formation and have demonstrated that cholinergic transmission in the pontine reticular formation induces REM sleep.[2,31] Electrically stimulating the LDT/PPT increases acetylcholine release in the pontine reticular formation[34] and increases REM sleep.[35] The release of endogenous acetylcholine in the pontine reticular formation is significantly greater during REM sleep than during wakefulness or NREM sleep.[36–38] Taken together, these data demonstrate that cholinergic projections from the LDT/PPT to the pontine reticular formation promote REM sleep.

Recent in vivo data obtained from normal rats demonstrate that the sedative-hypnotics zolpidem, diazepam, and eszopiclone differentially

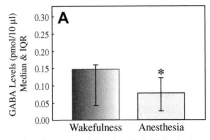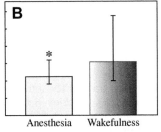

Fig. 2. Pontine reticular formation levels of GABA during wakefulness and isoflurane anesthesia. Consistent results were obtained when measuring GABA during the transition from wakefulness to anesthesia (*A*) and during the resumption of wakefulness after anesthesia (*B*). In both cases, GABA was significantly decreased during the loss of wakefulness caused by isoflurane anesthesia. (*Reprinted from* Vanini G, Watson CJ, Lydic R, et al. γ-aminobutyric acid-mediated neurotransmission in the pontine reticular formation modulates hypnosis, immobility, and breathing during isoflurane anesthesia. Anesthesiology 2008;109:978–88; with permission.)

alter acetylcholine release in the pontine reticular formation.[39] Intravenous administration of eszopiclone prevented the REM phase of sleep, increased electroencephalogram (EEG) delta power, and decreased acetylcholine release in rat pontine reticular formation (**Fig. 3**).[39] These data provide the first functional evidence for a heterogeneous distribution of GABA$_A$ receptor subtypes within the pontine reticular formation. The different effects of GABA$_A$ receptor agonists on sleep have been attributed to brain region-specific distributions of GABA$_A$ receptors and differences in sedative-hypnotic affinities for GABA$_A$ receptor subtypes.[40] These preclinical data can be contrasted with human psychopharmacology where there has been no study convincingly demonstrating differential GABA$_A$ subtype binding among benzodiazepine and nonbenzodiazepine sleeping medications.[40] To date, the nonbenzodiazepine, benzodiazepine-receptor agonist eszopiclone remains the only sleeping medication for which the long-term (6 months) effects have been characterized.[41,42]

Cholinergic neurons originating in the basal forebrain project throughout the entire cerebral cortex.[43] Acetylcholine release in the basal forebrain is highest during REM sleep, lower during quiet wakefulness, and lowest during NREM sleep.[44] Cortical acetylcholine release is increased during wakefulness[43,45,46] and REM sleep[45] as compared with NREM sleep. These data support the interpretation that cholinergic transmission from the basal forebrain promotes cortical activation during wakefulness and REM sleep.

ADENOSINE

Adenosine is a breakdown product of adenosine triphosphate (ATP). Increases in endogenous adenosine levels in a specific brain region during a period of prolonged wakefulness indicate that the region has been metabolically active. Direct biochemical measures show that ATP levels increase during sleep in areas of the brain that are most active during wakefulness.[47] This finding provides direct support for the hypothesis that sleep serves a restorative function.[48]

Four subtypes of adenosine receptors, A$_1$, A$_{2A}$, A$_{2B}$, and A$_3$, have been identified and are distributed widely throughout the brain. Adenosine A$_1$ and A$_{2A}$ receptors are antagonized by caffeine and the idea that adenosine promotes sleep is supported by the ubiquitous consumption of caffeine to maintain wakefulness and enhance alertness. In humans, oral administration of caffeine before nocturnal sleep increases sleep latency and reduces sleep efficiency.[49] Furthermore, morning caffeine ingestion has been shown to decrease sleep efficiency and overall sleep during the subsequent night.[50] No adenosine agonists are presently available to promote sleep. Adenosine, however, is relevant for sleep medicine, as insomnia can be caused by consumption of caffeine or by the respiratory stimulant theophylline. Interestingly, adenosine can have analgesic effects and this action shows promise for clinical use.[51]

Adenosinergic transmission in brain regions that regulate sleep and wakefulness has been

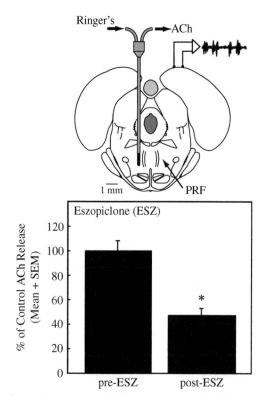

Fig. 3. Intravenous administration of eszopiclone to intact, behaving rats decreases acetylcholine (ACh) release in the pontine reticular formation (PRF). (*Top*) Coronal section of rat brain stem illustrates placement of a microdialysis probe in the PRF. Ringer's solution is pumped into the probe and samples are collected for quantification of ACh. (*Top right*) Electrodes and an amplifier for recording the cortical EEG and an EEG activity trace after intravenous administration of eszopiclone. (*Bottom*) Histograms summarize the significant decrease in ACh release within the PRF caused by intravenous administration of eszopiclone. (*From* Hambrecht-Wiedbusch VS, Gauthier EA, Baghdoyan HA, et al. Benzodiazepine receptor agonists cause drug-specific and state-specific alterations in EEG power and acetylcholine release in rat pontine reticular formation. Sleep 2010;33:909–18; with permission.)

extensively investigated.[2,52–54] Activating adenosine A_1 receptors causes neuronal inhibition, and A_1 is the most abundant adenosine receptor subtype in brain. This section highlights selected studies supporting the interpretation that adenosine promotes sleep, at least in part, by inhibiting neurons in several key wakefulness-promoting brain areas.

Prolonged wakefulness increases adenosine levels selectively in the basal forebrain (see **Fig. 1**) and cortex,[55] and increases adenosine A_1 receptor binding in human[56] and rat[57] brain. Pharmacologically increasing adenosine levels in the basal forebrain[58] or administering adenosine A_1 receptor agonists to the basal forebrain[54] causes an increase in sleep. Inactivating adenosine A_1 receptors in the basal forebrain decreases EEG delta power and NREM sleep time,[59] and immunohistochemical studies reveal that the basal forebrain contains A_1 receptors, but not A_{2A} receptors.[60] Cholinergic neurons in the basal forebrain project to the cortex and contribute to the EEG activation characteristic of wakefulness and REM sleep. Adenosine directly inhibits cholinergic neurons in the basal forebrain by activating A_1 receptors.[61] Adenosine indirectly inhibits wakefulness-promoting hypocretin (orexin)-containing neurons in the lateral hypothalamus (see **Fig. 1**) by activating A_1 receptors.[62] Blocking adenosine A_1 receptors in the lateral hypothalamus causes an increase in wakefulness and a decrease in sleep.[63] Histaminergic neurons in the tuberomammillary nucleus (see **Fig. 1**) express adenosine A_1 receptors, and activating those receptors increases NREM sleep.[64] These complementary data suggest that adenosine promotes sleep by inhibiting wakefulness-promoting neurons localized to the basal forebrain, lateral hypothalamus, and tuberomammillary nucleus.

Adenosine also exerts sleep-promoting effects by actions at the level of the prefrontal cortex (see **Fig. 1**) and the pontine reticular formation (see **Fig. 1**). In vivo microdialysis experiments in mouse[65] have shown that adenosine acting at A_1 receptors in the prefrontal cortex inhibits traits that characterize wakefulness (including acetylcholine release in the prefrontal cortex and activation of the EEG), as well as the state of wakefulness. Activation of adenosine A_1 receptors in the prefrontal cortex also causes a decrease in the release of acetylcholine in the pontine reticular formation. These findings demonstrate that in the prefrontal cortex, adenosine A_1 receptors mediate a descending inhibition of wakefulness-promoting systems. Within the pontine reticular formation, activation of adenosine A_{2A} receptors increases the time needed to recover from general anesthesia,[66] increases acetylcholine release,[66,67] and increases the amount of time spent in NREM sleep[67] and REM sleep.[67,68] The increase in REM sleep may be a result of the A_{2A}-mediated increase in acetylcholine release, because coadministration of a muscarinic receptor antagonist with the A_{2A} agonist blocks the REM sleep increase.[68] Studies examining the effects on sleep of adenosine receptor antagonists are required to conclude that endogenous adenosine within the pontine reticular formation modulates sleep. The finding that clinically used opioids, such as morphine and fentanyl, decrease adenosine levels in the pontine reticular formation[69] and disrupt REM sleep[70] suggests the possibility that adenosinergic transmission within the pontine reticular formation participates in REM sleep generation.

BIOGENIC AMINES

The monoamines have long been known to promote wakefulness. Serotonin (5-hydroxytryptamine; 5HT)-containing neurons of the dorsal raphé nucleus (see **Fig. 1**), norepinephrine-containing neurons of the locus coeruleus (see **Fig. 1**), and histamine-containing neurons of the tuberomammillary nucleus (see **Fig. 1**) discharge at their fastest rates during wakefulness, slow their firing in NREM sleep, cease discharging before and during REM sleep, and resume firing before the onset of wakefulness.[2] Dopaminergic neurons, by contrast, do not show major changes in firing rates across the sleep-wakefulness cycle.

Serotonin

Serotonin release in the dorsal raphé nucleus[71] and preoptic area[72] of rat is highest during wakefulness. Furthermore, electrical stimulation of the dorsal raphé nucleus increases wakefulness.[73] Serotonin receptors are divided into seven families ($5HT_1$-$5HT_7$).[74] Systemic administration of agonists for $5HT_{1A}$, $5HT_{1B}$, $5HT_{2A/2C}$ or $5HT_3$ receptors causes an increase in wakefulness and a decrease in sleep.[75] Local administration of a $5HT_{1A}$ receptor agonist to the dorsal raphé nucleus increases wakefulness in rat[76] but increases REM sleep in cat.[77] Microinjection of a $5HT_{2A/2C}$ receptor agonist into rat dorsal raphé nucleus also decreases REM sleep with no significant effect on wakefulness.[78] These incongruent findings may be due to species differences, or may indicate that in addition to promoting wakefulness, serotonin plays a permissive role in the generation of REM sleep. Systemic administration of antagonists for the $5HT_{2A}$ receptor or the $5HT_6$ receptor to rat decreases wakefulness, increases NREM sleep, and has no effect on REM sleep.[79]

These data are consistent with the view that serotonin is wakefulness-promoting. Genetically modified mice also have been used to explore the role of serotonin in sleep and wakefulness. Mice lacking the genes for the $5HT_{1A}$[80] or $5HT_{1B}$[81] receptor showed an increase in REM sleep. Administration of a $5HT_{1A}$,[80,82] a $5HT_{1B}$,[81] or a $5HT_{2A/2C}$[83] receptor agonist decreased REM sleep in rodent and human. These data indicate that serotonin acting at $5HT_{1A}$, $5HT_{1B}$, and $5HT_{2A/2C}$ receptors plays a role in suppressing REM sleep. The forgoing data underlie the fact that insomnia can be secondary to the use of selective serotonin reuptake inhibitors (SSRI) or serotonin, norepinephrine reuptake inhibitors (SNRI).

Norepinephrine

Noradrenergic cells of the locus coeruleus inhibit REM sleep, promote wakefulness, and project to a variety of other arousal-regulating brain regions (see **Fig. 1**) including the hypothalamus, thalamus, basal forebrain, and cortex.[84] Noradrenergic receptors include α_1-, α_2-, and β-adrenergic subtypes.[85] Administration of noradrenaline or α- and β-receptor agonists to the medial septal area[86,87] or the medial preoptic area[88,89] increases wakefulness. Stimulation of locus coeruleus neurons increases noradrenaline in the prefrontal cortex of anesthetized rat,[90,91] and contributes to cortical activation. These data are consistent with the view that noradrenaline promotes wakefulness. However, bilateral microinjection of an α_1-antagonist (prazosin), an α_2-agonist (clonidine), or a β-antagonist (propranolol) into the PPT increases REM sleep with little to no effect on NREM sleep or wakefulness.[92] The arousal-regulating effects of noradrenaline are brain-region specific. The treatment of hypertension with blockers of α- and/or β-adrenergic receptors can disrupt normal sleep.

Histamine

Histaminergic cell bodies, which are located in the tuberomammillary nucleus of the posterior hypothalamus have diffuse projections throughout the brain.[93] Data from posterior hypothalamic lesion studies and from single unit recordings indicate that the tuberomammillary nucleus promotes wakefulness.[93] Three histaminergic receptors, denoted H_1, H_2, and H_3, are present in the brain.[94] First generation H_1 receptor antagonists, such as diphenhydramine, cause drowsiness (sedation) and impaired performance in humans[95] and rats.[96] Newer antagonists that are relatively selective for the H_1 histamine receptor, such as the potent antagonist doxepin, improve subjective and objective measures of sleep in insomnia patients without causing sedation or psychomotor impairments the next day.[97] Systemic administration of the H_1 receptor antagonists mepyramine[98] and cyproheptadine[99] caused a significant increase in NREM sleep in cat and rat, respectively. Decreasing brain histamine levels by inhibiting synthesis significantly decreases wakefulness and increases NREM sleep in rat[100,101] and cat.[98] These data suggest that histaminergic signaling via the H_1 receptor promotes wakefulness. New therapies for sleep disorders and for maintaining vigilance include H_3 receptor antagonists and inverse agonists.[102–104]

Dopamine

Stimulants such as amphetamine, cocaine, and methylphenidate increase wakefulness and counter hypersomnia by increasing levels of endogenous dopamine.[105] In vivo imaging studies suggest that sleep deprivation increases dopamine levels in human brain.[106] The cell bodies of dopaminergic neurons that regulate arousal reside in the ventral tegmental area (see **Fig. 1**) and the substantia nigra pars compacta.[75] These dopaminergic neurons project to the dorsal raphé nucleus, basal forebrain, locus coeruleus, thalamus, and LDT.[107] There are also dopaminergic neurons in the ventrolateral periaqueductal gray that are active during wakefulness and have reciprocal connections with sleep-regulating brain areas.[108]

Five dopaminergic receptors have been cloned (D1–D5). Dopaminergic neurons of the substantia nigra and ventral tegmental area do not change firing rates as a function of states of sleep and wakefulness.[2] Dopamine does promote wakefulness and dopamine-transporter-knockout mice display increased wakefulness and decreased NREM sleep compared with controls.[109] Systemic administration of D1 receptor agonists or antagonists causes an increase or decrease, respectively, in wakefulness.[110] Intracerebroventricular administration of a D1 or D2 receptor agonist to rat increases wakefulness.[111] Systemic administration of a D2 receptor agonist causes biphasic effects with low doses decreasing wakefulness and high doses increasing wakefulness.[112,113] Systemic administration of D-amphetamine to rat increases wakefulness and decreases NREM sleep and REM sleep.[114] The mechanisms by which modafinil counters excessive daytime sleepiness remain to be specified. There is evidence that modafinil enhances synaptic release of dopamine and norepinephrine.[115]

GLUTAMATE

Glutamate is the main excitatory neurotransmitter in the brain and acts at α-amino-3-hydroxy-5-methyl-4-isoxazole propionic acid (AMPA), kainate, and N-methyl-D-aspartate (NMDA) ionotropic receptors. Surprisingly, little is known about glutamatergic regulation of sleep and wakefulness. Sleep state-dependent changes in levels of endogenous glutamate change differentially across the brain.[116] For example, glutamate levels in some areas of rat cortex show increases in concentration during wakefulness and REM sleep, and decreases during NREM sleep.[117] Microinjection and electrophysiological studies provide evidence that glutamate acts within the LDT/PPT[118–120] (see **Fig. 1**), the pontine reticular formation[121–123] (see **Fig. 1**), and medial portions of the medullary reticular formation[122,124] to modulate traits and states of arousal. Glutamatergic neurons are present in rat pontine reticular formation[125] and neurons in the pontine reticular formation are capable of synthesizing glutamate for use as a neurotransmitter.[126] Glutamate elicits excitatory responses from pontine reticular formation neurons,[127,128] and glutamatergic and cholinergic transmission in the pontine reticular formation interact synergistically to potentiate catalepsy.[129] Given individually, agonists for AMPA, kainate, and NMDA receptors evoke excitatory responses from pontine reticular formation neurons.[121] Dialysis delivery of the NMDA receptor antagonists ketamine or MK-801 to cat pontine reticular formation decreases acetylcholine release in the pontine reticular formation and disrupts breathing.[38]

PEPTIDES

Many peptides are known to modulate sleep.[130] This article focuses on hypocretin (orexin), leptin, and ghrelin because of their relevance for sleep disorders medicine.

Hypocretin-1 and -2

Numerous lines of evidence support a role for hypocretin-1 and -2 (also called orexin A and B) in the maintenance of wakefulness. The cell bodies of hypocretin-producing neurons are localized to the dorsolateral hypothalamus[131,132] and send projections to all the major brain regions that regulate arousal.[133,134] Hypocretinergic neurons discharge with the highest frequency during active wakefulness and show almost no discharge activity during sleep.[135,136] Hypocretin-1 levels in the hypothalamus of cat are greater during wakefulness and REM sleep than during NREM sleep.[137] Dogs displaying a narcoleptic phenotype have a mutation of the hypocretin receptor-2 gene,[138] and hypocretin mRNA and peptide levels are greatly reduced in human narcoleptic patients.[139,140] Patients presenting with narcolepsy-cataplexy also have greatly reduced levels of hypocretin in their cerebrospinal fluid compared with controls.[141] Preclinical studies have demonstrated that selective lesions of hypocretin-containing neurons[142,143] or genetic removal of the peptide[144] result in a narcoleptic phenotype. By what mechanisms might hypocretin enhance wakefulness?

Two receptors for the hypocretin peptides have been identified. Hypocretin-1 and -2 receptors have been localized to the LDT/PPT, pontine reticular formation, dorsal raphé nucleus, and locus coeruleus.[145–149] Electrophysiological studies demonstrate that hypocretin-1 or hypocretin-2 excite neurons in these same brain regions.[150–158] Hypocretin-1 and -2 also excite tuberomammillary neurons[159,160] and cholinergic neurons of the basal forebrain.[161]

Intracerebroventricular administration of hypocretin-1 increases wakefulness and decreases NREM sleep and REM sleep in rat.[162,163] When administered into the lateral preoptic area,[164] the LDT,[165] pontine reticular formation,[20,166] or basal forebrain,[167,168] hypocretin-1 causes an increase in wakefulness. In cat, microinjection of hypocretin-1 into the pontine reticular formation increases REM sleep if delivered during NREM sleep,[152] but suppresses REM sleep if delivered during wakefulness.[166] The wakefulness-promoting effect of hypocretin in the pontine reticular formation is further supported by evidence that delivery of antisense oligonucleotides against the hypocretin-2 receptor to the pontine reticular formation of rat enhances REM sleep and induces cataplexy.[169]

Measuring the effect of hypocretin-1 on the release of other arousal-regulating transmitters may provide insight into how hypocretin-1 promotes wakefulness. Microinjection of hypocretin-1 into the basal forebrain of rat increases cortical acetylcholine release.[170] Intracerebroventricular delivery of hypocretin-increases histamine in rodent frontal cortex[171] and anterior hypothalamus.[172] Microinjection of hypocretin-1 into the ventricles or the ventral tegmental area increases dopamine release in rat prefrontal cortex.[163] Hypocretin-1 delivered to rat dorsal raphé nucleus increases serotonin release in the dorsal raphé nucleus,[173] and dialysis delivery of hypocretin-1 to rat pontine reticular formation increases acetylcholine release[174] and GABA levels[20] in the pontine reticular formation. The increase in wakefulness produced by microinjecting hypocretin-1 into the pontine reticular formation is prevented by blocking GABA_A receptors.[175] This finding suggests that hypocretin may increase wakefulness, in part, by increasing GABA levels in the pontine reticular formation. Considered together, these data support the classification of hypocretin-1 as a wakefulness-promoting neuropeptide.

An alternative hypothesis is that a primary function of hypocretin is to enhance activity in motor systems and the increase in wakefulness is secondary. This hypothesis is supported by data showing that hypocretin-1 concentrations in the cerebrospinal fluid are significantly greater during active wakefulness with movement than during quiet wakefulness with no movement.[137] Hypocretinergic neurons also have very low firing rates during quiet wakefulness (without movement) compared with active wakefulness.[135,136] Oral administration of the hypocretin-1 and -2 receptor antagonist ACT-078573 increases NREM sleep and REM sleep in rat, dog, and human,[176] suggesting a direct, wakefulness-promoting effect of endogenous hypocretin.

Leptin and Ghrelin

Owing to the ongoing epidemic of obesity and the association between metabolic syndrome and sleep disorders, many studies aim to understand the sleep-related roles of leptin and ghrelin. Decreased levels of leptin (a hormone that suppresses appetite) and increased levels of ghrelin (a hormone that stimulates appetite) are associated with short sleep duration in humans.[177,178] The sleep of ob/ob mice (obese mice with reduced levels of leptin) is characterized by an increase in number of arousals and a decrease in the duration of sleep bouts compared with wild type controls.[179] The ob/ob mice also have an impaired response to the cholinergic enhancement of REM sleep.[180] Similarly, db/db mice (which are also obese but are resistant to leptin) have significant alterations in sleep architecture compared with wild type control mice that include, but are not limited to, increases in NREM sleep and REM sleep during the dark phase and decreases in wakefulness and NREM sleep bout duration.[181] Local administration of ghrelin into rat lateral hypothalamus, medial preoptic area, or paraventricular nucleus increases wakefulness, decreases NREM sleep, and increases food intake.[182] Together, these findings suggest that leptin and ghrelin, hormones that are important for appetite regulation, significantly influence sleep and are significantly modulated by sleep.

OPIOIDS

Opioids are the major class of drugs used to treat acute and chronic pain, and one side effect of opioids is sleep disruption. Sleep disruption, in turn, exacerbates pain[183,184] and increases the dose of opioids required for successful pain management.[69,70] Clinically relevant doses of opioids given to otherwise healthy humans disrupt sleep.[185] For example, a single intravenous infusion of morphine in healthy volunteers decreases stages 3 and 4 NREM sleep, decreases REM sleep, and increases stage 2 NREM sleep.[186] A nighttime dose of morphine or methadone also decreases stages 3 and 4 NREM sleep while increasing stage 2 NREM sleep.[187] Constant infusion of analgesic doses of remifentanil overnight decreases REM sleep in healthy volunteers.[188] The cycle of opioid-induced sleep disruption leading to increased pain and increased opioid requirement is recognized as a significant clinical problem that must be addressed at the mechanistic level.[189]

Opioid-induced disruption of REM sleep is mediated, at least in part, by decreasing acetylcholine release in the pontine reticular formation.[70] Opioids also decrease adenosine levels in the basal forebrain and in the pontine reticular formation,[69] two brain regions where adenosine has sleep-promoting effects. Local administration of morphine into the pontine reticular formation of cat[190] or rat[191] increases wakefulness and decreases REM sleep.

FUTURE DIRECTIONS

This selective overview was completed during the summer of 2010, a date also marking the 20th anniversary of the human genome project. The stunning successes—and unmet hopes—of genomic approaches to medicine were highlighted in the June 12th and 14th issues of The New York Times.[192,193] These two articles offer a sobering reminder that taking a molecule from preclinical discovery to commercially available drug typically requires 15 or more years. This time interval is without any mandate to understand the mechanisms of drug action. As a former director of research and development at Wyeth noted "Genomics did not speed up drug development. It gave us more rapid access to new molecular targets."[193] Potential molecular targets can be rapidly interrogated with high throughput screening programs that use a cell line transfected to contain a reporter construct. But identifying potential molecular targets leaves unanswered the question of whether the candidate targets will be druggable in vivo. This complexity is exemplified by sedative-hypnotic medications commonly used in sleep medicine. $GABA_A$ receptors are drug targets that promote a sleep-like state by unknown actions[40] when they are activated in some brain regions, yet $GABA_A$ receptors enhance wakefulness when activated selectively in the posterior hypothalamus[194] or pontine reticular formation.[18,19,21] As intricate as **Fig. 1** may seem, it barely hints at the complexity of data that must be logically integrated if we are to derive a coherent model of the endogenous neurochemical processes that regulate states of sleep and wakefulness.

Recent progress in understanding the basic neuropharmacology of sleep can be appreciated by comparing the 1990 and the 2005 editions of *Brain Control of Wakefulness and Sleep*.[2] The incorporation of basic neuropharmacology into sleep disorders medicine is readily apparent by comparing the first and most recent editions of *Principles and Practice of Sleep Medicine*.[195] Future progress is most likely to come from a systems biology approach that seeks to integrate genomic, cellular, network, and behavioral levels of analysis.[196] The focus on sleep medications in the Clinics of North America series demonstrates the cross-cutting relevance of sleep for the practice of medicine. The pressing clinical problem of sleep disorders medicine will continue to stimulate advances in understanding the neurochemical regulation of sleep.

ACKNOWLEDGMENTS

We thank Mary A. Norat and Sarah L. Watson for critical comments on this article.

REFERENCES

1. Watson CJ, Baghdoyan HA, Lydic R. A neurochemical perspective on states of consciousness. In: Hudetz AG, Pearce RA, editors. Suppressing the mind: anesthetic modulation of memory and consciousness. New York (NY): Springer/Humana Press; 2010. p. 33–80.
2. Steriade M, McCarley RW, editors. Brain control of wakefulness and sleep. New York: Kluwer Academic/Plenum Publishers; 2005. p. 1–728.
3. Datta S, MacLean RR. Neurobiological mechanisms for the regulation of mammalian sleep-wake behavior: reinterpretation of historical evidence and inclusion of contemporary cellular and molecular evidence. Neurosci Biobehav Rev 2007;31:775–824.
4. McCarley RW. Neurobiology of REM and NREM sleep. Sleep Med 2007;8:302–30.
5. Stenberg D. Neuroanatomy and neurochemistry of sleep. Cell Mol Life Sci 2007;64:1187–204.
6. Monti JM, Pandi-Perumal SR, Sinton CM, editors. Neurochemistry of sleep and wakefulness. New York: Cambridge University Press; 2008. p. 1–482.
7. Szymusiak R, McGinty D. Hypothalamic regulation of sleep and arousal. Ann N Y Acad Sci 2008;1129: 275–86.
8. Mallick BN, Pandi-Perumal SR, McCarley RW, et al, editors. Rapid eye movement sleep: regulation and function. New York: Cambridge University Press; 2010, in press.
9. Olsen RW, Sieghart W. International union of pharmacology. LXX. Subtypes of γ-aminobutyric acid$_A$ receptors: classification on the basis of subunit composition, pharmacology, and function. Update. Pharmacol Rev 2008;60:243–60.
10. Winsky-Sommerer R. Role of $GABA_A$ receptors in the physiology and pharmacology of sleep. Eur J Neurosci 2009;29:1779–94.
11. Fritschy J-M, Möhler H. $GABA_A$-receptor heterogeneity in the adult rat brain: differential regional and cellular distribution of seven major subunits. J Comp Neurol 1995;359:154–94.
12. Heldt SA, Ressler KJ. Forebrain and midbrain distribution of major benzodiazepine-sensitive $GABA_A$ receptor subunits in the adult C57 mouse as assessed with in situ hybridization. Neuroscience 2007;150:370–85.
13. Pirker S, Schwarzer C, Wieselthaler A, et al. $GABA_A$ receptors: immunocytochemical distribution of 13 subunits in the adult rat brain. Neuroscience 2000;101:815–50.
14. Farrant M, Nusser M. Variations on an inhibitory theme: phasic and tonic activation of $GABA_A$ receptors. Nat Rev Neurosci 2005;6:215–29.
15. Orser BA. Extrasynaptic $GABA_A$ receptors are critical targets for sedative-hypnotic drugs. J Clin Sleep Med 2006;2:S12–8.
16. Walsh JK, Deacon S, Dijk D-J, et al. The selective extrasynaptic $GABA_A$ agonist, gaboxadol, improves traditional hypnotic efficacy measures and enhances slow wave activity in a model of transient insomnia. Sleep 2007;30:593–602.
17. Camacho-Arroyo I, Alvarado R, Manjarrez J, et al. Microinjections of muscimol and bicuculline into the pontine reticular formation modify the sleep-waking cycle in the rat. Neurosci Lett 1991;129:95–7.
18. Flint R, Chang T, Lydic R, et al. $GABA_A$ receptors in the pontine reticular formation of C57BL/6J mouse modulate neurochemical, electrographic, and behavioral phenotypes of wakefulness. J Neurosci 2010;30:12301–9.
19. Xi M-C, Morales FR, Chase MH. Evidence that wakefulness and REM sleep are controlled by a GABAergic pontine mechanism. J Neurophysiol 1999;82:2015–9.

20. Watson CJ, Lydic R, Baghdoyan HA. Pontine reticular formation (PnO) administration of hypocretin-1 increases PnO GABA levels and wakefulness. Sleep 2008;31:453–64.

21. Vanini G, Watson CJ, Lydic R, et al. γ-aminobutyric acid-mediated neurotransmission in the pontine reticular formation modulates hypnosis, immobility, and breathing during isoflurane anesthesia. Anesthesiology 2008;109:978–88.

22. Vanini G, Wathen BL, Lydic R, et al. GABA levels in cat pontine reticular formation (PRF) are lower during rapid eye movement (REM) sleep and the neostigmine-induced REM sleep-like state (REM-Neo) than during wakefulness [abstract]. Sleep 2009;32(Suppl):0011.

23. Sanford LD, Tang X, Xiao J, et al. GABAergic regulation of REM sleep in reticularis pontis oralis and caudalis in rats. J Neurophysiol 2003;90:938–45.

24. Marks GA, Sachs OW, Birabil CG. Blockade of GABA, type A, receptors in the rat pontine reticular formation induces rapid eye movement sleep that is dependent upon the cholinergic system. Neuroscience 2008;156:1–10.

25. Vanini G, Torterolo P, McGregor R, et al. GABAergic processes in the mesencephalic tegmentum modulate the occurrence of active (rapid eye movement) sleep in guinea pigs. Neuroscience 2007;145:1157–67.

26. Vanini G, Baghdoyan HA, Lydic R. Relevance of sleep neurobiology for cognitive neuroscience and anesthesiology. In: Mashour GA, editor. Consciousness, awareness, and anesthesia. New York: Cambridge University Press; 2010. p. 1–23.

27. Vanini G, Lydic R, Baghdoyan HA. GABAergic modulation of REM sleep. In: Mallick BN, Pandi-Perumal R, McCarley RW, et al, editors. Rapid eye movement sleep—regulation and function. Cambridge University Press, in press.

28. Jouvet M. The role of monoamines and acetylcholine-containing neurons in the regulation of the sleep-waking cycle. Ergeb Physiol 1972;64:166–307.

29. Ishii M, Kurachi Y. Muscarinic acetylcholine receptors. Curr Pharm Des 2006;12:3573–81.

30. Baghdoyan HA, Lydic R. M2 muscarinic receptor subtype in the feline medial pontine reticular formation modulates the amount of rapid eye movement sleep. Sleep 1999;22:835–47.

31. Lydic R, Baghdoyan HA. Acetylcholine modulates sleep and wakefulness: a synaptic perspective. In: Monti JM, Pandi-Perumal SR, Sinton CM, editors. Neurochemistry of sleep and wakefulness. Cambridge (UK): Cambridge University Press; 2008. p. 109–43.

32. Baghdoyan HA. Location and quantification of muscarinic receptor subtypes in rat pons:

33. DeMarco GJ, Baghdoyan HA, Lydic R. Differential cholinergic activation of G proteins in rat and mouse brainstem: relevance for sleep and nociception. J Comp Neurol 2003;457:175–84.

34. Lydic R, Baghdoyan HA. Pedunculopontine stimulation alters respiration and increases ACh release in the pontine reticular formation. Am J Physiol 1993;264:R544–54.

35. Thakkar M, Portas C, McCarley RW. Chronic low-amplitude electrical stimulation of the laterodorsal tegmental nucleus of freely moving cats increases REM sleep. Brain Res 1996;723:223–7.

36. Kodama T, Takahashi Y, Honda Y. Enhancement of acetylcholine release during paradoxical sleep in the dorsal tegmental field of the cat brain stem. Neurosci Lett 1990;114:277–82.

37. Leonard TO, Lydic R. Pontine nitric oxide modulates acetylcholine release, rapid eye movement sleep generation, and respiratory rate. J Neurosci 1997;17:774–85.

38. Lydic R, Baghdoyan HA. Ketamine and MK-801 decrease acetylcholine release in the pontine reticular formation, slow breathing, and disrupt sleep. Sleep 2002;25:615–20.

39. Hambrecht-Wiedbusch VS, Gauthier E, Baghdoyan HA, et al. Zolpidem, eszopiclone, and diazepam differentially alter EEG delta power and acetylcholine release in the pontine reticular formation of Sprague-Dawley rat. Sleep 2010;33:909–18.

40. Krystal AD. In vivo evidence of the specificity of effects of GABA$_A$ receptor modulating medications. Sleep 2010;33:859–60.

41. Krystal AD, Walsh JK, Laska E, et al. Sustained efficacy of eszopiclone over 6 months of nightly treatment: results of a randomized, double-blind, placebo-controlled study in adults with chronic insomnia. Sleep 2003;26:793–8.

42. Walsh JK, Krystal AD, Amato DA, et al. Nightly treatment of primary insomnia with eszopiclone for six months: effect on sleep, quality of life, and work limitations. Sleep 2007;30:959–68.

43. Sarter M, Bruno JP. Cortical cholinergic inputs mediating arousal, attentional processing and dreaming: differential afferent regulation of the basal forebrain by telencephalic and brainstem afferents. Neuroscience 2000;95:933–52.

44. Vazquez J, Baghdoyan HA. Basal forebrain acetylcholine release during REM sleep is significantly greater than during waking. Am J Physiol Regul Integr Comp Physiol 2001;280:R598–601.

45. Marrosu F, Portas C, Mascia MS, et al. Microdialysis measurement of cortical and hippocampal acetylcholine release during sleep-wake cycle in freely moving cats. Brain Res 1995;671:329–32.

implications for REM sleep generation. Am J Physiol 1997;273:R896–904.

46. Materi LM, Rasmusson DD, Semba K. Inhibition of synaptically evoked cortical acetylcholine release by adenosine: an in vivo microdialysis study in the rat. Neuroscience 2000;97:219–26.

47. Dworak M, McCarley RW, Kim T, et al. Sleep and brain energy levels: ATP changes during sleep. J Neurosci 2010;30:9007–16.

48. Benington JH, Heller HC. Restoration of brain energy metabolism as the function of sleep. Prog Neurobiol 1995;45:347–60.

49. Landolt HP, Dijk DJ, Gaus SE, et al. Caffeine reduces low-frequency delta activity in the human sleep EEG. Neuropsychopharmacology 1995;12:229–38.

50. Landolt HP, Werth E, Borbely AA, et al. Caffeine intake (200 mg) in the morning affects human and EEG power spectra at night. Brain Res 1995;675:67–74.

51. Gan TJ, Habib AS. Adenosine as a non-opioid analgesic in the perioperative setting. Anesth Analg 2007;105:487–94.

52. Radulovacki M. Adenosine sleep theory: how I postulated it. Neurol Res 2005;27:137–8.

53. Basheer R, Strecker RE, Thakkar M, et al. Adenosine and sleep-wake regulation. Prog Neurobiol 2004;73:379–96.

54. Strecker RE, Moriarty S, Thakkar MM, et al. Adenosinergic modulation of basal forebrain and preoptic/anterior hypothalamic neuronal activity in the control of behavioral state. Behav Brain Res 2000;115:183–204.

55. Porkka-Heiskanen T, Strecker RE, McCarley RW. Brain site-specificity of extracellular adenosine concentration changes during sleep deprivation and spontaneous sleep: an in vivo microdialysis study. Neuroscience 2000;99:507–17.

56. Elmenhorst D, Meyer PT, Winz OH, et al. Sleep deprivation increases A_1 adenosine receptor binding in the human brain: a positron emission tomography study. J Neurosci 2007;27:2410–5.

57. Elmenhorst D, Basheer R, McCarley RW, et al. Sleep deprivation increases A_1 adenosine receptor density in the rat brain. Brain Res 2009;1258:53–8.

58. Porkka-Heiskanen T, Strecker RE, Thakkar M, et al. Adenosine: a mediator of the sleep-inducing effects of prolonged wakefulness. Science 1997;276:1265–8.

59. Thakkar MM, Winston S, McCarley RW. A_1 receptor and adenosine homeostatic regulation of sleep-wakefulness: effects of antisense to the A_1 receptor in the cholinergic basal forebrain. J Neurosci 2003;23:4278–87.

60. Basheer R, Halldner L, Alanko L, et al. Opposite changes in adenosine A_1 and A_{2A} receptor mRNA in the rat following sleep deprivation. Neuroreport 2001;12:1577–80.

61. Arrigoni E, Chamberlin NL, Saper CB, et al. Adenosine inhibits basal forebrain cholinergic and non-cholinergic neurons in vitro. Neuroscience 2006;140:403–13.

62. Liu Z-W, Gao XB. Adenosine inhibits activity of hypocretin/orexin neurons by the A1 receptor in the lateral hypothalamus: a possible sleep-promoting effect. J Neurophysiol 2007;97:837–48.

63. Thakkar MM, Engemann SC, Walsh KM, et al. Adenosine and the homeostatic control of sleep: effects of A1 receptor blockade in the perifornical lateral hypothalamus. Neuroscience 2008;153:875–80.

64. Oishi Y, Huang Z-L, Fredholm BB, et al. Adenosine in the tuberomammillary nucleus inhibits the histaminergic system via A1 receptors and promotes non-rapid eye movement sleep. Proc Natl Acad Sci U S A 2008;105:19992–7.

65. Van Dort CJ, Baghdoyan HA, Lydic R. Adenosine A_1 and A_{2A} receptors in mouse prefrontal cortex modulate acetylcholine release and behavioral arousal. J Neurosci 2009;29:871–81.

66. Tanase D, Baghdoyan HA, Lydic R. Dialysis delivery of an adenosine A_1 receptor agonist to the pontine reticular formation decreases acetylcholine release and increases anesthesia recovery time. Anesthesiology 2003;98:912–20.

67. Coleman CG, Baghdoyan HA, Lydic R. Dialysis delivery of an adenosine A_{2A} agonist into the pontine reticular formation of C57BL/6J mouse increases pontine acetylcholine release and sleep. J Neurochem 2006;96:1750–9.

68. Marks GA, Shaffery JP, Speciale SG, et al. Enhancement of rapid eye movement sleep in the rat by actions at A1 and A2a aednosine receptor subtypes with a differential sensitivity to atropine. Neuroscience 2003;116:913–20.

69. Nelson AM, Battersby AS, Baghdoyan HA, et al. Opioid-induced decreases in rat brain adenosine levels are reversed by inhibiting adenosine deaminase. Anesthesiology 2009;111:1327–33.

70. Lydic R, Baghdoyan HA. Neurochemical mechanisms mediating opioid-induced REM sleep disruption. In: Lavigne G, Sessle B, Choinière M, et al, editors. Sleep and pain. Seattle (WA): International Association for the Study of Pain Press; 2007. p. 99–122.

71. Portas CM, Bjorvatn B, Fagerland S, et al. On-line detection of extracellular levels of serotonin in dorsal raphé nucleus and frontal cortex over the sleep/wake cycle in the freely moving rat. Neuroscience 1998;83:807–14.

72. Python A, Steimer T, de Saint Hilaire Z, et al. Extracellular serotonin variations during vigilance states in the preoptic area of rats: a microdialysis study. Brain Res 2001;910:49–54.

73. Houdouin F, Cespuglio R, Jouvet M. Effects induced by the electrical stimulation of the nucleus

raphé dorsalis upon hypothalamic release of 5-hydroxyindole compounds and sleep parameters in the rat. Brain Res 1991;565:48—56.

74. Fink KB, Gothert M. 5-HT receptor regulation of neurotransmitter release. Pharmacol Rev 2007;59: 360—417.

75. Monti JM, Jantos H. The roles of dopamine and serotonin, and of their receptors, in regulating sleep and waking. Prog Brain Res 2008;172:625—46.

76. Monti JM, Jantos H. Dose-dependent effects of the 5-HT1A receptor agonist 8-OH-DPAT on sleep and wakefulness in the rat. J Sleep Res 1992;1:169—75.

77. Portas CM, Thakkar M, Rainnie D, et al. Microdialysis perfusion of 8-hydroxy-2-(di-n-propylamino) tetralin (8-OH-DPAT) in the dorsal raphé nucleus decreases serotonin release and increases rapid eye movement sleep in the freely moving cat. J Neurosci 1996;16:2820—8.

78. Monti JM, Jantos H. Effects of activation and blockade of 5-HT$_{2A/2C}$ receptors in the dorsal raphé nucleus on sleep and waking in the rat. Prog Neuropsychopharmacol Biol Psychiatry 2006;30:1189—95.

79. Moriarty S, Hedley L, Flores J, et al. Selective 5-HT$_{2A}$ and 5-HT$_6$ receptor antagonists promote sleep in rats. Sleep 2008;31:34—44.

80. Boutrel B, Monaca C, Hen R, et al. Involvement of 5-HT1A receptors in homeostatic and stress-induced adaptive regulations of paradoxical sleep: studies in 5-HT1A knock-out mice. J Neurosci 2002;22:4686—92.

81. Boutrel B, Franc B, Hen R, et al. Key role of 5-HT1B receptors in the regulation of paradoxical sleep as evidenced in 5-HT1B knock-out mice. J Neurosci 1999;19:3204—12.

82. Wilson SJ, Bailey JE, Rich AS, et al. The use of sleep measures to compare a new 5HT$_{1A}$ agonist with buspirone in humans. J Psychopharmacol 2005;19:609—13.

83. Monti JM, Jantos H. Effects of the serotonin 5-HT$_{2A/2C}$ receptor agonist DOI and of the selective 5-HT$_{2A}$ or 5-HT$_{2C}$ receptor antagonists EMD 281014 and SB-243213, respectively, on sleep and waking in the rat. Eur J Pharmacol 2006; 553:163—70.

84. Berridge CW, Waterhouse BD. The locus coeruleus-noradrenergic system: modulation of behavioral state and state-dependent cognitive processes. Brain Res Rev 2003;42:33—84.

85. Hein L. Adrenoceptors and signal transduction in neurons. Cell Tissue Res 2006;326:541—51.

86. Berridge CW, Foote SL. Enhancement of behavioral and electroencephalographic indices of waking following stimulation of noradrenergic beta-receptors within the medial septal region of the basal forebrain. J Neurosci 1996;16:6999—7009.

87. Berridge CW, Isaac SO, Espana RA. Additive wake-promoting actions of medial basal forebrain noradrenergic α1- and β-receptor stimulation. Behav Neurosci 2003;117:350—9.

88. Kumar VM, Datta S, Chhina GS, et al. Alpha adrenergic system in medial preoptic area in sleep-wakefulness in rats. Brain Res Bull 1986;16:463—8.

89. Sood S, Dhawan JK, Ramesh V, et al. Role of medial preoptic area beta adrenoceptors in the regulation of sleep-wakefulness. Pharmacol Biochem Behav 1997;57:1—5.

90. Berridge CW, Abercrombie ED. Relationship between locus coeruleus discharge rates and rates of norepinephrine release within the neocortex as assessed by in vivo microdialysis. Neuroscience 1999;93:1263—70.

91. Florin-Lechner SM, Druhan JP, Aston-Jones G, et al. Enhanced norepinephrine release in prefrontal cortex with burst stimulation of the locus coeruleus. Brain Res 1996;742:89—97.

92. Pal D, Mallick BN. Role of noradrenergic and GABA-ergic inputs in pedunculopontine tegmentum for regulation of rapid eye movement sleep in rats. Neuropharmacology 2006;51:1—11.

93. Haas HL, Sergeeva OA, Selbach O. Histamine in the nervous system. Physiol Rev 2008;88(3): 1183—241.

94. Haas HL, Panula P. The role of histamine and the tuberomamillary nucleus in the nervous system. Nat Rev Neurosci 2003;4:121—30.

95. Nicholson AN, Stine BM. Antihistamines: impaired performance and the tendency to sleep. Eur J Clin Pharmacol 1986;30:27—32.

96. Kaneko Y, Shimada K, Saitou K, et al. The mechanism responsible for the drowsiness caused by first generation H1 antagonists on the EEG pattern. Methods Find Exp Clin Pharmacol 2000; 22:163—8.

97. Roth T, Rogowski R, Hull S, et al. Efficacy and safety of doxepin 1 mg, 3 mg, and 6 mg in adults with primary insomnia. Sleep 2007;30:1555—61.

98. Lin JS, Sakai K, Jouvet M. Evidence for histaminergic arousal mechanisms in the hypothalamus of cats. Neuropharmacology 1988;27:111—22.

99. Tokunaga S, Takeda Y, Shinomiya K, et al. Effects of some H$_1$-antagonists on the sleep-wake cycle in sleep-disturbed rats. J Pharmacol Sci 2007; 103:201—6.

100. Monti JM, D'Angelo L, Jantos H, et al. Effects of a-fluoromethylhistidine on sleep and wakefulness in the rat. J Neural Transm 1988;72:141—5.

101. Kiyono S, Seo ML, Shibagaki M, et al. Effects of α-fluoromethylhistidine on sleep-waking parameters in rats. Physiol Behav 1985;34:615—7.

102. Parmentier R, Anaclet C, Guhennec C, et al. The brain H$_3$-receptor as a novel therapeutic target

for vigilance and sleep-wake disorders. Biochem Pharmacol 2007;73:1157–71.

103. Ligneau X, Perrin D, Landais L, et al. BF2.649 [1-{3-[3-(4-Chlorophenyl)propoxy]propyl}piperidine, hydrochloride], a nonimidazole inverse agonist/antagonist at the human histamine H3 receptor: preclinical pharmacology. J Pharmacol Exp Ther 2007;320:365–75.

104. Le S, Gruner JA, Mathiasen JR, et al. Correlation between ex vivo receptor occupancy and wake-promoting activity of selective H_3 receptor antagonists. J Pharmacol Exp Ther 2008;325:902–9.

105. Boutrel B, Koob GF. What keeps us awake: the neuropharmacology of stimulants and wakefulness-promoting medications. Sleep 2004;27:1181–94.

106. Volkow ND, Wang G-J, Telang F, et al. Sleep deprivation decreases binding of [^{11}C]raclopride to dopamine D_2/D_3 receptors in the human brain. J Neurosci 2008;28:8454–61.

107. Monti JM, Monti D. The involvement of dopamine in the modulation of sleep and waking. Sleep Med Rev 2007;11:113–33.

108. Lu J, Jhou TC, Saper CB. Identification of wake-active dopaminergic neurons in the ventral periaqueductal gray matter. J Neurosci 2006;26:193–202.

109. Wisor JP, Nishino S, Sora I, et al. Dopaminergic role in stimulant-induced wakefulness. J Neurosci 2001;21:1787–94.

110. Monti JM, Fernandez M, Jantos H. Sleep during acute dopamine D1 agonist SKF 38393 or D1 antagonist SCH 23390 administration in rats. Neuropsychopharmacology 1990;3:153–62.

111. Isaac SO, Berridge CW. Wake-promoting actions of dopamine D1 and D2 receptor stimulation. J Pharmacol Exp Ther 2003;307:386–94.

112. Monti JM, Hawkins M, Jantos H, et al. Biphasic effects of dopamine D-2 receptor agonists on sleep and wakefulness in the rat. Psychopharmacology (Berl) 1988;95:395–400.

113. Monti JM, Jantos H, Fernandez M. Effects of the selective dopamine D-2 receptor agonist, quinpirole on sleep and wakefulness in the rat. Eur J Pharmacol 1989;169:61–6.

114. Anderson ML, Margis R, Frey BN, et al. Electrophysiological correlates of sleep disturbance induced by acute and chronic administration of D-amphetamine. Brain Res 2009;1249:162–72.

115. Minzenberg MJ, Carter CS. Modafinil: a review of neurochemical actions and effects on cognition. Neuropsychopharmacology 2008;33:1477–502.

116. Brevig HN, Baghdoyan HA. Neurotransmitters and neuromodulators regulating sleep and wakefulness. In: Koob GF, Le Moa M, Thompson RF, editors. Encyclopedia of behavioral neuroscience, vol. 3: Oxford (UK): Academic Press; 2010. p. 456–63.

117. Dash MB, Douglas CL, Vyazovskiy VV, et al. Long-term homeostasis of extracellular glutamate in the rat cerebral cortex across sleep and waking states. J Neurosci 2009;29:620–9.

118. Datta S, Patterson EH, Spoley EE. Excitation of the pedunculopontine tegmental NMDA receptors induces wakefulness and cortical activation in the rat. J Neurosci Res 2001;66:109–16.

119. Datta S, Spoley EE, Patterson EH. Microinjection of glutamate into the pedunculopontine tegmentum induces REM sleep and wakefulness in the rat. Am J Physiol Regul Integr Comp Physiol 2001;280:R752–9.

120. Datta S, Spoley EE, Mavanji VK, et al. A novel role of pedunculopontine tegmental kainate receptors: a mechanism of rapid eye movement sleep generation in the rat. Neuroscience 2002;114:157–64.

121. Stevens DR, McCarley RW, Greene RW. Excitatory amino acid-mediated responses and synaptic potentials in medial pontine reticular formation neurons of the rat in vitro. J Neurosci 1992;12:4188–94.

122. Lai YY, Siegel JM. Pontomedullary glutamate receptors mediating locomotion and muscle tone suppression. J Neurosci 1991;11:2931–7.

123. Onoe H, Sakai K. Kainate receptors: a novel mechanism in paradoxical (REM) sleep generation. Neuroreport 1995;6:353–6.

124. Lai YY, Siegel JM. Medullary regions mediating atonia. J Neurosci 1988;8:4790–6.

125. Kaneko T, Itoh K, Shigemoto R, et al. Glutaminase-like immunoreactivity in the lower brainstem and cerebellum of the adult rat. Neuroscience 1989;32:79–98.

126. Jones BE. Arousal states. Front Biosci 2003;8:S438–51.

127. Núñez A, Buño W, Reinoso-Suárez F. Neurotransmitter actions on oral pontine tegmental neurons of the rat: an in vitro study. Brain Res 1998;804:144–8.

128. Greene RW, Carpenter DO. Actions of neurotransmitters on pontine medial reticular formation neurons of cat. J Neurophysiol 1985;54:520–31.

129. Elazar Z, Berchanski A. Glutamatergic-cholinergic synergistic interaction in the pontine reticular formation. Effects on catalepsy. Naunyn Schmiedebergs Arch Pharmacol 2001;363:569–76.

130. De Lecea L. Neuropeptides and sleep-wake regulation. In: Monti JM, Pandi-Perumal R, Sinton CM, editors. Neurochemistry of sleep and wakefulness. New York: Cambridge University Press; 2008. p. 387–401.

131. de Lecea L, Kilduff TS, Peyron C, et al. The hypocretins: hypothalamus-specific peptides with

neuroexcitatory activity. Proc Natl Acad Sci U S A 1998;95:322–7.

132. Sakurai T, Amemiya A, Ishii M, et al. Orexin and orexin receptors: a family of hypothalamic neuro-peptides and G protein-coupled receptors that regulate feeding behavior. Cell 1998;92:572–95.

133. Peyron C, Tighe DK, van den Pol AN, et al. Neurons containing hypocretin (orexin) project to multiple neuronal systems. J Neurosci 1998;18: 9996–10015.

134. Zhang J-H, Sampogna S, Morales FR, et al. Distri-bution of hypocretin (orexin) immunoreactivity in the feline pons and medulla. Brain Res 2004;995: 205–17.

135. Lee MG, Hassani OK, Jones BE. Discharge of identified orexin/hypocretin neurons across the sleep-waking cycle. J Neurosci 2005;25:6716–20.

136. Mileykovskiy BY, Kiyashchenko LI, Siegel JM. Behavioral correlates of activity in identified hypo-cretin/orexin neurons. Neuron 2005;46:787–98.

137. Kiyashchenko LI, Mileykovskiy BY, Maidment N, et al. Release of hypocretin (orexin) during waking and sleep states. J Neurosci 2002;22: 5282–6.

138. Lin L, Faraco J, Li R, et al. The sleep disorder canine narcolepsy is caused by a mutation in the hypocretin (orexin) receptor 2 gene. Cell 1999;98: 365–76.

139. Thannickal TC, Moore RY, Nienhuis R, et al. Reduced number of hypocretin neurons in human narcolepsy. Neuron 2000;27:469–74.

140. Peyron C, Faraco J, Rogers W, et al. A mutation in a case of early onset narcolepsy and a generalized absence of hypocretin peptides in human narco-leptic brains. Nat Med 2000;6:991–7.

141. Nishino S, Kanbayashi T. Symptomatic narcolepsy, cataplexy, and hypersomnia, and their implications in the hypothalamic hypocretin/orexin system. Sleep Med Rev 2005;9:269–310.

142. Beuckmann CT, Sinton CM, Williams SC, et al. Expression of a poly-glutamine-ataxin-3 transgene in orexin neurons induces narcolepsy-cataplexy in the rat. J Neurosci 2004;24:4469–77.

143. Murillo-Rodriguez E, Liu M, Blanco-Centurian C, et al. Effects of hypocretin (orexin) neuronal loss on sleep and extracellular adenosine levels in the rat basal forebrain. Eur J Neurosci 2008;28: 1191–8.

144. Willie JT, Chemelli RM, Sinton CM, et al. Distinct narcolepsy syndromes in orexin receptor-2 and orexin null mice: molecular genetic dissection of non-REM and REM sleep regulatory processes. Neuron 2003;38:715–30.

145. Bernard R, Lydic R, Baghdoyan HA. Hypocretin-1 causes G protein activation and increases ACh release in rat pons. Eur J Neurosci 2003;18: 1775–85.

146. Greco MA, Shiromani PJ. Hypocretin receptor protein and mRNA expression in the dorsolateral pons of rats. Brain Res Mol Brain Res 2001;88: 176–82.

147. Hervieu GJ, Cluderay JE, Harrison DC, et al. Gene expression and protein distribution of the orexin-1 receptor in the rat brain and spinal cord. Neurosci-ence 2001;103:777–92.

148. Marcus JN, Aschenasi CN, Lee CE, et al. Differen-tial expression of orexin receptors 1 and 2 in the rat brain. J Comp Neurol 2001;435:6–25.

149. Brischoux F, Mainville L, Jones BE. Muscarinic-2 and orexin-2 receptors on GABAergic and other neurons in the rat mesopontine tegmentum and their potential role in sleep-wake control. J Comp Neurol 2008;510:607–30.

150. Burlet S, Tyler CJ, Leonard CS. Direct and indirect excitation of laterodorsal tegmental neurons by hy-pocretin/orexin peptides: implications for wakeful-ness and narcolepsy. J Neurosci 2002;22: 2862–72.

151. Takahashi K, Koyama Y, Kayama Y, et al. Effects of orexin on the laterodorsal tegmental neurones. Psychiatry Clin Neurosci 2002;56:335–6.

152. Xi M-C, Fung SJ, Yamuy J, et al. Induction of active (REM) sleep and motor inhibition by hypocretin in the nucleus pontis oralis of cat. J Neurophysiol 2002;87:2880–8.

153. Liu R-J, van den Pol AN, Aghajanian GK. Hypocre-tins (orexins) regulate serotonin neurons in the dorsal raphé nucleus by excitatory direct and inhibitory indirect actions. J Neurosci 2002;22: 9453–64.

154. Soffin EM, Gill CH, Brough SJ, et al. Pharmacolog-ical characterization of the orexin receptor subtype mediating postsynaptic excitation in the rat dorsal raphé nucleus. Neuropharmacology 2004;46: 1168–76.

155. Brown RE, Sergeeva O, Eriksson KS, et al. Conver-gent excitation of dorsal raphe serotonin neurons by multiple arousal systems (orexin/hypocretin, histamine and noradrenaline). J Neurosci 2002; 22:8850–9.

156. Bourgin P, Huitron-Resendiz S, Spier AD, et al. Hy-pocretin-1 modulates rapid eye movement sleep through activation of locus coeruleus neurons. J Neurosci 2000;20:7760–5.

157. Hagan JJ, Leslie RA, Patel S, et al. Orexin A acti-vates locus coeruleus cell firing and increases arousal in the rat. Proc Natl Acad Sci U S A 1999; 96:10911–6.

158. Horvath TL, Peyron C, Diano S, et al. Hypocretin (orexin) activation and synaptic innervation of the locus coeruleus noradrenergic system. J Comp Neurol 1999;415:145–59.

159. Eriksson KS, Sergeeva O, Brown RE, et al. Orexin/ hypocretin excites the histaminergic neurons of the

tuberomammillary nucleus. J Neurosci 2001;21: 9273–9.

160. Bayer L, Eggerman E, Serafin M, et al. Orexins (hypocretins) directly excite tuberomammillary neurons. Eur J Neurosci 2001;14:1571–5.

161. Eggerman E, Serafin M, Bayer L, et al. Orexins/hypocretins excite basal forebrain cholinergic neurones. Neuroscience 2001;108:177–81.

162. Piper DC, Upton N, Smith MI, et al. The novel brain neuropeptide, orexin-A, modulates the sleep-wake cycle of rats. Eur J Neurosci 2000;12:726–30.

163. Vittoz NM, Berridge CW. Hypocretin/orexin selectively increases dopamine efflux within the prefrontal cortex: involvement of the ventral tegmental area. Neuropsychopharmacology 2006; 31:384–95.

164. Methippara MM, Alam MN, Szymusiak R, et al. Effects of lateral preoptic area application of orexin-A on sleep-wakefulness. Neuroreport 2000; 11:3423–6.

165. Xi M-C, Morales FR, Chase MH. Effects on sleep and wakefulness on the injection of hypocretin-1 (orexin-A) into the laterodorsal tegmental nucleus of the cat. Brain Res 2001;901:259–64.

166. Moreno-Balandran ME, Garzon M, Bodalo C, et al. Sleep-wakefulness effects after microinjections of hypocretin-1 (orexin A) in cholinoceptive areas of the cat oral pontine tegmentum. Eur J Neurosci 2008;28:331–41.

167. Espana RA, Baldo BA, Kelley AE, et al. Wake-promoting and sleep-suppressing actions of hypocretin (orexin): basal forebrain sites of action. Neuroscience 2001;106:699–715.

168. Thakkar M, Ramesh V, Strecker RE, et al. Microdialysis perfusion of orexin-A in the basal forebrain increases wakefulness in freely behaving rat. Arch Ital Biol 2001;139:313–28.

169. Thakkar M, Ramesh V, Cape EG, et al. REM sleep enhancement and behavioral cataplexy following orexin (hypocretin)-II receptor antisense perfusion in the pontine reticular formation. Sleep Res Online 1999;2:113–20.

170. Dong H-L, Fukuda S, Murata E, et al. Orexins increase cortical acetylcholine release and electro-encephalographic activation through orexin-1 receptor in the rat basal forebrain during isoflurane anesthesia. Anesthesiology 2006;104:1023–32.

171. Hong Z-Y, Huang Z-L, Qu W-M, et al. Orexin A promotes histamine, but not norepinephrine or serotonin, release in frontal cortex of mice. Acta Pharmacol Sin 2005;26:155–9.

172. Ishizuka T, Yamamoto Y, Yamatodani A. The effect of orexin-A and -B on the histamine release in the anterior hypothalamus in rats. Neurosci Lett 2002; 323:93–6.

173. Tao R, Ma Z, McKenna JT, et al. Differential effect of orexins (hypocretins) on serotonin release in the dorsal and median raphé nuclei of freely behaving rats. Neuroscience 2006;141:1101–5.

174. Bernard R, Lydic R, Baghdoyan HA. Hypocretin (orexin) receptor subtypes differentially enhance acetylcholine release and activate G protein subtypes in rat pontine reticular formation. J Pharmacol Exp Ther 2006;317:163–71.

175. Brevig HN, Watson CJ, Lydic R, et al. Hypocretin and GABA interact in the pontine reticular formation to increase wakefulness. Sleep 2010;33: 1285–93.

176. Brisbare-Roch C, Dingemanse J, Koberstein R, et al. Promotion of sleep by targeting the orexin system in rats, dogs, and humans. Nat Med 2007;13:150–5.

177. Taheri S, Lin L, Austin D, et al. Short sleep duration is associated with reduced leptin, elevated ghrelin, and increased body mass index. PLoS Med 2004; 1:210–7 (e62).

178. Spiegel K, Tasali E, Penev P, et al. Brief communication: sleep curtailment in healthy young men is associated with decreased leptin levels, elevated ghrelin levels, and increased hunger and appetite. Ann Intern Med 2004;141:846–50.

179. Laposky AD, Shelton J, Bass J, et al. Altered sleep regulation in leptin-deficient mice. Am J Physiol Regul Integr Comp Physiol 2006;290: R894–903.

180. Douglas CL, Bowman GN, Baghdoyan HA, et al. C57BL/6J and B6.V-LEP^{OB} mice differ in the cholinergic modulation of sleep and breathing. J Appl Physiol 2005;98:918–29.

181. Laposky AD, Bradley MA, Williams DL, et al. Sleep-wake regulation is altered in leptin-resistant (db/db) genetically obese and diabetic mice. Am J Physiol Regul Integr Comp Physiol 2008;295: R2059–66.

182. Szentirmai E, Kapás L, Krueger JM. Ghrelin micro-injection into forebrain sites induces wakefulness and feeding in rats. Am J Physiol Regul Integr Comp Physiol 2007;292:R575–85.

183. Roehrs T, Hyde M, Blaisdell B, et al. Sleep loss and REM sleep loss are hyperalgesic. Sleep 2006;29: 145–51.

184. Chhangani BS, Roehrs TA, Harris EJ, et al. Pain sensitivity in sleepy pain-free normals. Sleep 2009;32:1011–7.

185. Lavigne G, Sessle BJ, Choinière M, et al, editors. Sleep and pain. Seattle: International Association for the Study of Pain; 2007. p. 1–473.

186. Shaw IR, Lavigne G, Mayer P, et al. Acute intravenous administration of morphine perturbs sleep architecture in healthy pain-free young adults: a preliminary study. Sleep 2005;28:677–82.

187. Dimsdale JE, Norman D, DeJardin D, et al. The effect of opioids on sleep architecture. J Clin Sleep Med 2007;15:33–6.

188. Bonafide CP, Aucutt-Walter N, Divittore N, et al. Remifentanil inhibits rapid eye movement sleep but not the nocturnal melatonin surge in humans. Anesthesiology 2008;108:627–33.

189. Moore JT, Kelz MB. Opiates, sleep, and pain. The adenosinergic link. Anesthesiology 2009;111: 1175–6.

190. Keifer JC, Baghdoyan HA, Lydic R. Sleep disruption and increased apneas after pontine microinjection of morphine. Anesthesiology 1992;77: 973–82.

191. Watson CJ, Lydic R, Baghdoyan HA. Sleep and GABA levels in the oral part of rat pontine reticular formation are decreased by local and systemic administration of morphine. Neuroscience 2007; 144:375–86.

192. Wade N. A decade later, genetic map yields few new cures. NY Times. June 12, 2010;2010.

193. Pollack A. Awaiting the genome payoff. NY Times. June 14, 2010;2010.

194. Lin JS, Sakai K, Vanni-Mercier G, et al. A critical role of the posterior hypothalamus in the mechanisms of wakefulness determined by microinjection of muscimol in freely moving cats. Brain Res 1989; 479:225–40.

195. Kryger MH, Roth T, Dement WC, editors. Principles and practice of sleep medicine. 5th edition. Philadelphia (PA): W.B. Saunders; 2010. p. 1–1505.

196. Klipp E, Herwig R, Kowald A, et al. Systems biology in practice: concepts, implementation and application. Weinheim (Germany): Wiley-VCH; 2005.

Pharmacotherapy for Insomnia

Thomas Roth, PhD[a,b,*], Timothy Roehrs, PhD[a,b]

KEYWORDS
- Insomnia • Sleep disorders • Pharmacotherapy
- Therapeutics

DIAGNOSTIC CRITERIA AS THERAPEUTIC TARGETS FOR INSOMNIA

Insomnia is a disorder characterized by chronic difficulty with sleep and associated impairments in daytime function. There are 3 diagnostic systems that provide diagnostic criteria for insomnia.[1–3] These are the International Classification of Sleep Disorders (ICSD II), the International Classification of Diseases 10 (ICD-10), and the Diagnostic and Statistical Manual of Mental Disorders, Fourth edition (DSM-IV). Although these vary to some extent, they all require (1) a report of disturbed sleep, (2) a report of impaired daytime function, and (3) some indication of frequency and or chronicity.

As such, these nosologies provide the clinical researcher with therapeutic targets or study end points. In terms of nocturnal symptoms, the investigator is afforded 3 sets of end points: difficulty falling asleep, difficulty staying asleep, and nonrestorative sleep (NRS). It is also important to recognize that many of these outcomes can be measured either by patient report using post sleep questionnaires (PSQ) or electrophysiological measures of sleep-wake (polysomnography [PSG]). There are several studies reporting the differential prevalence of these symptoms. It is generally felt that younger individuals typically report sleep-onset problems, whereas the elderly report more sleep maintenance problems.[4] Also, although the data are limited, NRS is more frequently found in younger populations. Importantly, in most cases more than one of these symptoms are present. In fact, if an individual has only a sleep-onset or a sleep-offset problem, it is often indicative of a circadian rhythm disorder: a phase delay in the case of sleep onset and phase advance in the case of early morning awakenings.

Difficulty Falling Asleep

Efficacy in sleep induction is evidenced by a reduction in reports of time needed to fall asleep on PSQ, or a reduction in latency to persistent sleep (LPS) on PSG. In most clinical trials the entry criteria is 30 or more minutes to fall asleep and hence a responder is often operationalized as fewer than 30 minutes to fall asleep. Although the results of patient report studies and sleep laboratory studies are similar in terms of determining efficacy, patient reports tend to overestimate the actual sleep latency, on both drug and placebo, as determined by PSG.

Difficulty Maintaining Sleep

Efficacy in maintenance is evident by the response to the question, "how long were you awake during the night" on the post sleep questionnaire and wake time after sleep onset (WASO) on PSG. However, it is important to recognize that WASO is a nonspecific measure of sleep maintenance. There are 3 distinct sleep problems subsumed under WASO: frequency of nocturnal awakenings, time to fall back to sleep after the awakening, and the presence and duration of early morning awakenings.

a Department of Internal Medicine, Sleep Disorders & Research Center, Henry Ford Hospital, Henry Ford Health System, 2799 West Grand Boulevard, Detroit, MI 48202, USA
b Department of Psychiatry and Behavioral Neuroscience, Wayne State University, School of Medicine, 2751 East Jefferson, Detroit, MI 48207, USA
* Corresponding author. Sleep Disorders & Research Center, Henry Ford Hospital, 2799 West Grand Boulevard, Detroit, MI 48202.
E-mail address: Troth1@hfhs.org

Sleep Med Clin 5 (2010) 529–539
doi:10.1016/j.jsmc.2010.09.002

Number of awakenings

An integral part of sleep maintenance insomnia is frequent awakenings during the night. The question arises as to how to operationalize an awakening. In terms of patient reports that seems straightforward, it is simply the answer to the question "how often did you wake up last night." However, in sleep laboratory studies the question arises as to how long should one be awake before it is called an awakening? Sleep recordings are scored as to stage in 30-second units.[5] However, there is little question that individuals can be awake for shorter durations, seconds, as evidenced in changes in physiology (eg, enervation of upper airway muscles, auditory awakening threshold, and presence of cough reflex). On the other hand, individuals do not report brief awakenings. Although patients with insomnia tend to overestimate the sleep problem by overestimating time to sleep onset and underestimating total sleep time, they underestimate the number of nocturnal awakenings. As a convention, in insomnia research, an awakening is defined as having duration of 1 minute or longer. There is no validation for this number, and ultimately this criterion needs to be determined by looking at different wake durations and determining which best predicts insomnia morbidity and distress.

Duration of awakenings

Another component of sleep maintenance is the duration of wake time during the night. Two individuals can have 100 minutes of WASO where one awakens 4 times and takes an average of 25 minutes to fall back to sleep, whereas another awakens 100 times and always returns to sleep within a minute. The causes, consequences, and even the treatment of these two WASO elevations are different. One can speculate that the long latencies back to sleep, like long latency to initial sleep onset, are mediated by some sort of hyperarousal. In contrast, the frequent brief awakenings are triggered by internal stimuli (eg, respiratory events, pain) or external events (noise, an uncomfortable sleep environment). The rapid return to sleep is mediated by normal homeostatic processes. There are data that suggest these two types of sleep maintenance sleep disturbances have different etiologies, different consequences, and are amenable to different treatments. Although further research is warranted to confirm these differences, there is no question that efficacy trials must evaluate the effects of treatment on each of these two types of sleep maintenance difficulties separately.

Early morning awakenings

The final manifestation of sleep maintenance difficulties is early morning awakenings; that is, arising before the desired time. It is important to differentiate early morning awakenings as an isolated symptom, as opposed to it coexisting with other sleep problems. Earlier morning awakenings, when they occur in association with other sleep disturbances, are thought to be associated with depressive disorders. In contrast, early morning awakening as an isolated symptom is most often associated with a circadian rhythm disorder (ie, phase advance).

Wake after sleep has rarely been studied in clinical trials. In fact, how to operationalize it in the sleep laboratory or in patient report studies has not evolved. In laboratory studies, where time in bed is typically fixed and predetermined, it is defined as the minutes of wake after the last epoch of sleep; however, the reliability of this definition has never been determined. If a subject is awake for 2 hours and then falls asleep for 1 minute before the predetermined rise time, should that be considered no early morning awakening time? This issue in home studies is equally complex. In their home environment, when a person awakens too early, he or she will often simply get out of bed. So, determining how early this premature awakening was needs to be somehow operationalized. One might speculate that the lack of attention to early morning awakenings can be traced to the fact that studies on the pharmacologic management of insomnia have almost exclusively focused on benzodiazepine receptor agonists (BzRAs). With these medications, sedative activity is related to blood levels of the drug.[6] Thus, if you have blood levels in hour 7 or 8 of the night, there is a high probability that some subjects (ie, slower metabolizers) would experience residual effects upon arising. As we move to drugs that work at other receptors (eg, histamine, orexin, serotonin, and melatonin), the duration of sedative activity may be influenced by variables other than blood levels of the drug.

Other Measures

Aside from these traditional measures of insomnia-related symptoms, there are other end points, both in the sleep laboratory and on PSQ that are routinely evaluated. In PSG studies, information is obtained not only about sleep initiation and continuity, but also about sleep stage distribution. Sleep stage distribution is often referred to as sleep architecture. There is a considerable literature on the effects of drugs on sleep stage distribution. For many years, there was interest in drug effects on rapid-eye movement (REM) sleep, with the hypothesis that REM suppression was a significant negative drug effect. Many drugs of abuse, such as alcohol, stimulants, and barbiturates, suppress REM sleep, further "supporting" this view. However, it became clear that virtually all antidepressants are very potent REM suppressants and were not associated with abuse or any other known side effects. In fact, some hypothesized that REM suppression was a mechanism of antidepressant effects.[7]

More recently, the focus has turned to positive aspects of sleep stage alterations, in particular on enhancement of stages 3 and 4 or sleep-wave sleep. A variety of gamma aminobutyric acid ($GABA_A$) agonists and serotonin antagonists have been shown to increase time in stages 3 and 4 sleep, as well as the amount of slow-wave activity as determined by spectral analysis.[8] The basic assumption of these studies is that slow-wave activity represents sleep that is in some way "better" or "more restorative" than other aspects of sleep. Thus, increasing time in slow-wave sleep has therapeutic value. There is little question that stages 3 and 4 sleep is much more consolidated than other non-REM (NREM) or REM stages; however, cause and effect is very unclear. Does enhancing slow-wave sleep decrease sleep fragmentation, does decreasing sleep fragmentation increase slow-wave sleep, or both?

In patient reports, there is an increasing interest in "sleep quality." PSQs routinely ask subjects to rate the "quality of their sleep," "depth of their sleep," and the "refreshing nature of their sleep." These types of questions seem to be important, as one of the symptoms of insomnia is "nonrestorative sleep." The difficulty with these questions is that they have not been validated. In fact, the question remains as to what would be the external criteria for their validation. It has been hypothesized that time spent in stages 3 and 4 NREM or the amount of slow-wave activity would be an appropriate validation criteria. However, although some studies have shown a correlation between slow-wave sleep and ratings of sleep quality, others have failed to demonstrate this relation. In addition, current data, albeit minimal, suggest there is no relation between the amount of slow-wave sleep and the diagnosis NRS. Many medications that have been shown to be effective in inducing and maintaining sleep have also been shown to be improve ratings of sleep quality. However, the question remains as to whether this reported improvement in "sleep quality" reflects any improvement in sleep beyond an improvement in sleep initiation and maintenance.

Future Directions in Evaluating Efficacy of Hypnotics

As research in insomnia pharmacotherapy advances, we can see some emerging trends. It is important to remember that criteria B for an insomnia diagnosis requires the individual report experiencing daytime impairment or distress associated with the sleep difficulty. Daytime impairment can be measured in terms of laboratory assays of some type of cognitive or psychomotor performance. This certainly has been the case in sleep deprivation research, which has consistently demonstrated performance impairments associated with sleep loss.[9] However, with few exceptions, laboratory studies have failed to differentiate between patients with insomnia and those with normal sleep in terms of their performance.[10] In contrast, patient reports of daytime impairment or distress consistently show differences between patients with insomnia and matched controls. Patient reports of quality of life, work impairment, absenteeism, daytime fatigue, and daytime sleepiness have all been found to be impaired among patients with insomnia. These impairments have been demonstrated using valid scales, as well as after controlling for demographic variables and co-morbid conditions.[11] Clearly, these measures represent potential outcomes for future insomnia clinical trials. Finally, another outcome that has also been shown to be affected by insomnia in elderly populations is falls. It is critically important to determine if resolving insomnia decreases the number of falls among patients with insomnia, especially elderly patients with insomnia.

Thus far, all of the end points discussed have focused on a single symptom of insomnia. They have not focused on the entire constellation of symptoms needed to meet diagnostic criteria for insomnia. In other symptom-based disorders, such as depression and schizophrenia, efficacy is defined by looking at the disorder-related symptom complex, not any single symptom. This approach is clearly needed in insomnia research. Scales, such as the Insomnia Severity Index, evaluate the totality of insomnia symptoms and can categorize patients as to the severity of their insomnia.[12] Clinical trials of sleep-promoting agents have begun using this scale. Aside from getting a global picture of the improvement in overall insomnia, these types of scales better enable the clinician to look at responder and remission rates rather than simply mean response on one aspect of the disorder.

The final new direction in insomnia clinical trials is the selection of insomnia populations for inclusion into the clinical trials. The vast majority of hypnotic trials have been performed in patients with primary insomnia. These are subjects who have insomnia that is not associated with any co-morbid condition, even though it is estimated that 85% to 90% of patients meeting diagnostic criteria for insomnia have a comorbid condition.[13] Comorbid conditions include psychiatric disorders (the most common), medical disorders, other sleep disorders, and circadian rhythm disorders. In studying these conditions it will not only be important to determine whether the sleep agent is effective in treating the sleep disturbances, but also how the improvements in insomnia affect the comorbid condition.

In terms of efficacy, it is highly likely the agents that work in primary insomnia will also work in co-morbid insomnia, as the current pharmacologic treatments of insomnia are nonspecific. The more relevant question is the dose necessary for efficacy. Does a given dose of a hypnotic have the same benefit in primary insomnia as insomnia comorbid with depression or comorbid with a pain condition? Although there are no direct studies to answer this question, comparisons across studies suggest that at least some comor-bid insomnias may require a higher dose. Given the frequency of use of hypnotics in comorbid insomnia, dose response studies in these popula-tions are needed.

The second issue in comorbid insomnia is what is the impact on improving sleep on the status of the comorbid condition? Increasingly, studies are appearing in the literature addressing this ques-tion. For example, the use of gabapentin and zolpi-dem (both drugs known to improve sleep) has been shown to decrease the use of opioids for pain management postoperatively.[14,15] In another series of studies, eszopiclone plus a selective serotonin reuptake inhibitor (SSRI) has been shown to augment antidepressant response in insomnia patients with comorbid depression and anxiolytic response in insomnia patients with co-morbid general anxiety disorder.[16,17] The question then arises as to whether the comorbid condition improvement is a direct drug effect or is mediated by the improved sleep. In the pain studies, gaba-pentin, but not zolpidem, has known analgesic effects. The fact that they both decreased opioid use suggests that this effect may be mediated by the improvement in sleep associated with both these drugs. In terms of the augmentation of depression and anxiety, there is a different picture. Although augmentation has been demonstrated with eszopiclone studies, there was no augmenta-tion demonstrated in zolpidem studies.[18,19] This suggests that the augmentation was not mediated by the improved sleep, as both drugs improved

sleep, but rather by differential binding properties of the two drugs. It is much too early to make any definitive conclusion of the effects of any sleep-promoting agent on any comorbid condi-tion, much less the mechanism of that effect. However, these studies clearly demonstrate the need for further research in a variety of comorbid insomnias. Finally, it is important to point out that insomnia is comorbid with many medical condi-tions including hypertension and ulcers. Does consolidating sleep improve these conditions? Such studies will not only inform us about insomnia therapy, but also insomnia pathophysiology.

THERAPEUTICS FOR INSOMNIA

Physicians use a variety of different pharma-cologic agents to treat insomnia, both those that have been approved by the Food and Drug Administration (FDA) for the treatment of insomnia, as well as sedating medications that have not been systematically studied for insomnia management (ie, off-label use). Interestingly, very few people seek treatment for their insomnia. In fact, in a representative study, it was estimated that only about 21% of patients with insomnia discuss their sleep problem with their physician and only 5% of insomnia patients receive treatment.[20–22] In contrast, patients with insomnia very commonly self-medicate for insomnia. In different population-based studies, rates of over-the-counter (OTC) sleep aid use have been found to range from 10% to 29% and rates of alcohol use to help promote sleep is between 10% and 28%. Many of these individ-uals report using both.

Self-Medication

Alcohol is the most available sedative compound, and in fact was the chemical basis of early sleep-promoting agents. Alcohol at low doses is often used to self-medicate for insomnia. The reason for this is that alcohol, even at low doses, improves sleep in the first part of the night, by improving rapidity of sleep onset, and by increasing stages 3 and 4 sleep. However, although it increases stages 3 and 4 sleep, it suppresses REM sleep.[23] In the second half of the night, alcohol produces a dose-related increase in sleep disruption. This is evident in an increase of number of awakenings, longer awakenings, and REM rebound. Interest-ingly, among alcoholic individuals these effects have been shown to persist even after they have stopped drinking. Aside from the second-half sleep fragmentation, the use of alcohol as a sleep aid, even at low doses, is problematic. First, within 6 nights, tolerance to alcohol develops and there is a resultant sleep disturbance beyond basal levels of insomnia and additional alcohol doses are consumed to try to achieve the positive effects on sleep.[24] Future research is needed to determine if this type of alcohol consumption leads to daytime alcohol consumption. Finally, in one population-based study, insomnia patients who reported hypnotic alcohol use reported greater levels of daytime sleepiness than individuals using prescription or OTC sleep aids.[25]

OTC agents represent the other major route of insomnia self-management. OTC sleep aids are either an H1 antihistamine alone, or an H1 antihistamine in combination with an analgesic. The H1 antihistamine is typically diphenhydramine 25 mg or 50 mg. Although diphenhydramine is thought of as a pure antihistamine, it is important to remember that it also possesses anticholinergic properties. In fact, many of the side effects associated with their use (eg, dry mouth) are mediated by their anticholinergic activity. In terms of efficacy, although there are reports that diphenhydramine increases total sleep time during the night,[26] there are virtually no parallel group placebo-controlled trials evaluating the hypnotic efficacy of these agents. In daytime administration studies, diphenhydramine has been shown to lose its sedative properties, as measured by sleep latency, after 2 or 3 administrations.[27] Finally, diphenhydramine has a half-life of 10 to 15 hours and hence results in reports of residual sedation in the morning.

The final self-treatment modality is herbal medication. According to the National Health Interview of the general population, 5% of patients with insomnia reported "alternative treatments," primarily herbal medications.[28] The most common of the many herbal medications taken for insomnia is valerian root. In a recent review of the literature, 29 trials in insomnia patients were identified . The conclusion of the review is that valerian root does not improve the sleep of patients with insomnia, whether assayed by patient report or PSG.[29] The other herbal used to treat insomnia, as well as other conditions like depression, is St John's Wart. Again, there are no consistent data demonstrating its efficacy. Finally, as these are herbal medications, it is assumed that they are safe. In fact, there are few data evaluating their safety. The FDA in 1999 issued a warning that St John's Wart interacts with other drugs via cytochrome 450.[30] Importantly, patients should always consult their clinician before undertaking ANY treatment for their insomnia.

Prescription Medications

Drugs indicated for the treatment of insomnia

With the introduction of flurazepam, the benzodiazepine receptor agonists (BzRAs) have been the drugs of choice for the treatment of insomnia for the past 50 years. These medications are termed BzRAs because their mechanism of action involves occupation of the benzodiazepine (alpha) receptors on the GABA$_A$ receptor complex resulting in the opening of the chloride ion channel and thereby facilitating GABA inhibition. Importantly, these medications act allosterically, requiring GABA to be present for them to exert their effects on the ion channel.[31] This affords them a wide, relative to efficacy, safety margin.[32] This is in sharp contrast to the medications they replaced: the barbiturates and barbiturate derivatives. These medications do not require GABA to be present, and as a result they are lethal in high doses. Among the BzRAs are the those medications that have a benzodiazepine structure (ie, flurazepam, temazepam, triazolam, estazolam, and quazepam), as well as other drugs that bind at these receptors but are not benzodiazepines (ie, zolpidem, zaleplon, eszopiclone, and zolpidem CR).

These drugs vary on 2 dimensions. First, these medications vary in terms of pharmacokinetic parameters and, second, in terms of which of the benzodiazepine receptor subtypes they have binding affinity for. As for kinetics, all of these medications are rapidly absorbed and, thus, at therapeutic doses they all hasten sleep onset (ie, decrease sleep latency). Specifically, they all have a Cmax of 1.0 to 1.5 hours. This is not the case for some of the BzRA anxiolytics (eg, oxazepam), which has a longer Tmax and thus no sleep-inducing properties. In contrast, there are dramatic differences between the BzRAs in terms of their half-lives. As a general rule, with single-compartment kinetics, drugs with a half-life longer than 6 hours are likely to result in residual effects when used at doses that have demonstrated hypnotic properties. Among the benzodiazepines, only triazolam has a short half-life. Temazepam and estazolam have intermediate half-lives, whereas flurazepam and quazepam have long half-lives. All of the intermediate and long-acting drugs have been shown to exhibit residual effects. Among the non-benzodiazepines, zolpidem and zaleplon have short half-lives, whereas eszopiclone has an intermediate half-life. The efficacy of the BzRAs has been well documented with these medications having been shown to exhibit dose-dependent hypnotic activity.[33,34] Depending on Tmax, T1/2, and dose, these medications induce and maintain sleep. Among the non-benzodiazepines, based on FDA labeling, zaleplon and zolpidem are indicated for sleep induction, whereas eszopiclone and zolpidem CR are indicated for sleep induction, as well as sleep maintenance.

The development of tolerance to the hypnotic activity of these drugs has been a controversial area. Tolerance is defined as a loss of efficacy with continued nightly use, or the need to escalate dose to sustain efficacy. Clinical lore has been that with long-term nightly use, there is a loss of efficacy (ie, tolerance). However, the vast majority of the literature indicates with clinical doses there is no loss of efficacy over the periods studied. There have been individual studies that have been thought to indicate the development of tolerance. However, careful inspection of these studies indicates that the drug shows a stable response across time, whereas the placebo group shows an improvement in sleep across time.[35] This can result in a loss of statistical significance when comparing drug with placebo. However, this is more appropriately interpreted as a placebo response, or a sleep hygiene response in the placebo group. In fact, recently, several BzRAs have been shown to have efficacy with 6 months of nightly use.[36,37]

The other major difference among the BzRAs relates to binding affinity. All of the benzodiazepines demonstrate similar affinity to 4 benzodiazepine receptor subtypes (alpha 1, 2, 3, and 5) located on the GABA$_A$ complex. In contrast, zolpidem and zaleplon have higher affinity to the alpha 1 subtype than the other subtypes. Eszopiclone shows a decreased preference for the alpha 1 complex, having affinity to alpha 2 and 3, as well. Although knock-in genetic data from animal studies suggest differential effects associated with different receptor subtypes, this has not been clearly demonstrated in human studies. The current speculation is that alpha 1 mediates the sleep-promoting effects, whereas alpha 2 and 3 are involved in anxiolytic and possibly antidepressant effects.[38]

There are 2 medications indicated for insomnia that do not bind at the GABA$_A$ complex. Ramelteon is a melatonin receptor agonist. The suprachiasmatic nucleus (SCN) contains both MT1 and MT2 receptors. The MT1 receptor is thought to attenuate the SCN's alerting signal and thereby decreases sleep latency, whereas the MT2 receptor has been hypothesized to have phase-shifting properties.[39] Ramelteon 8 mg has been shown to decrease sleep latency and is therefore indicated for sleep-onset insomnia.[40] It has not been shown to posses sleep maintenance properties. The drug most recently approved for insomnia is doxepin. Doxepin is a tricyclic antidepressant. The usual dosage of doxepin for treatment of depression is 75 to 150 mg per day. At this dosage, and even at lower dosages, such as 25 mg per day, doxepin has antihistaminic, antimuscarinic, antiadrenergic, and antiserotonergic effects.[41] Its affinity for H1 receptors, which is thought to be largely responsible for its sedating effect, is much higher than its affinity for the other receptors. At the dosages indicated for insomnia, doxepin is felt to be a pure H1 antagonist. In fact, in clinical trials there were no anticholinergic side effects. At 3 and 6 mg, doxepin has been shown to maintain sleep throughout the night. In contrast to the BzRAs, it has been shown to increase sleep during the last 2 hours of the night without having morning residual effects.[42] It is hypothesized that the circadian raise in histamine in the morning overrides the sedative effects of doxepin in the morning. Doxepin is indicated for sleep maintenance insomnia only as, at these dosages, it has had inconsistent effects on sleep latency.

Although the BzRAs have clearly demonstrated acute and chronic efficacy, the major concern with them has been safety. With the introduction of flurazepam, a drug with a 50-hour half-life, there has always been a concern about residual effects. Residual effects have been demonstrated with laboratory tests like digit symbol substitution and reaction time, sleep laboratory tests like the Multiple Sleep Latency Test, as well as with on-the-road driving tests.[43,44] It is important to recognize that all BzRAs impair many aspects of human performance after ingestion. Early in the night when peak plasma concentrations occur, the degree of impairment relates to drug concentrations,[10] which is a result of dose and time since ingestion. In contrast, the duration of impairment relates to half-life and dose.[45]

In studies looking at equipotent doses of BzRAs, that is they exhibited comparable impairment at peak plasma and/or had comparable effects on sleep latency, the drugs with longer half-lives were associated with greater residual effects. However, it is important to recognize that every drug, even those with short half lives, when taken at supra therapeutic doses, can result in residual effects. Thus, whereas both triazolam and zolidem have half-lives of 2 to 4 hours, they have been shown to be associated with residual effects when "higher doses" have been used (eg, 0.5 triazolam and 20 mg zolpidem).

Aside from residual effects, BzRAs also affect memory. Specifically the BzRAs produce anterograde amnesia.[46] Anterograde amnesia refers to the loss of information for materials presented after the ingestion of medication. The degree of amnesia has been related to dose and timing of stimulus information in relation to time of drug ingestion.[47] Take together, these clearly indicate that amnesia relates to drug concentrations. Data indicate that the amnestic properties of BzRAs are mediated by 3 mechanisms. First, amnesia is mediated by the sedative properties of drugs. All sedative drugs, including BzRAs, barbiturates, and antidepressants, produce amnesia.[48] Second, sleep itself is amnestic. People routinely fail to recall information presented during sleep. Thus, to the degree to which BzRAs produce sleep, they inhibit memory consolidation and therefore produce amnesia. Finally, amnesia is also associated with receptor selectivity at the alpha 1 subunit of the GABA$_A$ complex. Animal knock-out data have demonstrated that the alpha 1 subunit mediates both sleep and anterograde amnesia.[49] As currently there are no BzRAs that do not bind to the alpha 1 subunit, all currently available BzRAs have been associated with amnesia. Interestingly, the 2 non-BzRA hypnotics, ramelteon and doxepin, have not have not been shown to have anterograde amnesia to the same extent as BzRAs.

Discontinuation of hypnotic medications is associated with 3 distinct discontinuation phenomena. The first is recrudescence, which is a return of symptoms to baseline (pretreatment) levels. Recrudescence occurs as currently available hypnotics seem to provide symptomatic relief and thus when they are discontinued, the insomnia symptoms reoccur. It is important that this conclusion has been drawn from relatively short therapeutic trials of 5 weeks or less. More recent trials of 6 months have shown some benefit even after the discontinuation of medication. The possibility of insomnia attenuation beyond nights of medication use warrants further investigation.

The second discontinuation phenomenon is rebound insomnia. This is the most common discontinuation effect of BzRAs seen in clinical practice. Rebound insomnia is defined as a worsening of insomnia to levels beyond those seen at baseline. Rebound has been reported as longer sleep latencies, decreased total sleep time, and greater WASO lasting for 1 to 2 nights after discontinuation. Rebound is highly dose dependent.[50] The lowest doses that have consistently shown to posses hypnotic properties have not produced rebound, whereas higher doses of these medications routinely produce rebound. In contrast to dose, duration of use has not been shown to be determinant of rebound. However, long-term trials with multiple doses evaluating rebound have not been performed systematically. Most importantly, rebound is associated with half-life. Rebound is

seen with short- and intermediate-acting BzRAs, but not long acting. The reason for the lack of rebound with long-acting medication is because they self-taper across time, thereby precluding an abrupt drug-free state. In this same way, clinicians can prevent the occurrence of rebound by gradually tapering medication across nights rather than abruptly discontinuing them. In any case, there are no data to suggest that rebound insomnia is associated with dependence.

Finally, withdrawal has been reported with the use of BzRAs when used as anxiolytics. Withdrawal refers to the appearance of a cluster of symptoms after discontinuation of medication, that were not seen before initiating medication. These symptoms are unpleasant and include anxiety, tachycardia, palpitations, muscle cramps, and occasionally even seizures. These effects have been reported with both short-acting and long-acting medications. In the case of longer-acting medications, there is a delay in the occurrence of these symptoms until the drug has cleared the system. The duration of withdrawal varies from several days to several weeks. Unlike rebound, withdrawal symptoms have been reported even with clinical doses of these medications.

The abuse of BzRAs has been a topic of much clinical discussion.[51] There is little question that drug abusers will abuse these medications. The more important question is whether use of these medications will lead to abuse in patients. From an epidemiologic point of view, it is important to point out that most hypnotic users use hypnotics continuously for 2 weeks or less. Second, patients who use these medications rarely escalate dosage beyond that which was prescribed for them.[52] However, the question arises about the long-terms users. Is long-term use indicative of behavioral or physical dependence or is it reflective of therapy-seeking behavior. Efficacy studies of 6 months of nightly use have failed to uncover any signs or symptoms of physical dependence. However, the question arises about behavioral dependence. Short-term self-administration studies indicate the risk of behavioral dependence is low. First, they show that whereas patients with insomnia will self-administer these medications, they will do so at the same rate as they self-administer placebo. Second, over 2 weeks of access to multiple pills nightly, subjects self-administering placebo increase the number of pills they take, those taking active medication do not.[53] In fact, there is a slight trend to decrease them. Second, most patients with insomnia, when given an opportunity to self-administer these medications during the day, do not.[54] Thus, the pattern of use of these medications (ie, taken only at the therapeutic dosage and only in a clinical context) suggests they are being used for therapeutic purposes rather than reflecting dependence.

Recently there has been a concern about an increased incidence of complex behaviors in sleep associated with BzRAs. Among the behaviors reported are sleep eating, sleep walking, sleep driving, and even violent behaviors.[55] These have been reported with the use of zolpidem, zaleplon, and zopiclone (not available in the United States). These reports are from case series and their true incidence, and what mediates them, is unknown. Although there are no systematic data on these phenomena, it is believed that their occurrence is associated with higher doses, sleep deprivation, and coingestion with alcohol and other central nervous system depressant medications.

Drugs used off-label for the treatment of insomnia

The most commonly used off-label drugs for the treatment of insomnia are the antidepressants. Trazodone, amitriptyline, and mirtazepine are the 3 most widely used antidepressant medications, used at "lower doses" for the management of insomnia.[56] Although these medications each have different binding profiles, it is generally accepted that their activity as serotonin antagonists and as H1 antihistamines mediate their sleep-promoting properties.[57,58] The major problem with the use of these medications is the lack of information on the dose-related efficacy and safety of these medications when used to treat insomnia in nondepressed patients. Although it is always asserted that "low doses of sedating antidepressants" can be used to mange insomnia, there are no studies to define what low dose means. A review of the literature indicates that there are no studies in primary insomnia with amitriptyline or mirtazepine and only 2 studies with trazodone. In one study, a trazodone dose 150 mg was studied whereas in the other study it was 50 mg. That is a threefold difference in dose while both are referred to as "low dose." Also, the typically suggested hypnotic doses of trazodone are 25 to 50 mg. In the 150-mg study performed in "poor sleepers" over a 3-week period, trazodone decreased WASO as well as stage 1 NREM sleep; however, it failed to significantly increase total sleep time or decrease sleep latency.[59] In the 50-mg study, trazodone did decrease sleep latency, but the effect on total sleep time was present for only 1 week of administration.[60] Clearly, there is an inconsistency, as a 150-mg dose failed to increase total sleep time sleep, whereas 50 mg did. Thus, the concern about dose-related efficacy for these medications is critical.

The issue of dose is most clearly demonstrated with doxepin. Traditionally, it was recommended that low-dose doxepin (ie, 25–50 mg) can be used to treat insomnia.[41] When systematic dose-response studies were performed, it was discovered that the therapeutic doses for insomnia were as low as 3 to 6 mg.[42] Also, it has generally been accepted that patients develop tolerance for the daytime sedative effects of these drugs after 1 to 2 weeks of use. Thus, we are left with the question of not only what is the therapeutic dose, but also for how long is this efficacy maintained. Clinical lore suggests that the dose needs to be adjusted over time. The most important question relates to the safety of low-dose sedating antidepressants. A variety of side effects of these drugs ranging from suicidality, residual effects, anticholinergic effects, and cardiac conduction abnormalities have been associated with the antidepressant doses of these medications.[61–63] What the risks associated with the hypnotic doses of these medications are remains unexplored. In the absence of systematic data, it is generally concluded that the risk-benefit ratio of these medications is not as favorable as the drugs currently indicated for insomnia therapy.[13]

The atypical antipsychotics quetiapine and olazepine are also frequently used for the management of insomnia in nonpsychiatric patients. Although these medications bind at multiple receptors, their sleep-promoting activity is felt to be mediated primarily by their antihistaminic activity. The concern with the use of these medications is again related to dose and safety. The antihistaminic activity of the atypical antipsychotics is felt to contribute to weight gain. Does this also apply to "hypnotic doses"? In the case of atypical antipsychotics, there are no data on efficacy or safety in primary insomnia.

The final category of drugs used off label for the treatment of insomnia is the benzodiazepine anxiolytics. Of these, the most commonly used are clonazepam, alprazolam, and lorazepam. These medications have the same mechanism of action as the BzRAs indicated for insomnia. The 2 major concerns with these medications is that they have longer half-lives than the hypnotics in the same class. Also, like all of the other off-label-use drugs, there are little or no dose-response safety and efficacy data for these medications when used as hypnotics.

New Therapeutic Targets and Approaches

Given the track record of BzRAs, there are further attempts to identify molecules that possess superior kinetics and or a "better" biding profile for

GABA a receptor subtypes. Among medications in this class are indiplon and adipiplon.[64,65] Both of these medications have encountered issues that have stalled their development. In addition to new molecules, companies have attempted to develop new formulations of currently available medications. These attempts fall into 2 categories. First, there are several new formulations (eg, sublingual, spray, inhalation) being developed to decrease time to getting therapeutic blood levels and hence a faster sleep onset. One sublingual formulation is being developed at a lower dose of zolpidem (3.5 mg) intended for as-needed treatment of awakening during the night with difficulty falling back to sleep.[66] Second, there are several attempts to extend the duration of action of zaleplon by developing delayed-release or sustained-release formulations. The goal here, given the rapid offset of zaleplon, would be to develop a formulation of zaleplon that maintains sleep through the night without causing morning residual effects.

Aside from new BzRAs, there are increasing attempts to identify new therapeutic targets.

The orexin system is a relatively small number of neurons located in the lateral hypothalamus with extensive projections to many brain regions, but importantly ones involved in the regulation of sleep and wake. Activation of orexin neurons promotes wakefulness. Orexin neurons serve a controller function for other wake-promoting systems in the brain, including histamanergic neurons in the tubero-mamillary nucleus (TMN) and cholinergic neurons in the basal forebrain, noradrenergic neurons in the locus coeruleus, and serotonergic neurons in the dorsal raphe.[67] It is an absence of orexin that has been identified as the pathophysiology of narcolepsy.[68] There are 2 orexin receptors, and work is just starting to differentiate the functions of these receptors. Although there are currently no orexin agonists being studied for the treatment of sleepiness, orexin antagonists (for both receptors) are being evaluated for their efficacy in the management of insomnia.[69] Although there are few data currently in the literature, presentations at various meetings have suggested dual orexin antagonists have the potential for both inducing as well as maintaining sleep without residual effects. Some of the compounds in this class also seem to enhance REM sleep. Research is needed to determine the clinical significance, if any, of REM enhancement. Finally, given the various projections, there are lots of questions about the possible side effects.

Serotonin is an important transmitter in the regulation of sleep-wake function. Serotonergic neurons in the dorsal raphe play an important role in the control of sleep-wake states.[70] Firing rates of these neurons are maximal in wake, decline in NREM sleep, and are absent in REM sleep. The use of serotonergic compounds is complicated by the heterogeneity of the various receptor subtypes. The significance of these medications for sleep is evidenced by the high rate of sleep disturbance associated with the use of SSRIs. In contrast, antidepressant medications, which are serotonin antagonists, are the ones most typically used off-label for the management of insomnia. Specifically, those that are 5HT2a or 5HT2c are the ones most likely to promote sleep. There are several 5HT2a receptor agonists that are being developed for insomnia. These medications do not seem to have sedative activity and hence do not induce sleep, nor do they have any of the side effects associated with sedation (eg, psychomotor impairment, amnesia, ataxia, abuse liability in at-risk populations). These medications are effective in sleep maintenance. They are especially effective in sleep consolidation. It is hypothesized that this sleep consolidation is mediated by the robust enactment of slow-wave sleep exhibited by these medications. Finally, drugs that are serotonin antagonists and have other activities are also being investigated for the treatment of insomnia. Serotonin antagonists that also bind to the MT1 receptor, those that also are histamine antagonists, and those that are dopamine modulators are also being investigated in insomnia clinical trials. Although for the past 50 years we have been focused on the $GABA_A$ system, these new therapies hold promise for advances in the management of insomnia.

REFERENCES

1. Edinger JD, Bonnet MH, Bootzin RR, et al. Derivation of research diagnostic criteria for insomnia: report of an American Academy of Sleep Medicine work group. Sleep 2004;27:1567–96.
2. World Health Organization. International classification of diseases (ICD-10). Geneva (Switzerland): World Health Organization; 1991.
3. American Psychiatric Association. Diagnostic and statistical manual of mental disorders (DSM-IV-TR). Text Revision. 4th edition. Washington, DC: American Psychiatric Association; 2000.
4. Roehrs T, Zorick F, Sicklesteel J, et al. Age-related sleep-wake disorders at a sleep disorder center. J Am Geriatr Soc 1983;31(6):364–70.
5. Rechtschaffen A, Kales A, editors. A manual of standardized terminology, techniques and scoring system for sleep stages of human subjects. Los Angeles (CA): Brain Information Service/Brain Research Institute, UCLA; 1968.

6. Greenblatt DJ, von Moltke LL, Harmatz JS, et al. Kinetic and dynamic interaction study of zolpidem and ketoconazole, itraconazole, and fluconazole. Clin Pharmacol Ther 1998;64(6):661–71.

7. Vogel GW, Buffenstein A, Minter K, et al. Drug effects on REM sleep and on endogenous depression. Neurosci Biobehav Rev 1990;14:49–63.

8. Walsh JK, Zammit G, Schweitzer PK, et al. Tiagabine enhances slow wave sleep and sleep maintenance in primary insomnia. Sleep Med 2006;6:155–61.

9. Drake C, Roehrs T, Burduvali E, et al. Effects of rapid versus slow accumulation of eight hours of sleep loss. Psychophysiology 2001;38:979–87.

10. Riedel BW, Lichstein KL. Insomnia and daytime functioning. Sleep Med Rev 2000;4(3):277–98.

11. Ancoli-Israel A, Roth T. Characteristics of insomnia in the United States: results of the 1991 National Sleep Foundation survey I. Sleep 1999;22(2):S347–53.

12. Bastein CH, Vallieres A, Morin CM. Validation of the insomnia severity index as an outcome measure for insomnia research. Sleep Med 2001;2:297–307.

13. National Institutes of Health. State of the science conference statement on manifestations and management of chronic insomnia in adults June 13–15, 2005. Sleep 2005;28(9):1049–57.

14. Tashjian RZ, Banerjee R, Bradley MP, et al. Zolpidem reduces postoperative pain, fatigue, and narcotic consumption following knee arthroscopy: a prospective randomized placebo-controlled double-blinded study. J Knee Surg 2006;19(2):105–11.

15. Dirks J, Fredensborg BB, Christensen D, et al. A randomized study of the effects of single-dose gabapentin versus placebo on postoperative pain and morphine consumption after mastectomy. Anesthesiology 2002;97(3):560–4.

16. Fava M, McCall WV, Krystal A, et al. Eszopiclone co-administered with fluoxetine in patients with insomnia coexisting with major depressive disorder. Biol Psychiatry 2006;59:1052–60.

17. Drake CL, Scofield H, Roth T. Vulnerability to insomnia: the role of familial aggregation. Sleep Med 2008;9:297–302.

18. Gumenyuk V, Roth T, Moran JE, et al. Cortical locations of maximal spindle activity: magnetoencephalography (MEG) study. J Sleep Res 2009;18(2):245–53.

19. Roth T, Ancoli-Israel. Daytime consequences and correlates of insomnia in the United States: results of the 1991 National Sleep Foundation survey. II. Sleep 1999;22(2):S354–8.

20. Gallup. Sleep in America. Princeton (NJ): Gallup; 1995. p. 1–78.

21. Johnson EO, Roehrs T, Roth T, et al. Epidemiology of alcohol and medication as aids to sleep in early adulthood. Sleep 1998;21:178–86.

22. Roehrs T, Roth T. Sleep, sleepiness, sleep disorders and alcohol use and abuse. Sleep Med Rev 2001;5:287–97.

23. Roehrs T, Papineau K, Rosenthal L, et al. Ethanol as a hypnotic in insomniacs: self administration and effects of sleep and mood. Neuropsychopharmacology 1999;20:279–86.

24. Roehrs T, Blaisdel B, Cruz N, et al. Tolerance to hypnotic effects of ethanol in insomniacs [abstract]. Sleep 2004;27:A52.

25. Roehrs T, Hollebeek E, Drake C, et al. Substance use for insomnia in metropolitan Detroit. J Psychosom Res 2003;53:571–6.

26. Rickels K, Morris RJ, Newman H, et al. Diphenhydramine in insomnia family practice patients: a double-blind study. J Clin Pharmacol 1983;23(5–6):234–42.

27. Richardson GS, Roehrs TA, Rosenthal L, et al. Tolerance to daytime sedative effects of H1 antihistamines. J Clin Psychopharmacol 2002;22:511–5.

28. Pearson NJ, Johnson LL, Nahin RL. Insomnia, trouble sleeping, and complementary and alternative medicine. Arch Intern Med 2006;166:1775–82.

29. Taibi DM, Landis CA, Petry H, et al. A systematic review of valerian as a sleep aid: safe but not effective. Sleep Med Rev 2007;11:209–30.

30. Clinical Practice Review Committee. American Academy of Sleep Medicine. Oral nonprescription treatment for insomnia: an evaluation of products with limited evidence. J Clin Sleep Med 2005;1:173–87.

31. Mohler H, Fritschy JM, Rudolph U. A new benzodiazepine pharmacology. J Pharmacol Exp Ther 2002;300:2–8.

32. Mendelson WB, Thompson C, Franko T. Adverse reactions to sedative hypnotics: three years' experience. Sleep 1996;19:702–6.

33. Merlotti L, Roehrs T, Koshorek G, et al. The dose effects of zolpidem on the sleep of healthy normals. J Clin Psychopharm 1989;9(1):9–14.

34. Lamphere JK, Roehrs TA, Zorick FJ, et al. The dose effects of zopiclone. Hum Psychopharmacol 1989;4:41–6.

35. Karin A, Tolbert D, Cao C. Disposition kinetics and tolerance of escalating single doses of remelteon, a high-affinity MT_1 and MT_2 melatonin receptor agonist indicated for treatment of insomnia. J Clin Pharmacol 2006;46:140–8.

36. Krystal A, Walsh J, Roth T, et al. Evaluation of the efficacy and safety of eszopiclone over six months of treatment in patients with insomnia [abstract]. Poster presented at sleep 2006. Salt Lake City (UT): Associated Professional Sleep Societies, June 17–26, 2006.

37. Walsh JK, Krystal AD, Amato DA, et al. Nightly treatment of primary insomnia with eszopiclone for six months: effect on sleep, quality of life and work limitations. Sleep 2007;30:959–68.

38. Milter MM, Seidel WF, Van Den Hoed J, et al. Comparative hypnotic effects of flurazepam, triazolam, and placebo: a long-term simultaneous

nighttime and daytime study. J Clin Psychopharmacol 1984;4:2–13.

39. Kato K, Hirai K, Nichiyama K, et al. Neurochemical properties of ramelteon (TAK-375), a selective MT_1 and MT_2 receptor agonist. Neuropharmacology 2005;48:301–10.

40. Roth T, Stubbs C, Walsh JK. Ramelteon (TAK-375), a selective MT1/MT2-receptor agonist, reduces latency to persistent sleep in a model of transient insomnia related to a novel sleep environment. Sleep 2005;28(3):303–7.

41. Hajak G, Rodenbeck A, Voderholzer U, et al. Doxepin in the treatment of primary insomnia: a placebo-controlled, double-blind, polysomnographic study. J Clin Psychiatry 2001;62:453–63.

42. Roth T, Rogowski R, Hull S. Efficacy and safety of doxepin 1 mg, 3 mg, and 6 mg in adults with primary insomnia. Sleep 2007;30:1555–61.

43. Carskadon MA, Seidel WF, Greenblatt DJ, et al. Daytime carryover of triazolam and flurazepam in elderly insomniacs. Sleep 1982;5:362–71.

44. Rush CR, Griffiths RR. Zolpidem, triazolam and temazepam: behavioral and subject-rated effects in normal volunteers. J Clin Psychopharmacol 1996;16:146–57.

45. Danjou P, Fruncillo PR, Worthington P, et al. A comparison of the residual effects of zaleplon and zolpidem following administration 5 to 2 h before awakening. Br J Clin Pharmacol 1999;48:367–74.

46. Roehrs T, Merlotti L, Zorick F, et al. Sedative, memory and performance effects of hypnotics. Psychopharmacology (Berl) 1994;116:130–4.

47. Roehrs T, Zorick F, Sicklesteel J, et al. Effects of hypnotics on memory. J Clin Psychopharmacol 1983;3:310–3.

48. Green JF, McElholm A, King DJ. A comparison of the sedative and amnestic effects of chlorpromazine and lorazepam. Psychopharmacology (Berl) 1996; 128:67–73.

49. Mohler H, Crestani F, Rudolph U. GABA-A receptor subtypes: a new pharmacology. Curr Opin Pharmacol 2001;1:22–5.

50. Roehrs TA, Vogel G, Roth T. Rebound insomnia: its determinants and significant. Am J Med 1990;88: 43S–6S.

51. Woods JH, Winger G. Current benzodiazepine issues. Psychopharmacology (Berl) 1995;118:107–15.

52. Mellinger GD, Balter MB, Uhlenhuth EH. Insomnia and its treatment. Arch Gen Psychiatry 1985;42:225–32.

53. Roehrs T, Pedrosi B, Rosenthal L, et al. Hypnotic self administration and dose escalation. Psychopharmacology (Berl) 1996;127:150–4.

54. Roehrs T, Bonahoom A, Pedrosi B, et al. Nighttime versus daytime hypnotic self-administration. Psychopharmacology (Berl) 2002;161:137–42.

55. Lisko B, Pikalov A. Zaleplon overdose associated with sleepwalking and complex behavior. J Am Acad Child Adolesc Psychiatry 2004;43:927–8.

56. Walsh JK. Drugs used to treat insomnia in 2002: regulatory-based rather than evidence-based medicine. Sleep 2004;27:1441–2.

57. Jenck F, Moreau JL, Mutel V, et al. Evidence for a role of 5-HT1C receptors in the antiserotonergic properties of some antidepressant drugs. Eur J Pharmacol 1993;231:223–9.

58. Richelson E. The pharmacology of antidepressants at the synapse: focus on newer compounds. J Clin Psychiatry 1994;55(Suppl A):34–9.

59. Montgomery I, Oswald I, Morgan K, et al. Trazodone enhances sleep in subjective quality but not in objective duration. Br J Clin Pharmacol 1983;16:139–44.

60. Walsh JK, Erman M, Erwin CW, et al. Subjective hypnotic efficacy of trazodone and zolpidem in DSM-III-R primary insomnia. Hum Psychopharmacol 1998;13:191–8.

61. Golden RN, Dawkins K, Nicholas L. Trazodone and nefazone. In: Schatzberg A, Nemeroff C, editors. The American psychiatric textbook of psychopharmacology. Washington, DC: American Psychiatric Textbook, Inc; 2004. p. 315–25.

62. Levenson JL. Prolonged QT interval after trazodone overdose. Am J Psychiatry 1999;156:969–70.

63. Haria M, Fitton A, McTavish D. Trazodone. A review of its pharmacology, therapeutic use in depression and therapeutic potential in other disorders. Drugs Aging 1994;4:331–55.

64. Lydiard RB, Lankford DA, Seiden DJ, et al. Efficacy and tolerability of modified-release indiplon in elderly patients with chronic insomnia: results of a 2-week double-blind, placebo-controlled trial. J Clin Sleep Med 2006;2(3):309–15.

65. Roth T, Lankford A, Accomando WP, et al. Sleep onset and maintenance in patients with chronic insomnia treated with adipiplon in a cross-over study. Sleep 2008;31(Suppl):A40–1 [abstract].

66. Roth T, Hull SG, Lankford DA, et al. Low-dose sublingual zolpidem tartrate is associated with dose-related improvement in sleep onset and duration in insomnia characterized by middle-of-the-night (MOTN) awakenings. Sleep 2008;31(9):1277–84.

67. Sakurai T, Amemiya A, Ishii M, et al. Orexins and orexin receptors: a family of hypothalamic neuropeptides and G protein-coupled receptors that regulate feeding behavior. Cell 1998;92(4):573–85.

68. Lin L, Faraco J, Li R, et al. The sleep disorder canine narcolepsy is caused by a mutation in the hypocretin (orexin) receptor 2 gene. Cell 1999;98(3):365–76.

69. Brisbare-Roch C, Dingemanse J, Kobertsein R, et al. Promotion of sleep by targeting the orexin system in rats, dogs, and humans. Nat Med 2007;13(2): 150–5.

70. Landolt HP, Meier V, Burgess HJ, et al. Serotonin-2 receptors and human sleep: effect of a selective antagonist on EEG power spectra. Neuropsychopharmacology 1999;21(3):455–66.

Allergy/Respiratory and Cardiovascular Drugs

Paula K. Schweitzer, PhD

KEYWORDS

- Allergy • Asthma • Chronic obstructive pulmonary disease
- Antihistamines • Antihypertensives • Theophylline
- Corticosteroids

Individuals with allergic rhinitis or asthma commonly report increased daytime sleepiness and decreased sleep quality, as well as decrements in cognitive function, quality of life, and work productivity as compared with asymptomatic individuals.[1–3] Controlled clinical trials have also demonstrated that patients with seasonal rhinitis[4,5] or asthma,[6] including clinically stable asthma,[7] have more microarousals during sleep, increased daytime sleepiness, and poorer quality of life than normal individuals. Asthmatics also show objective sleep disruption and impaired cognitive function during the daytime.[8,9] Patients with chronic obstructive pulmonary disease (COPD) show frequent arousals during sleep,[10,11] which correlate with subjective complaints of daytime sleepiness[12] but not necessarily with objective sleepiness as measured by the Multiple Sleep Latency Test (MSLT).[13] In addition, both hypoxemic and nonhypoxemic patients with COPD show decrements in cognitive performance.[14] These impairments in sleep and waking function in individuals with allergic rhinitis, asthma, or COPD may be caused or exacerbated by the disease and/or treatment with drugs that affect the central nervous system (CNS). On the other hand, CNS-active drug treatment that improves disease symptoms may result in better sleep and daytime function.[6,15]

The relationship between sleep and cardiovascular disease is complex. Individuals with sleep disorders are more likely to develop cardiovascular disease and, conversely, individuals with cardiovascular disease are more likely to have sleep disorders.[16–19] Sleep complaints and daytime sleepiness are commonly reported by untreated hypertensive males but are even more frequently reported by treated hypertensive males.[20] Cognitive impairment is common in patients with heart failure and may be at least partially related to sleep disturbances associated with sleep apnea or Cheyne-Stokes breathing.[21,22] As with respiratory diseases, sleep disturbance, daytime sleepiness, or cognitive impairment may be caused by disease or its treatment.

This article reviews drugs used to treat allergy and respiratory disorders as well as cardiovascular disease, and which have effects on sleep and/or waking function.

ALLERGY AND RESPIRATORY DRUGS

Drugs used to treat allergic rhinitis, asthma, and COPD include antihistamines, decongestants, corticosteroids, bronchodilators (including β-agonists and anticholinergic drugs), leukotriene antagonists, mast cell stabilizers, monoclonal antibodies, and theophylline. Their effects on sleep and waking function are summarized in **Table 1**.

Antihistamines

Histamine, which is widely present throughout the CNS and body, interacts with other transmitter systems in the control of sleep-wake regulation, circadian and feeding rhythms, immunity, learning, and memory.[23,24] Histaminergic neurons fire

Sleep Medicine and Research Center, St Luke's Hospital, 232 South Woods Mill Road, Chesterfield, MO 63017, USA
E-mail address: paula.schweitzer@stlukes-stl.com

Sleep Med Clin 5 (2010) 541–557
doi:10.1016/j.jsmc.2010.08.004
1556-407X/10/$ — see front matter © 2010 Elsevier Inc. All rights reserved.

sleep.theclinics.com

Table 1
Effects of allergy and respiratory drugs on sleep and waking behavior[a]

Drug Class	Drug Example	Subjective	PSG	MSLT	Performance	Comments
H$_1$ antagonists: first-generation	Chlorpheniramine, clemastine, cyproheptadine, diphenhydramine, doxylamine, hydroxyzine, promethazine, triprolidine	Sedation	Variable, may ↓ SL & ↑ TST	↓	↓	Tolerance to some of the sedating effects may develop
H$_1$ antagonists: second-generation	Cetirizine, desloratadine, fexofenadine, levocetirizine, loratadine	Nonsedating	No data	↔	↔	Cetirizine is more sedating than other drugs; loratadine impairs performance at high doses; fexofenadine does not increase sleepiness or impair performance even at high doses
Decongestants	Pseudoephedrine	Insomnia	↑ wake	No data	?↑	
Corticosteroids: oral	Dexamethasone, hydrocortisone, prednisone	Insomnia	↓ REM ↑ wake	?↑	?↓	
Corticosteroids: inhaled	Budesonide, flunisolide, fluticasone	Rare insomnia	No data	No data	?	Improvements in sleep quality, daytime sleepiness, and performance accompany symptom improvement

Methylxanthine	Theophylline	Insomnia	↑ wake	↑	↔	
Bronchodilators: inhaled anticholinergics	Ipratropium, tiotropium	No sleep complaints	No data	No data	See comments	Improved sleep quality accompanies symptom improvement
Bronchodilators: β_2 agonists	Terbutaline, salmeterol, fomoterol	Restlessness	No data	No data	See comments	Improved sleep quality accompanies symptom improvement
Leukotriene antagonists	Montelukast	Case reports of insomnia	No data	No data	See comments	Improvements in sleep quality, daytime sleepiness, and performance accompany symptom improvement
Mast cell stabilizers	Cromolyn sodium, nedocromil	No sleep complaints	No data	No data	No data	
Monoclonal antibodies	Omalizumab	No sleep complaints	No data	No data	See comments	Improvements in sleep quality and daytime activities accompany symptom improvement

Abbreviations: MSLT, multiple sleep latency test; PSG, polysomnography; REM, rapid eye movement sleep; SL, sleep latency; TST, total sleep time.

[a] ↓ = decrease; ↑ = increase; ↔ = no change.

actively during wakefulness, reinforced by excitatory input from orexin/hypocretin neurons, and are inhibited by γ-aminobutyric acid (GABA) input during sleep. Four types of histamine receptors have been described (H_1–H_4). H_1 receptors are present throughout the body, particularly in the CNS, vascular endothelial cells, and smooth muscle. In the CNS, H_1 receptors appear to mediate the waking effect of histamine while in the periphery they affect vasodilation, bronchoconstriction, and capillary permeability. H_2 receptors mediate gastric acid secretion, which is blocked by H_2 antihistamines such as cimetidine. H_3 receptors are presynaptic autoreceptors that mediate release of histamine and other transmitters including acetylcholine, glutamate, and GABA. H_4 receptors are found primarily in the periphery and may be involved in inflammation. Histamine H_1 antagonists are a mainstay in the treatment of allergic rhinitis.

Drugs currently classified as H_1 antagonists are not truly histamine antagonists but inverse agonists, as they stabilize the receptor in its inactive state.[25] Among the classic antihistamines, drugs have been divided into 2 groups by their sedative potential. First-generation H_1 antihistamines (see **Table 1**) are lipophilic molecules that easily cross the blood-brain barrier, demonstrating H_1 receptor occupancy of 60% or more.[26,27] In addition to H_1 antagonism they show muscarinic cholinergic, α-adrenergic, and serotonergic (5-HT) antagonism, which may also influence sedation. Elimination half-lives range from 4 to 8 hours for diphenhydramine to 20 to 27 hours for hydroxyzine and chlorpheniramine; doxylamine has a half-life of 10 hours. Second-generation antihistamines (see **Table 1**) are hydrophilic molecules that do not easily penetrate the CNS. Although they are much more selective than the first generation antihistamines, H_1 receptor occupancy varies from almost negligible (fexofenadine) to as high as 30% (cetirizine 20 mg).[28] Elimination half-lives range from 7 to 27 hours. The second-generation drugs astemizole and terfenadine have been withdrawn from the United States market because of cardiotoxicity.

The effects of H_1-antihistamines on sleepiness and performance are well reviewed in several articles.[29–36] Both the incidence and degree of subjective sleepiness during daytime administration is significantly higher with the first-generation antihistamines than with the second-generation compounds.[35,37] MSLT studies in normal[38–43] and atopic individuals[44] generally confirm that diphenhydramine, hydroxyzine, promethazine, and triprolidine are sedating whereas cetirizine, desloratadine, fexofenadine, loratadine, and terfenadine are not. On the other hand, bedtime administration of first-generation drugs has variable effects on nocturnal sleep. Diphenhydramine, widely used as an over-the-counter hypnotic, sometimes results in improved subjective measures of sleep latency, sleep duration, and sleep quality,[45,46] and sometimes has no significant effect on subjective sleep estimates[47,48] in individuals with insomnia. Polysomnography (PSG) data are also inconsistent. A study of 184 insomniacs treated with diphenhydramine showed no improvement in sleep and no effects on sleep architecture,[48] while a study of 12 poor sleepers treated with promethazine showed increased total sleep time (TST).[49] Two small studies on normal individuals showed decreased sleep latency and increased TST with hydroxyzine[50] but increased sleep latency and decreased rapid eye movement (REM) with chlorpheniramine.[51] Nonetheless, it is clear that when administered during the daytime, first-generation drugs result in increased sleepiness both subjectively and objectively in most individuals when used acutely.

In addition, controlled studies evaluating psychomotor skills, memory, attention, and actual driving performance confirm that the first-generation H_1 antagonists impair performance whereas the second-generation drugs are much less likely to do so.[44,52–54] First-generation drugs have been associated with injuries[55,56] and traffic accidents[57] as well. Even when administered at night, sedation and psychomotor impairment may be present the following morning.[58] A review of 212 studies with both positive and placebo controls concluded that the risk of performance impairment was minimal and similar among astemizole, cetirizine, loratadine, and terfenadine, whereas the risk of impairment was significantly higher for the first-generation drugs, with triprolidine offering the highest risk followed by diphenhydramine, clemastine, and chlorpheniramine.[59] Shamsi and Hindmarch[29] confirmed these findings in a review of 76 well-controlled studies by computation of a proportional impairment ratio, which allowed antihistamines to be ranked with respect to their ability to cause impairments in cognitive or psychomotor function. However, they also indicated that impairment was present with some second-generation drugs, particularly mizolastine (not available in the United States), cetirizine, and loratadine, especially when used in higher doses. On the other hand, fexofenadine did not impair cognitive, psychomotor, or driving performance even with doses in excess of the clinical dose.[60–62] Studies on desloratadine and levocetirizine also suggest they do not impair cognition, memory, or driving performance.[43,63,64] Further examination of data on cetirizine indicates that whereas most MSLT[40,44] and performance studies[65-67] demonstrate that cetirizine is nonsedating, several studies suggest it is more subjectively sedating and more likely to impair performance than most other second-generation drugs, particularly when used in high doses or in combination with alcohol.[35,62,68,69] This result is consistent with the observation that H_1 receptor occupancy is higher with cetirizine than with other second-generation drugs, and doubles with a 20-mg dose compared with 10 mg.[70]

There is evidence that tolerance to some of the sedating effects of antihistamines may develop with repeated use over time. Increased MSLT-measured sleepiness and impaired performance present on the first day of treatment with diphenhydramine were diminished by the third or fourth day of treatment in both atopic individuals[44] and normals.[71] Several other placebo-controlled studies on normals showed less impairment in subjective sleepiness and/or performance after 3 to 7 days of diphenhydramine or hydroxyzine compared with the first or second day.[66,72-74] However, in some cases performance was still poorer than with placebo, particularly in studies of driving performance,[73] and in other cases no tolerance was found.[75]

Decongestants

Decongestants may be given alone or in combination with antihistamines for the treatment of rhinitis. Decongestants decrease blood flow to mucous membranes by direct effect on α-adrenergic receptors and cause vasoconstriction indirectly by releasing norepinephrine, which in turn acts on α-adrenergic receptors. Phenylephrine, phenylpropanolamine, and oxymetazoline (a topical decongestant) are direct agonists whereas pseudoephedrine acts indirectly. Phenylephrine is selective for α_1 receptors, phenylpropanolamine is selective for α_2 receptors, and pseudoephedrine and oxymetazoline are nonselective.[76] Phenylpropanolamine is no longer available for human use in the United States. Although the structural formulas of decongestants are similar to those of both epinephrine and amphetamine, these drugs are much less lipophilic and the frequency of CNS adverse reactions is fairly low.[77] These drugs have been reported to cause insomnia, but data are limited.[78] Insomnia complaints occurred in 10% to 27% of patients given pseudoephedrine alone or in combination with second-generation antihistamines for the treatment of allergic or vasomotor rhinitis and appeared to be more frequent with higher doses and some extended-release formulations.[79-84] In a PSG study, the administration of pseudoephedrine in the evening (as part of either a 60-mg 4 times daily or sustained-release 120-mg twice-daily dosing regimen) produced increased wake time during sleep compared with the morning administration of a once-daily controlled-release formulation (240 mg).[85] Phenylpropanolamine has been reported to increase plasma caffeine levels,[86] possibly adding to the stimulant effect of caffeine. Several studies have documented improvement in psychomotor and driving performance with use of decongestants given alone or in combination with first-generation or second-generation antihistamines.[87-89]

Corticosteroids

Corticosteroids are used in the treatment of allergies, asthma, and COPD. Their potent anti-inflammatory effects are the result of up-regulation of anti-inflammatory proteins and inhibition of proinflammatory proteins following binding to glucocorticoid receptors.[90] Glucocorticoids are lipophilic and readily penetrate the CNS.

Oral corticosteroids are widely believed to disrupt sleep, but the results of objective studies are inconsistent. Differences in receptor affinities between synthetic and endogenous corticosteroids, dosage, methodologic issues associated with the study of patient populations, and the variety of organ systems affected by corticosteroids, as well as the variety of side effects reported,[91] all contribute to this confusion.

In patient populations, corticosteroids have frequently been associated with sleep disturbance. Insomnia rates in several studies range from 20% to 70% of patients receiving steroid medication for treatment of asthma,[92] optic neuritis,[93] or inflammatory ulcerative disease.[94] Parent ratings of sleep disturbance increased when steroids were added to the chemotherapy regimen of children with leukemia or other types of cancer. Behavioral observations of 12 healthy subjects given prednisone 80 mg/d for 5 days showed decreased sleep in 25% and mild hypomania in 67%.[95]

The most consistent effect of systemic corticosteroids on PSG-recorded sleep in normal subjects is a marked decrease in REM sleep.[96,97] Although less consistent, there is good evidence for increased waking during the night with cortisol, dexamethasone, and prednisone. Dexamethasone, administered before bedtime, resulted in increased daytime alertness the next day as measured with MSLT.[98]

In a single study evaluating performance in healthy subjects, prednisone 80 mg/d given for 5 days produced increased frequency of errors of commission on a verbal memory task.[99] Predni-sone was associated with decreased cognitive functioning in a study of patients with systemic lupus erythematosus.[100]

Intranasal corticosteroids do not appear to have the same negative effects as oral corticosteroids, likely the result of significantly lower systemic potency. However, systemic absorption is possible especially when used long term and in higher doses. There have been case reports of hyperactivity, insomnia, and psychosis with these drugs. Improvement in allergy symptoms with use of budenoside,[101] flunisolide,[102] or fluticasone[103–105] is associated with improved sleep quality, decreased daytime sleepiness, and increased cognitive performance.[106] Similarly, improvement in functional status and sleep quality accompanies amelioration of asthma symptoms treated with fluticasone.[107,108]

Theophylline

Theophylline, a respiratory stimulant and weak bronchodilator, is used in the treatment of asthma and COPD. Theophylline is used relatively infre-quently because of side effects and lower efficacy compared with inhaled anticholinergics, β_2-agonists, and corticosteroids.[109] However, at low doses it may have both anti-inflammatory and immunomodulatory effects. Theophylline is chemi-cally related to caffeine. Proposed mechanisms of action include adenosine receptor antagonism (which may be responsible for sleep complaints as well as arrhythmias), phosphodiesterase inhibi-tion (which may explain the side effects of nausea and headache), increased histone deacetylase activity (which suppresses the expression of inflammatory genes and may increase efficacy of corticosteroids), increased interleukin-10 release, stimulation of norepinephrne release, and inhibi-tion of intracellular calcium and kinases.[109] Peak plasma concentration is usually reached within 2 hours, but the half-life varies by preparation and is typically shorter in children (3.5 hours) and longer in adults (8–9 hours). Absorption is lower at night than in the morning[110] and may be greatly affected by food.[111]

Disturbed sleep is a common complaint among patients taking theophylline. In a prospective study, patients with asthma treated with theophyl-line were more likely to complain of sleep mainte-nance difficulty (55%) than were patients treated with other asthma medications (31%).[112] In a retro-spective study of treated patients with asthma, 46% of whom complained of insomnia, only theophylline or corticosteroid therapy was associ-ated with the complaint of insomnia.[92] Most of the

studies purporting that theophylline does not adversely affect sleep are limited by the lack of a placebo control or other methodologic difficul-ties. Because theophylline improves asthma-related symptoms, there have also been reports of improved sleep continuity and daytime function associated with its use.[6,113]

Theophylline, administered for up to 3 weeks, has been shown to disturb PSG-recorded sleep in healthy subjects,[114,115] children with cystic fibrosis,[116] and patients with asthma,[117] sleep apnea,[118] or COPD.[119] Several studies have shown more PSG-recorded sleep disturbance as well as lower sleep quality and quality-of-life measures in asthma patients treated with oral theophylline compared with inhaled β_2-agonists.[120–122] Dose-dependent increases in MSLT latency and performance were noted with short-term administration of theophylline in normals.[115] Asthmatic children were more likely to exhibit behavioral or attentional problems when receiving sustained-release theophylline for 4 weeks than when on placebo[123] However, a meta-analysis of 12 studies of theophylline did not indicate impairment in cognition or behavior.[124] Furthermore, academic achievement did not differ between 72 asthmatic patients who were treated with theophylline and siblings without asthma.[125]

Bronchodilators

Bronchodilators used in the treatment of asthma and COPD include anticholinergics as well as short-acting and long-acting β_2-agonists. These drugs have a direct relaxation effect on airway smooth muscle cells. Anticholinergics mediate smooth muscle contraction through parasympa-thetic stimulation via antagonism of muscarinic receptors M_1 and M_3. β_2-agonists bind to β_2-adrenergic receptors, which are present in high density in airway smooth muscle cells as well as in mast cells, submucosal glands, vascular endothelium, and circulating inflamma-tory cells.[126] The most common side effects are nervousness and restlessness, particularly with the long-acting β_2-agonists. Difficulty sleeping is rarely reported.

Both short-acting (ipratropium) and long-acting (tiotropium) inhaled anticholinergics improve oxygen saturation during sleep concomitant with improvements in lung function.[127,128] Sleep quality was also improved by ipratropium although the only change in PSG was an increase in REM sleep, likely the result of improved disease, not a direct effect of the drug on sleep.[127] Salmeterol, a long-acting β_2-agonist, has been associated with improved sleep quality and less wake time as well as fewer awakenings and arousals in PSG studies, particularly when compared with theophylline.[120–122]

Leukotriene Modifiers

Leukotriene modifiers either prevent leukotrienes from binding to their receptors or block the production of leukotrienes, lipid mediators that promote airway inflammation. These drugs are used in the treatment of asthma and allergic rhinitis. Clinical studies indicate that improvement in disease symptoms is accompanied by improved ratings of sleep quality and daytime somnolence and fatigue[129,130] as well as improved performance.[131] However, postmarketing reports have documented insomnia, restlessness, dream abnormalities, and somnambulism, and the subsequent Food and Drug Administration review of clinical trials indicated that sleep disorders (primarily insomnia) were reported more frequently with these drugs than with placebo.[132]

CARDIOVASCULAR DRUGS

Drugs used in the treatment of cardiovascular disease include antihypertensives, antiarrhythmics, antithrombotics, diuretics, inotropic and vasopressor agents, lipid-lowering drugs, and vasodilators. Several antihypertensive drugs also have antiarrhythmic properties. The effects of cardiovascular drugs on sleep and waking function are summarized in **Table 2**.

Antihypertensives

β-Antagonists

β-blockers are used in the treatment of hypertension, arrhythmia, heart failure, and myocardial infarction, as well as glaucoma and migraine. Information on pharmacologic characteristics of β-antagonists relevant to CNS sleep-wake function is given in **Table 3**. These drugs differ with regard to several pharmacologic factors including selectivity for β_1/β_2-adrenergic receptors, α_1 antagonism, intrinsic sympathomimetic activity, and vasodilating properties. CNS side effects reported include tiredness, fatigue, sedation, insomnia, nightmares, vivid dreams, depression, mental confusion, and psychomotor impairment.[133] Although these complaints seem to be more common with the more lipophilic drugs, high β_2 and/or 5-HT receptor occupancy may be more important factors in causing sleep disruption.[134] Nebivolol, a highly lipophilic compound that is highly selective for β_1 receptors, appears to be less disruptive of sleep than other

β-blockers, although fatigue is variably reported.[135,136] Fatigue or sedation has been reported, at least transiently, in β-antagonists with vasodilating properties that also block α_1 receptors (eg, carvedilol, labetolol).[137] Drugs that are more selective for β_1 receptors have lower affinity for 5-HT receptors. In addition, some β-antagonists decrease melatonin release via inhibition of β_1 receptors, which could affect sleep.[138,139] Because plasma concentration is also a factor,[140] drug dose is important. Except for nebivolol, most β_1-selective drugs are less selective at higher doses. Sleep disturbance is most commonly associated with propranolol (high lipid solubility, nonselective) and less commonly associated with atenolol (low lipid solubility, high β_1 selectivity) and nebivolol (high lipid solubility, very high β_1 selectivity). Both subjective and PSG data of normals[141,142] and hypertensive males[143] demonstrate increased wake with propranolol, metoprolol, and pindolol, but not with atenolol. REM is also decreased particularly at higher doses. Although cognitive and psychomotor performance deficits have been reported in several studies, these drugs appear to produce few consistent neuropsychological deficits.[133,144] In a review of 55 studies on neuropsychological effects of β-blockers, Dimsdale and colleagues[145] concluded that β-blockers improved cognitive function in 16% of observations, worsened it in 17%, and caused no change in 67%, with no significant difference between lipophilic and nonlipophilic drugs.

α_2-Agonists

Sedation is the most common side effect of both clonidine and methyldopa, occurring in 30% to 75% of patients, but the severity appears to diminish with time, suggesting that tolerance may develop.[146] There are also reports of insomnia and nightmares with these drugs. Intravenous clonidine, which has been used in the clinical practice of pain management,[147] results in suppression of alpha and increases in delta by electroencephalographic spectral analysis,[148] as well as subjective drowsiness and acute performance impairment.[149] Placebo-controlled PSG studies of clonidine in healthy subjects[150–152] and individuals with bruxism[153] or hypertension[154,155] show increased TST and decreased REM. No MSLT studies exist to quantify daytime sedation objectively. However, a single morning dose of clonidine resulted in microsleeps in 6 of 8 healthy subjects despite efforts of study personnel to keep them awake.[156] The same subjects showed increased stage 2 and decreased REM during a 3-hour daytime nap.

Table 2
Effects of cardiovascular drugs on sleep and waking behavior[a]

Drug Class	Drug Example	Subjective	PSG	MSLT	Performance	Comments
α₁-Antagonists	Prazosin Terazosin	Transient sedation	↑ TST ? ↑ REM	No data	Limited data	Prazosin used to treat PTSD
α₂-Agonists	Clonidine Methyldopa	Sedation Nightmares	↑ TST ↓ REM	No data	↓	
Angiotensin-converting enzyme inhibitors	Captopril Lisinopril		↔	No data	↔	Dry cough may disturb sleep
Angiotensin II blockers	Losartan Valsartan	No sleep-related complaints	No data	No data	No data	Subjective reports of improved performance
β-Antagonists	See **Table 3**	Fatigue, sedation, nightmares, insomnia	↑ wake ↓ REM	No data	↑ ↓ ↔	Sleep disturbance more likely with propranolol, less likely with atenolol, nebivolol; see **Table 3**
Calcium Antagonists	Verapamil Nifedipine	Rare sedation	No data	No data	Limited data	
Diuretics	Hydrochlorothiazide	No sleep-related complaints	No data	No data	No data	
Lipid-lowering drugs	Atorvastatin Lovastatin Simvastatin	Case reports of insomnia	↔ to ↑ wake (lovastatin)	↔	? ↓	
Vasodilators	Hydralazine	Rare fatigue	No data	No data	No data	

Abbreviations: MSLT, multiple sleep latency test; PSG, polysomnography; REM, rapid eye movement sleep; TST, total sleep time.
[a] ↓ = decrease; ↑ = increase; ↔ = no change.

Table 3
β-Antagonists: selected pharmacologic characteristics

Drug	Lipid Solubility[a]	β Selectivity[b]	Affinity for 5-HT Receptors	Comments
Propranolol	High	Nonselective	High	
Timolol	High	Nonselective	High	
Nadolol	Low	Nonselective	High	
Sotalol	Low	Nonselective	High	
Atenolol	Low	β_1	Low	
Bisoprolol	Moderate	β_1	Low	
Metoprolol	Moderate	β_1	Low	
Pindolol	Moderate	Nonselective	High	Intrinsic sympathomimetic activity[c]
Acebutolol	Moderate	β_1	Low	Intrinsic sympathomimetic activity[c]
Labetolol	Moderate	Nonselective	Low	α_1 antagonism
Carvedilol	Low	β_1	Low	α_1 antagonism
Nebivolol	High	β_1	Low	Endothelial nitric oxide release

Abbreviation: 5-HT, serotonin.

[a] Although lipophilic compounds appear to be more disruptive of sleep than hydrophilic compounds, high β_2- and/or 5-HT—receptor occupancy is probably more important.

[b] Nonselective β-antagonists appear to have more CNS-related side effects. They also have higher affinity for 5-HT receptors.

[c] β-antagonists with intrinsic sympathomimetic activity act as partial agonists at β_2 receptors.

Clonidine has been shown to cause deficits in attention, vigilance, working memory, and reaction time in normals[157,158] and in elderly hypertensive patients.[159] Verbal memory impairment and poorer workplace performance have been reported in patients receiving methyldopa.[160]

Other antihypertensives

The α_1-antagonists (eg, prazosin, terazosin) are sometimes associated with transient sedation. Prazosin has been used in the treatment of nightmares and sleep disturbance in combat-related posttraumatic stress disorder.[161] In placebo-controlled studies prazosin increased TST, REM, and subjective sleep quality, and reduced nightmares.[162,163]

Reports of sleep disturbance or wake dysfunction are rare with the calcium channel blockers (eg, verapamil, nifedipine), although fatigue is occasionally reported.[164] However, these drugs decrease the effectiveness of hypnotics and potentiate the effects of stimulants, at least in studies in animals.[165] Studies on small numbers of normals have shown slight increases in subjective sleepiness and impairment of memory with single doses

of amlodipine,[166] but no decrements in alertness or performance with single doses of nifedipine.[167]

Whereas most angiotensin-converting enzyme inhibitors are hydrophilic compounds, captopril and lisinopril both have some CNS activity. Fatigue, drowsiness, and insomnia have been rarely reported. However, a dry, irritating cough is a common side effect[168] that may contribute to sleep apnea possibly related to rhinopharyngeal inflammation.[169] PSG-recorded sleep was not affected by 14-day administration of cilazapril compared with the positive control, metoprolol, which produced increased awakenings.[170] There was no evidence of impairment in alertness or performance in studies of captopril.[171,172]

Angiotensin-II blockers do not appear to have sleep-related side effects. There are reports of improved cognitive function in hypertensive patients treated with losartan[173] or valsartan.[174]

Vasodilators (eg, hydralazine) are rarely associated with fatigue.[175] Diuretics, anticoagulants, antiplatelets, and thrombolytics do not directly impair sleep or waking function,[175] although one might expect more frequent awakenings for micturition with diuretics.

Antiarrhythmic Drugs

Fatigue is the most common CNS complaint of patients taking antiarrhythmic drugs, with placebo-adjusted incidence from clinical trials generally ranging from 5% to 10%,[176] except for the β-antagonists where rates may be higher. Nightmares and insomnia have been rarely reported. There are few objective data available.

Lipid-Lowering Drugs

The 2 primary classes of lipid-lowering drugs are statins and fibrates. Statins lower cholesterol by suppressing cholesterol biosynthesis via inhibition of 3-hydroxy-3-methylglutaryl coenzyme A (HMG-CoA) reductase. Fibrates decrease fatty acid and triglyceride levels by activating peroxisomal pathways.[177]

Atorvastatin, lovastatin, and simvastatin have been associated with subjective reports of insomnia.[178–180] However, placebo-controlled clinical trials and PSG studies have in general failed to show increased sleep disturbance even with the more lipophilic compounds.[181–185] One PSG study in normals showed increased wake after sleep onset with lovastatin while pravastatin did not differ from placebo.[186] Roth and colleagues[187] reported performance decrements with lovastatin even though nocturnal sleep and daytime sleep tendency (measured by MSLT) were not affected. Two other randomized trials demonstrated small but significant deficits in cognitive performance with both lovastatin[188] and simvastatin.[189] Several other studies have failed to show neuropsychological deficits.[184,190–193] Although there have been case reports of short-term memory loss associated with statin use, a meta-analysis of observational studies suggests that these drugs may actually lower the odds for development of cognitive impairment.[184]

SUMMARY

Sleep disturbance, daytime sleepiness, and decrements in cognitive function occur in individuals with allergic rhinitis, respiratory disorders, and cardiovascular disease. These impairments may be caused or exacerbated by disease or by treatment with drugs that affect the CNS. First-generation H_1 antihistamines produce both subjective and objective sleepiness in most individuals when used acutely. While tolerance may develop to some of the sedating effects, performance, including driving, may continue to be impaired. Second-generation H_1 antagonists are much less likely to cause sleepiness or performance impairment when used in recommended doses. Theophylline, oral corticosteroids, and decongestants may produce sleep disturbance. CNS side effects associated with β-blockers include fatigue, insomnia, and nightmares. These complaints are more common among drugs with high β_2- or 5-HT–receptor occupancy. Sedation is frequently reported with use of the α_2-agonists clonidine and methyldopa.

REFERENCES

1. Meltzer EO, Nathan R, Derebery J, et al. Sleep, quality of life, and productivity impact of nasal symptoms in the United States: findings from the burden of Rhinitis in America survey. Allergy Asthma Proc 2009;30(3):244–54.
2. Mullol J, Maurer M, Bousquet. Sleep and allergic rhinitis. J Investig Allergol Clin Immunol 2008;18:415–9.
3. Janson C, De Backer W, Gislason T, et al. Increased prevalence of sleep disturbances and daytime sleepiness in subjects with bronchial asthma: a population study of young adults in three European countries. Eur Respir J 1996;9(10):2132–8.
4. Stuck BA, Czajkowski J, Hagner AE, et al. Changes in daytime sleepiness, quality of life, and objective sleep patterns in seasonal allergic rhinitis: a controlled clinical trial. J Allergy Clin Immunol 2004;113(4):663–8.
5. Lavie P, Gertner R, Zomer, et al. Breathing disorders in sleep associated with 'microarousals' in patients with allergic rhinitis. Acta Otolarynygol 1981;92:529–33.
6. Mastronarde JG, Wise RA, Shade DM, et al. Sleep quality in asthma: results of a large prospective clinical trial. J Asthma 2008;45(3):183–9.
7. Vir R, Bhagat R, Shah A. Sleep disturbances in clinically stable young asthmatic adults. Ann Allergy Asthma Immunol 1997;79(3):251–5.
8. Fitzpatrick MF, Engleman H, Whyte KF, et al. Morbidity in nocturnal asthma: sleep quality and daytime cognitive performance. Thorax 1991;46(8):569–73.
9. Janson C, De Backer W, Gislason T, et al. Increased prevalences of sleep disturbances and daytime sleepiness in subjects with bronchial asthma: a population study of young adults in three European countries. Eur Respir J 1969;9:2132–8.
10. Brezinova V, Catterall JR, Douglas NJ, et al. Night sleep of patients with chronic ventilatory failure and age matched controls: number and duration of the EEG episodes of intervening wakefulness and drowsiness. Sleep 1982;5(2):123–30.

11. Fleetham J, West P, Mezon B, et al. Sleep, arousals, and oxygen desaturation in chronic obstructive pulmonary disease. The effect of oxygen therapy. Am Rev Respir Dis 1982;126(3): 429–33.

12. Arand DL, McGinty DJ, Littner MR. Respiratory patterns associated with hemoglobin desaturation during sleep in chronic obstructive pulmonary disease. Chest 1981;80(2):183–90.

13. Orr WC, Shamma-Othman Z, Levin D, et al. Persistent hypoxemia and excessive daytime sleepiness in chronic obstructive pulmonary disease (COPD). Chest 1990 Mar;97(3):583–5.

14. Liesker JJ, Postma DS, Beukema RJ, et al. Cognitive performance in patients with COPD. Respir Med 2004;98(4):351–6.

15. Spaeth J, Klimek L, Mösges R. Sedation in allergic rhinitis is caused by the condition and not by antihistamine treatment. Allergy 1996;51(12):893–906.

16. Taylor DJ, Mallory LJ, Lichstein KL, et al. Comorbidity of chronic insomnia with medical problems. Sleep 2007;30:213–8.

17. Schwartz S, McDowell Anderson W, Cole SR, et al. Insomnia and heart disease: a review of epidemiologic studies. J Psychosom Res 1999;47:313–33.

18. Mallon L, Broman JE, Hetta J. Sleep complaints predict coronary artery disease mortality in males: a 12-year follow-up study of a middle-aged Swedish population. J Intern Med 2002;1:207–16.

19. Broström A, Strömberg A, Dahlström U, et al. Sleep difficulties, daytime sleepiness, and health-related quality of life in patients with chronic heart failure. J Cardiovasc Nurs 2004;19(4):234–42.

20. Siegrist J, Matschinger H, Motz W. Untreated hypertensives and their quality of life. J Hypertens Suppl 1987;5(1):S15–20.

21. Bédard MA, Montplaisir J, Richer F, et al. Obstructive sleep apnea syndrome: pathogenesis of neuropsychological deficits. J Clin Exp Neuropsychol 1991;13(6):950–64.

22. Staniforth AD, Kinnear WJ, Starling R, et al. Effect of oxygen on sleep quality, cognitive function and sympathetic activity in patients with chronic heart failure and Cheyne-Stokes respiration. Eur Heart J 1998;19(6):922–8.

23. Haas HL, Sergeeva OA, Selbach O. Histamine in the nervous system. Physiol Rev 2008;88(3): 1183–241.

24. Huang Z, Mochizuki T, Qu W, et al. Altered sleep characteristics and lack of arousal response to H3 receptor antagonist in histamine H1 receptor knockout mice. Proc Natl Acad Sci U S A 2006; 103:4687–92.

25. Timmerman H, Leurs R, Brann MR, et al. In vitro pharmacology of clinically used central nervous system-active drugs as inverse H1 receptor agonists. J Pharmacol Exp Ther 2007;322:172–9.

26. Okamura N, Yanai K, Higuchi M, et al. Functional neuroimaging of cognition impaired by a classical antihistamine, d-chlorpheniramine. Br J Pharmacol 2000;129:115–23.

27. Tashiro M, Mochizuki H, Iwabuchi K, et al. Roles of histamine in regulation of arousal and cognition: Functional neuroimaging of histamine H1 receptors in human brain. Life Sci 2002;72:409–14.

28. Tashiro M, Sakurada Y, Iwabuchi K, et al. Central effects of fexofenadine and cetirizine: measurement of psychomotor performance, subjective sleepiness, and brain histamine H1-receptor occupancy using ^{11}C-doxepin positron emission tomography. J Clin Pharmacol 2004;44:890–900.

29. Shamsi Z, Hindmarch I. Sedation and antihistamines: a review of inter-drug differences using proportional impairment ratios. Human Psychopharmacol 2000;15:S3–30.

30. Estelle F, Simons R. H1-receptor antagonists comparative tolerability and safety. Drug Saf 1994;10:350–80.

31. Passalacqua G, Bousquet J, Bachert C, et al. The clinical safety of H1-receptor antagonists. An EAACI position paper. Allergy 1996;51:666–75.

32. Meltzer EO. Performance effects of antihistamines. J Allergy Clin Immunol 1990;86:613–9.

33. Nolen TM. Sedative effects of antihistamines: safety, performance, learning, and quality of life. Clin Therapeutics 1997;19:39–55.

34. Rombaut NEI, Hindmarch I. Psychometric aspects of antihistamines: a review. Human Psychopharmacol 1994;9:157–69.

35. Moskowitz H, Wilkinson C. Antihistamines and driving-related behavior: A review of the evidence for impairment. (Report No. DOT HS 809 714). Washington, DC: National Highway Traffic Safety Administration; 2004.

36. Bender B, Berning S, Dudden R, et al. Sedation and performance impairment of diphenhydramine and second-generation antihistamines: a meta-analysis. J Allergy Clin Immunol 2003;111:770–6.

37. Izumi N, Mizuguzhi H, Umehara H, et al. Analysis of disease-dependent sedative profiles of H1-antihistamines by large-scale surveillance using the visual analog scale. Methods Find Exp Clin Pharmacol 2008;225–30.

38. Roth T, Roehrs T, Koshorek G, et al. Sedative effects of antihistamines. J Allergy Clin Immunol 1987;80:94–8.

39. Roehrs TA, Tietz EI, Zorick FJ, et al. Daytime sleepiness and antihistamines. Sleep 1984;7:137–41.

40. Seidel WF, Cohen S, Bliwise NG, et al. Cetirizine effects on objective measures of daytime sleepiness and performance. Ann Allergy 1987;59:58–62.

41. Nicholson AN, Turner C. Central effects of the H1-antihistamine, cetirizine. Aviat Space Environ Med 1998;69:166–71.

42. Nicholson AN, Stone BM, Turner C, et al. Antihistamines and aircrew: usefulness of fexofenadine. Aviat Space Environ Med 2000;71:2–6.

43. Nicholson AN, Handford AD, Turner C, et al. Studies on performance and sleepiness with the H1-antihistamine, desloratadine. Aviat Space Environ Med 2003;74(8):809–15.

44. Schweitzer PK, Muehlbach MJ, Walsh JK. Sleepiness and performance during three-day administration of cetirizine or diphenhydramine. J Allergy Clin Immunol 1994;94:716–24.

45. Rickels K, Morris RJ, Newman H, et al. Diphenhydramine in insomniac family practice patients: a double- blind study. J Clin Pharmacol 1983; 23(5–6):234–42.

46. Kudo Y, Kurihara M. Clinical evaluation of diphenhydramine hydrochloride for the treatment of insomnia in psychiatric patients: a double-blind study. J Clin Pharmacol 1990;30(11):1041–8.

47. Glass JR, Sproule BA, Herrmann N, et al. Effects of 2-week treatment with temazepam and diphenhydramine in elderly insomniacs: a randomized, placebo-controlled trial. J Clin Psychopharmacol 2008;28(2):182–8.

48. Morin CM, Koetter U, Bastien C, et al. Valerian-hops combination and diphenhydramine for treating insomnia: a randomized placebo-controlled clinical trial. Sleep 2005;28(11):1465–71.

49. Adam K, Oswald I. The hypnotic effects of an antihistamine: promethazine. Br J Clin Pharmacol 1986;22(6):715–7.

50. Alford C, Rombaut N, Jones J, et al. Acute effects of hydroxyzine on nocturnal sleep and sleep tendency the following day: a C-EEG study. Human Psychopharmacol 1992;7:25–35.

51. Boyle J, Eriksson M, Stanley N, et al. Allergy medication in Japanese volunteers; treatment effect of single doses on nocturnal sleep architecture and next day residual effects. Curr Med Res Opin 2006;22:1343–51.

52. Aso T, Sakai Y. Effects of terfenadine on actual driving performance. Jpn J Clin Pharmacol Ther 1988;19:681–8.

53. Betts T, Markham D, Debenham S, et al. Effects of two antihistamine drugs on actual driving performance. BMJ 1984;288:281–2.

54. Walsh JK, Muehlbach MJ, Schweitzer PK. Simulated assembly line performance following ingestion of cetirizine or hydroxyzine. Ann Allergy 1992;69:195–200.

55. Gilmore TM, Alexander BH, Mueller BA, et al. Occupational injuries and medication use. Am J Ind Med 1996;30:234–9.

56. Finkle WD, Adams JL, Greenland S, et al. Increased risk of serious injury following an initial prescription for diphenhydramine. Ann Allergy Asthma Immunol 2002;89(3):244–50.

57. Starmer G. Antihistamines and highway safety. Accid Anal Prev 1985;17:311–7.

58. Soldatos CR, Dikeos DG. Neuroleptics, antihistamines and antiparkinsonian drugs: effects on sleep. In: Kales A, editor. Pharmacology of Sleep. Berlin: Springer-Verlag; 1995. p. 443–64.

59. Hindmarch I. Psychometric aspects of antihistamines. Allergy 1990;50:48–54.

60. Vermeeren A, O'Hanlon JF. Fexofenadine's effects, alone and with alcohol, on actual driving and psychomotor performance. J Allergy Clin Immunol 1998;101(3):306–11.

61. Hindmarch I. CNS effects of antihistamines: is there a third generation of non-sedative drugs? Clin Exp Allergy Rev 2002;2:26–31.

62. Verster JC, Volkerts ER. Antihistamines and driving ability: evidence from on-the-road driving studies during normal traffic. Ann Allergy Asthma Immunol 2004;92:294–303.

63. Verster JC, de Weert AM, Bijtjes SI, et al. Driving ability after acute and sub-chronic administration of levocetirizine and diphenhydramine: a randomized, double-blind, placebo-controlled trial. Psychopharmacology (Berl) 2003;169(1):84–90.

64. Vuurman EF, Rikken GH, Muntjewerff ND, et al. Effects of desloratadine, diphenhydramine, and placebo on driving performance and psychomotor performance measurements. Eur J Clin Pharmacol 2004;60(5):307–13.

65. Gengo FM, Manning C. A review of the effects of antihistamines on mental processes related to automobile driving. J Allergy Clin Immunol 1990; 86:1034–9.

66. Volkerts ER, van Willigenburg APP, van Laar MW, et al. Does cetirizine belong to the new generation of antihistamines? An investigation into its acute and subchronic effects on highway driving, psychometric test performance and daytime sleepiness. Human Psychopharmacology 1992;7: 227–38.

67. Spencer CM, Faulds D, Peters DH. Cetirizine. A reappraisal of its pharmacological properties and therapeutic use in selected allergic disorders. Drugs 1993;46:1055–80.

68. Simons FER, Fraser TG, Reggin JD, et al. Comparison of the central nervous system effects produced by six H1 -receptor antagonists. Clin Exp Allergy 1996;26:1092–7.

69. Ramaekers JG, Uiterwijk MM, O'Hanlon JF. Effects of loratadine and cetirizine on actual driving and psychometric test performance, and EEG during driving. Eur J Clin Pharmacol 1992;42:363–9.

70. Tashiro M, Kato M, Miyake M, et al. Dose dependency of brain histamine H(1) receptor occupancy following oral administration of cetirizine hydrochloride measured using PET with [^{11}C]doxepin. Hum Psychopharmacol 2009;24(7):540–8.

71. Richardson GS, Roehrs TA, Rosenthal L, et al. Tolerance to daytime sedative effects of H1 antihistamines. J Clin Psychopharmacol 2002;22(5):511–5.

72. O'Hanlon JF, Ramaekers JG. Antihistamines effects on actual driving performance in a standardized test: a summary of Dutch experience, 1989–94. Allergy 1995;50:234–42.

73. Kay GG, Berman B, Mockoviak SH, et al. Initial and steady-state effects of diphenhydramine and loratadine on sedation, cognition, mood, and psychomotor performance. Arch Intern Med 1997;157:2350–6.

74. Levander S, Stahle-Backdahl M, Hagermark O. Peripheral antihistamine and central sedative effects of single and continuous oral doses of cetirizine and hydroxyzine. Eur J Clin Pharmacol 1991;41:435–9.

75. Goetz DW, Jacobson JM, Murnane JE, et al. Prolongation of simple and choice reaction time in a double-blind comparison of twice-daily hydroxyzine versus terfenadine. J Allergy Clin Immunol 1989;84:316–22.

76. Corboz M, Rivelli M, Mingo G, et al. Mechanism of decongestant activity of α2-adrenoceptor agonists. Pulm Pharmacol Ther 2008;21:449–54.

77. Noble R. A controlled clinical trial of the cardiovascular and psychological effects of phenylpropanaolamine and caffeine. Drug Intell Clin Pharm 1988;22:296–9.

78. Bye CE, Hill HM, Hughes DTD, et al. A comparison of blood levels of L (+)-pseudoephedrine following different formulations and their relation to cardiovascular and subjective effects in man. Eur J Clin Pharmacol 1975;8:47–53.

79. Stroh JE Jr, Ayars GH, Bernstein IL, et al. A comparative tolerance study of terfenadine-pseudoephedrine combination tablets and pseudoephedrine tablets in patients with allergic or vasomotor rhinitis. J Int Med Res 1988;16(6):420–7.

80. Segal AT, Falliers CJ, Grant JA, et al. Safety and efficacy of terfenadine/pseudoephedrine versus clemastine/ phenylpropanolamine in the treatment of seasonal allergic rhinitis. Ann Allergy 1993;70(5):389–94.

81. Bertrand B, Jamart J, Arendt C. Cetirizine and pseudoephedrine retard alone and in combination in the treatment of perennial allergic rhinitis: a double-blind multicentre study. Rhinology 1996;34:91–6.

82. Bronsky E, Boggs P, Findlay S, et al. Comparative efficacy and safety of a once-daily loratadine-pseudoephedrine combination versus its components alone and placebo in the management of seasonal allergic rhinitis. J Allergy Clin Immunol 1995;96(2):139–47.

83. Kaiser HB, Banov CH, Berkowitz RR, et al. Comparative efficacy and safety of once-daily versus twice-daily loratadine-pseudoephedrine combinations versus placebo in seasonal allergic rhinitis. Am J Ther 1998;5(4):245–51.

84. Moinuddin R, deTineo M, Maleckar B, et al. Comparison of the combinations of fexofenadine-pseudoephedrine and loratadine-montelukast in the treatment of seasonal allergic rhinitis. Ann Allergy Asthma Immunol 2004;92(1):73–9.

85. Rombaut NEI, Alford C, Hindmarch I. Effects of oral administration of different formulations of pseudoephedrine on day- and night-time CNS activity. Med Sci Res 1989;17:831–3.

86. Lake CR, Rosenberg DB, Gallant S, et al. Phenylpropanolamine increases plasma caffeine levels. Clin Pharmacol Ther 1990;47:675–85.

87. Seppälä T, Nuotto E, Korttila K. Single and repeated dose comparison of three antihistamines and phenylpropanolamine: psychomotor performance and subjective appraisals of sleep. Br J Clin Pharmacol 1981;12(2):179–88.

88. Stanley N, Alford CA, Rombaut NE, et al. Comparison of the effects of astemizole/pseudoephedrine and triprolidine/pseudoephedrine on CNS activity and psychomotor function. Int Clin Psychopharmacol 1996;11(1):31–6.

89. Gaillard AW, Verduin CJ. The combined effects of an antihistamine and pseudoephedrine on human performance. J Drug Res. 1983;8:1929–36.

90. Barnes PJ. Anti-inflammatory actions of glucocorticoids: molecular mechanisms. Clin Sci (Lond) 1998;94(6):557–72.

91. Searle JP, Compton MR. Side-effects of corticosteroid agents. Med J Aust 1986;144:139–42.

92. Bailey WC, Richards JM, Manzella BA, et al. Characteristics and correlates of asthma in a university clinic population. Chest 1990;98:821–8.

93. Chrousos GA, Kattah JC, Beck RW, et al. Side effects of glucocorticoid treatment: Experience of the optic neuritis treatment trial. JAMA 1993;269:2110–2.

94. Lozada F, Silverman S, Migliorati C. Adverse side effects associated with prednisone in the treatment of patients with oral inflammatory ulcerative diseases. J Am Dent Assoc 1984;109:269–70.

95. Wolkowitz OM, Rubinow D, Doran AR, et al. Prednisone effects on neurochemistry and behavior: Preliminary findings. Arch Gen Psychiatry 1990;47:963–8.

96. Born J, Zwick A, Roth G, et al. Differential effects of hydrocortisone, fluocortolone, and aldosterone on nocturnal sleep in humans. Acta Endocrinol 1987;116:129–37.

97. Young AH, Sharpley AL, Campling GM, et al. Effects of hydrocortisone on brain 5-HT function and sleep. J Affect Disord 1994;32(2):139–46.

98. Rosenthal L, Folkerts M, Helmus T, et al. Administration of dexamethasone and its effects on sleep and daytime alertness. Sleep Res 1995;24:58.

99. Wolkowitz OM, Reus VI, Weingartner H, et al. Cognitive effects of corticosteroids. Am J Psychiatry 1990;147:1297–303.

100. McLaurin E, Holliday S, Williams P, et al. Predictors of cognitive dysfunction in patients with systemic lupus erythematosus. Neurology 2005;64(2):297–303.

101. Hughes K, Glass C, Ripchinski M, et al. Efficacy of the topical nasal steroid budesonide on improving sleep and daytime somnolence in patients with perennial allergic rhinitis. Allergy 2003;58(5):380–5.

102. Craig T, Teets S, Lehman E, et al. Nasal congestion secondary to allergic rhinitis as a cause of sleep disturbance and daytime fatigue and the response to topical nasal corticosteroids. J Allergy Clin Immunol 1998;101:633–7.

103. Craig T, Mende C, Hughes K, et al. The effect of topical nasal fluticasone on objective sleep testing and the symptoms of rhinitis, sleep, and daytime somnolence in perennial allergic rhinitis. Allergy Asthma Proc 2003;24:53–8.

104. Martin BG, Andrews CP, van Bavel JH, et al. Comparison of fluticasone propionate aqueous nasal spray and oral montelukast for the treatment of seasonal allergic rhinitis symptoms. Ann Allergy Asthma Immunol 2006;96(6):851–7.

105. Meltzer EO, Lockey RF, Friedman BF, et al. Efficacy and safety of low-dose fluticasone propionate compared with montelukast for maintenance treatment of persistent asthma. Mayo Clin Proc 2002;77(5):437–45.

106. Mansfield LE, Posey CR. Daytime sleepiness and cognitive performance improve in seasonal allergic rhinitis treated with intranasal fluticasone propionate. Allergy Asthma Proc 2007;28(2):226–9.

107. Mahajan P, Pearlman D, Okamoto L. The effect of fluticasone propionate on functional status and sleep in children with asthma and on the quality of life of their parents. J Allergy Clin Immunol 1998;102(1):19–23.

108. Mahajan P, Okamoto LJ, Schaberg A, et al. Impact of fluticasone propionate powder on health-related quality of life in patients with moderate asthma. J Asthma 1997;34(3):227–34.

109. Barnes PJ. Theophylline in chronic obstructive pulmonary disease: new horizons. Proc Am Thorac Soc 2005;2(4):334–9.

110. Scott PH, Tabachnik E, MacLeod S, et al. Sustained release theophylline for childhood asthma: Evidence for circadian variation of theophylline pharmacokinetics. J Pediatr 1981;99:476–9.

111. Hendeles L, Massanari M, Weinberger M. Update on the pharmacodynamics and pharmacokinetics of theophylline. Chest 1985;88(Suppl):103S–11S.

112. Janson C, Gislason T, Boman G, et al. Sleep disturbances in patients with asthma. Respir Med 1990;84:37–42.

113. Kraft M, Wenzel SE, Bettinger CM, et al. The effect of salmeterol on nocturnal symptoms, airway function, and inflammation in asthma. Chest 1997;111:1249–54.

114. Kaplan J, Fredrickson PA, Renaux SA, et al. Theophylline effect on sleep in normal subjects. Chest 1993;103:193–5.

115. Roehrs T, Merlotti L, Halpin D, et al. Effects of theophylline on nocturnal sleep and daytime sleepiness/alertness. Chest 1995;108(2):382–7.

116. Avital A, Sanchez I, Holbrow J, et al. Effect of theophylline on lung function tests, sleep quality, and nighttime SaO_2 in children with cystic fibrosis. Am Rev Respir Dis 1991;144:1245–9.

117. Rhind GB, Connaughton JJ, McFie J, et al. Sustained release choline theophyllinate in nocturnal asthma. BMJ 1985;291:1605–7.

118. Saletu B, Oberndorfer S, Anderer P, et al. Efficiency of continuous positive airway pressure versus theophylline therapy in sleep apnea: Comparative sleep laboratory studies on objective and subjective sleep and awakening quality. Neuropsychobiology 1999;39:151–9.

119. Mulloy E, McNicholas WT. Theophylline improves gas exchange during rest, exercise, and sleep in severe chronic obstructive pulmonary disease. Am Rev Respir Dis 1993;148:1030–6.

120. Selby C, Engleman HM, Fitzpatrick MF, et al. Am J Inhaled salmeterol or oral theophylline in nocturnal asthma? Respir Crit Care Med 1997;155(1):104–8.

121. Wiegand L, Mende CN, Zaidel G, et al. Salmeterol vs theophylline: sleep and efficacy outcomes in patients with nocturnal asthma. Chest 1999;115(6):1525–32.

122. Fitzpatrick MF, Mackay T, Driver H, et al. Salmeterol in nocturnal asthma: a double blind, placebo controlled trial of a long acting inhaled beta 2 agonist. BMJ 1990;301(6765):1365–8.

123. Rachelefsky GS, Wo J, Adelson J, et al. Behavior abnormalities and poor school performance due to oral theophylline use. Pediatrics 1986;78:1133–8.

124. Stein MA, Krasowski M, Leventhal BL, et al. Behavioral and cognitive effects of methylxanthines: a meta-analysis of theophylline and caffeine. Arch Pediatr Adolesc Med 1996;150:284–8.

125. Lindgren S, Lokshin B, Stronmquist A, et al. Does asthma or treatment with theophylline limit children's academic performance? N Engl J Med 1992;327:926–30.

126. Hanania N, Donohue J. Pharmacologic interventions in chronic obstructive pulmonary disease: bronchodilators. Proc Am Thorac Soc. 2007;4:526–34.

127. Martin RJ, Bartelson BL, Smith P, et al. Effect of ipratropium bromide treatment on oxygen saturation and sleep quality in COPD. Chest 1999; 115(5):1338–45.

128. McNicholas WT, Calverley PM, Lee A, et al. Tiotropium Sleep Study in COPD Investigators. Long-acting inhaled anticholinergic therapy improves sleeping oxygen saturation in COPD. Eur Respir J 2004;23(6):825–31.

129. Santos CB, Hanks C, McCann J, et al. The role of montelukast on perennial allergic rhinitis and associated sleep disturbances and daytime somnolence. Allergy Asthma Proc 2008;29(2):140–5.

130. Virchow JC, Bachert C. Efficacy and safety of montelukast in adults with asthma and allergic rhinitis. Respir Med 2006;100(11):1952–9.

131. Valk PJ, Simons M. Effects of loratadine/montelukast on vigilance and alertness task performance in a simulated cabin environment. Adv Ther 2009; 26(1):89–98.

132. Food and Drug Administration. Updated Information on Leukotriene Inhibitors: Montelukast (marketed as Singulair), Zafirlukast (marketed as Accolate), and Zileuton (marketed as Zyflo and Zyflo CR). Available at: http://www.fda.gov/Drugs/DrugSafety/PostmarketDrugSafetyInformationfor PatientsandProviders/DrugSafetyInformationfor HeathcareProfessionals/ucm165489.htm. Accessed April 1, 2010.

133. McAinsh J, Cruickshank JM. Beta-blockers and central nervous system side effects. Pharmacol Ther 1990;46:163–97.

134. Yamada Y, Shibuya F, Hamada J, et al. Prediction of sleep disorders induced by β-adrenergic receptor blocking agents based on receptor occupancy. J Pharmacokinet Biopharm 1995;23:131–45.

135. Van Bortel L, Fici F, Mascagni F. Efficacy and tolerability of nebivolol compared with other antihypertensive drugs: a meta analysis. Am J Cardiovasc Drugs 2008;8:35–44.

136. Yilmaz M, Erdem A, Yalta K, et al. Impact of beta-blockers on sleep in patients with mild hypertension: a randomized trial between nebivolol and metoprolol. Adv Ther 2008;25:871–83.

137. Pearce CJ, Wallin JD. Labetalol and other agents that block both alpha- and beta-adrenergic receptors. Cleve Clin J Med 1994;61:59–69.

138. Stoschitzky K, Sakotnik A, Lercher P, et al. Influence of beta-blockers on melatonin release. Eur J Clin Pharmacol 1999;55(2):111–5.

139. Stoschitzky K, Stoschitzky G, Brussee H, et al. Comparing beta-blocking effects of bisoprolol, carvedilol and nebivolol. Cardiology 2006;106(4): 199–206.

140. Dahlöf C, Dimenäs E. Side effects of beta-blocker treatments as related to the central nervous system. Am J Med Sci 1990;299(4):236–44.

141. Betts TA, Alford C. Beta-blockers and sleep: a controlled trial. Eur J Clin Pharmacol 1985; 28(Suppl):65–8.

142. Kostis JB, Rosen RC. Central nervous system effects of beta-adrenergic-blocking drugs: the role of ancillary properties. Circulation 1987;75(1):204–12.

143. Kostis JB, Rosen RC, Holzer BC, et al. CNS side effects of centrally-active antihypertensive agents: a prospective, placebo-controlled study of sleep, mood state, and cognitive and sexual function in hypertensive males. Psychopharmacology (Berl) 1990;102(2):163–70.

144. Muldoon MF, Manuck SB, Shapiro AP, et al. Neurobehavioral effects of antihypertensive medications. J Hypertens 1991;9(6):549–59.

145. Dimsdale JE, Newton RP, Joist T. Neuropsychological side effects of beta-blockers. Arch Intern Med 1989;149(3):514–25.

146. Paykel ES, Fleminger R, Watson JP. Psychiatric side effects of antihypertensive drugs other than reserpine. J Clin Psychopharmacol 1982;2:14–39.

147. Bernard JM, Hommeril JL, Passuti N, et al. Postoperative analgesia by intravenous clonidine. Anesthesiology 1991;75(4):577–82.

148. Bischoff P, Scharein E, Schmidt GN, et al. Topography of clonidine-induced electroencephalographic changes evaluated by principal component analysis. Anesthesiology 2000;92(6): 1545–52.

149. Hall JE, Uhrich TD, Ebert TJ. Sedative, analgesic and cognitive effects of clonidine infusions in humans. Br J Anaesth 2001;86(1):5–11.

150. Kanno O, Clarenbach P. Effects of clonidine and yohimbine on sleep in man: Polygraphic study and EEG analysis by normalized slope descriptors. Electroencephalogr Clin Neurophysiol 1985;60: 478–84.

151. Gentili A, Godschalk MF, Gheorghiu D, et al. Effect of clonidine and yohimbine on sleep in healthy men: a double-blind, randomized, controlled trial. Eur J Clin Pharmacol 1996;50(6):463–5.

152. Miyazaki S, Uchida S, Mukai J, et al. Clonidine effects on all-night human sleep: opposite action of low- and medium-dose clonidine on human NREM-REM sleep proportion. Psychiatry Clin Neurosci 2004;58(2):138–44.

153. Huynh N, Lavigne GJ, Lanfranchi PA, et al. The effect of 2 sympatholytic medications—propranolol and clonidine—on sleep bruxism: experimental randomized controlled studies. Sleep 2006;29(3): 307–16.

154. Kostis JB, Rosen RC, Holzer BC, et al. CNS side effects of centrally-active antihypertensive agents: A prospective, placebo-controlled study of sleep, mood state, and cognitive and sexual function in hypertensive males. Psychopharmacology 1990; 102:163–70.

155. Danchin N, Genton P, Atlas P, et al. Comparative effects of atenolol and clonidine on polygraphically recorded sleep in hypertensive men: a randomized, double-blind, crossover study. Int J Clin Pharmacol Ther 1995;33(1):52–5.

156. Carskadon MA, Cavallo A, Rosekind MR. Sleepiness and nap sleep following a morning dose of clonidine. Sleep 1989;12:338–44.

157. Tiplady B, Bowness E, Stien L, et al. Selective effects of clonidine and temazepam on attention and memory. J Psychopharmacol 2005;19(3): 259–65.

158. Jäkälä P, Riekkinen M, Sirviö J, et al. Clonidine, but not guanfacine, impairs choice reaction time performance in young healthy volunteers. Neuropsychopharmacology 1999;21(4):495–502.

159. Denolle T, Sassano P, Allain H, et al. Effects of nicardipine and clonidine on cognitive functions and electroencephalography in hypertensive patients. Fundam Clin Pharmacol 2002;16(6): 527–35.

160. Croog SH, Levine S, Testa MA, et al. The effects of antihypertensive therapy on the quality of life. N Engl J Med 1986;314:1657–64.

161. Dierks MR, Jordan JK, Sheehan AH. Prazosin treatment of nightmares related to posttraumatic stress disorder. Ann Pharmacother 2007;41:1013–7.

162. Raskind M, Peskind E, Hoff D, et al. A parallel group placebo controlled study of prazosin for trauma nightmares and sleep disturbance in combat veterans with post-traumatic stress disorder. Biol Psychiatry 2007;15:928–34.

163. Taylor F, Martin P, Thompson C, et al. Prazosin effects on objective sleep measures and clinical symptoms in civilian trauma posttraumatic stress disorder: a placebo-controlled study. Biol Psychiatry 2008;63:629–32.

164. Talbert RL, Bussey HI. Update on calcium-channel blocking agents. Clin Pharm 1983;2(5):403–16.

165. Monti J. Minireview: Disturbances of sleep and wakefulness associated with the use of antihypertensive agents. Life Sci 1987;41:1979–88.

166. Nicholson AN, Roberts DP, Stone BM, et al. Antihypertensive therapy in critical occupations: studies with an angiotensin II antagonist. Aviat Space Environ Med 2001;72(12):1096–101.

167. McDevitt DG, Currie D, Nicholson AN, et al. Central effects of the calcium antagonist, nifedipine. Br J Clin Pharmacol 1991;32(5):541–9.

168. Israili ZH, Hall WD. Cough and angioneurotic edema associated with angiotensin-converting enzyme inhibitor therapy. A review of the literature and pathophysiology. Ann Intern Med 1992;117: 234–42.

169. Cicolin A, Mangiardi L, Mutani R, et al. Angiotensin-converting enzyme inhibitors and obstructive sleep apnea. Mayo Clin Proc 2006;81:53–5.

170. Dietrich B, Herrmann WM. Influence of cilazapril on memory functions and sleep behaviour in comparison with metoprolol and placebo in healthy subjects. Br J Clin Pharmacol 1989;27(Suppl 2): 249S–61S.

171. Currie D, Lewis RV, McDevitt DG, et al. Central effects of the angiotensin-converting enzyme inhibitor, captopril. I. Performance and subjective assessments of mood. Br J Clin Pharmacol 1990; 30(4):527–36.

172. McDevitt DG, Currie D, Nicholson AN, et al. Central effects of repeated administration of atenolol and captopril in healthy volunteers. Eur J Clin Pharmacol 1994;46(1):23–8.

173. Tedesco MA, Ratti G, Mennella S, et al. Comparison of losartan and hydrochlorothiazide on cognitive function and quality of life in hypertensive patients. Am J Hypertens 1999;12(11 Pt 1): 1130–4.

174. Fogari R, Mugellini A, Zoppi A, et al. Effects of valsartan compared with enalapril on blood pressure and cognitive function in elderly patients with essential hypertension. Eur J Clin Pharmacol 2004;59(12):863–8.

175. Huffman JC, Stern TA. Neuropsychiatric consequences of cardiovascular medications. Dialogues Clin Neurosci 2007;9(1):29–45.

176. Kruyer WB, Hickman JR Jr. Medication-induced performance decrements: Cardiovascular medications. J Occup Med 1990;32:342–9.

177. Pahan K. Lipid-lowering drugs. Cell Mol Life Sci 2006;63:1165–78.

178. Ditschuneit HH, Kuhn K, Ditschuneit H. Comparison of different HMG-CoA reductase inhibitors. Eur J Clin Pharmacol 1991;40(Suppl 1):S27–32.

179. Tobert JA, Shear CL, Chremos AN, et al. Clinical experience with lovastatin. Am J Cardiol 1990;65: 23–6.

180. Rosenson RS, Goranson NL. Lovastatin-associated sleep and mood disturbances. Am J Med 1993;95: 548–9.

181. Keech AC, Armitage JM, Wallendszus, et al. Absence of effects of prolonged simvastatin therapy on nocturnal sleep in a large randomized placebo-controlled study. Br J Clin Pharmacol 1996;42:483–90.

182. Ehrenberg BL, Lamon-Fava S, Corbett KE, et al. Comparison of the effects of pravastatin and lovastatin on sleep disturbance in hypercholesterolemic subjects. Sleep 1999;22:117–21.

183. Eckernäs SA, Roos BE, Kvidal P, et al. The effects of simvastatin and pravastatin on objective and subjective measures of nocturnal sleep: a comparison of two structurally different HMG CoA reductase inhibitors in patients with primary moderate hypercholesterolaemia. Br J Clin Pharmacol 1993; 35(3):284–9.

184. Kostis JB, Rosen RC, Wilson AC. Central nervous system effects of HMG CoA reductase inhibitors: lovastatin and pravastatin on sleep and cognitive performance in patients with hypercholesterolemia. J Clin Pharmacol 1994;34(10):989—96.

185. Partinen M, Pihl S, Strandberg T, et al. Comparison of effects on sleep of lovastatin and pravastatin in hypercholesterolemia. Am J Cardiol 1994;73(12): 876—80.

186. Vgontzas A, Kales A, Bixler E, et al. Effects of lovastatin and pravastatin on sleep efficiency and sleep stages. Clin Pharmacol Ther 1991;50:730—7.

187. Roth T, Richardson GR, Sullivan JP, et al. Comparative effects of pravastatin and lovastatin on nighttime sleep and daytime performance. Clin Cardiol 1992;15:426—32.

188. Muldoon MF, Barger SD, Ryan CM, et al. Effects of lovastatin on cognitive function and psychological well-being. Am J Med 2000;108(7): 538—46.

189. Muldoon MF, Ryan CM, Sereika SM, et al. Randomized trial of the effects of simvastatin on cognitive functioning in hypercholesterolemic adults. Am J Med 2004;117(11):823—9.

190. Wagstaff LR, Mitton MW, Arvik BM, et al. Statin-associated memory loss: analysis of 60 case reports and review of the literature. Pharmacotherapy 2003;23:871—80.

191. Etminan M, Gill S, Samii A. The role of lipid-lowering drugs in cognitive function: a meta-analysis of observational studies. Pharmacotherapy 2003;23: 726—30.

192. Harrison RW, Ashton CH. Do cholesterol-lowering agents affect brain activity? A comparison of simvastatin, pravastatin, and placebo in healthy volunteers. Br J Clin Pharmacol 1994;37(3):231—6.

193. Gibellato MG, Moore JL, Selby K, et al. Effects of lovastatin and pravastatin on cognitive function in military aircrew. Aviat Space Environ Med 2001; 72(9):805—12.

Drug-Related Sleep Stage Changes: Functional Significance and Clinical Relevance

Timothy Roehrs, PhD[a,b],*, Thomas Roth, PhD[a,b]

- Slow wave sleep • REM sleep • Drug effects
- Sleep deprivation effects

With the discovery of rapid eye movement (REM) sleep by Aserinsky and Kleitman in the early 1950s and the description of the non—rapid eye movement (NREM)-REM cycle by Dement, it became clear that sleep is not a unitary state. Sleep is organized into distinct brain states (REM and NREM), each having identifiable and characteristic physiologic patterns, that vary cyclically across the night. Although significant reductions or disruptions of a sleep stage are inevitably followed on a recovery night by a rebound in the disrupted sleep stage, the functional significance and clinical relevance of sleep stage variations are still not clear. Newer drugs are being developed that have been shown to enhance NREM, specifically slow wave sleep, as well as REM sleep. This article reviews and discusses the clinical relevance and functional significance of drug-related sleep stage effects.

NORMAL SLEEP STAGING

Polysomnographic (PSG) studies, which refers to the simultaneous recording of multiple electrophysiologic parameters (ie, electro-oculogram [EOG], electromyogram [EMG], and electroencephalogram [(EEG]) during sleep, have shown that sleep is a complex, highly organized biologic state composed of 2 distinct brain states, REM and NREM sleep.[1,2] In terms of EEG activity, NREM sleep is characterized by EEG slowing and increased voltage relative to the low voltage (10–30 μV) and fast frequency (16–26 Hz) of activated wakefulness. Relaxed wakefulness with eyes closed exhibits an α (8–12 Hz) EEG pattern of 20 to 40 μV, which further slows to 3 to 7 Hz and decreases in amplitude during drowsy, stage 1 NREM sleep. Stage 2 NREM sleep is characterized by phasic events of sleep spindles (12–14 Hz) and K-complexes (negative sharp waves of 0.5 Hz and greater) and increased arousal thresholds relative to stage 1 NREM sleep. When arousal threshold is highest, the EEG of NREM stage 3 and 4 sleep has 0.5 to 2 Hz waves of 75 μV and greater, termed slow waves. NREM stages 3 and 4 are merely differentiated by the quantity of slow wave activity on a given epoch (20%–50% vs >50%) and often, to maintain scoring reliability, are not differentiated in visual sleep scoring. In contrast, the EEG of REM sleep reverts to the

This work was in part supported by Grant #R01-DA17355.

[a] Department of Internal Medicine, Sleep Disorders & Research Center, Henry Ford Hospital, Henry Ford Health System, 2799 West Grand Boulevard, Detroit, MI 48202, USA

[b] Department of Psychiatry and Behavioral Neuroscience, Wayne State University, School of Medicine, 2751 East Jefferson, Detroit, MI 48207, USA

* Corresponding author. Department of Internal Medicine, Sleep Disorders & Research Center, Henry Ford Hospital, 2799 West Grand Boulevard, Detroit, MI 48202.

E-mail address: troehrs1@hfhs.org

Sleep Med Clin 5 (2010) 559–570

doi:10.1016/j.jsmc.2010.08.002

low-voltage, mixed-frequency pattern seen in stage 1 NREM sleep. The EOG of REM displays bursts of rapid eye movements, for which this stage is named. In contrast with this aroused EEG, the EMG shows a total atonia of voluntary muscles.

Sleep is entered through NREM stage 1, which normally lasts 1 to 7 minutes before the sleep spindles and K-complexes of NREM stage 2 begin.[1,2] As stage 2 progresses, a gradual appearance of high-voltage slow wave activity occurs, eventually reaching criteria for scoring stage 3 and 4 NREM sleep. This first episode of NREM stages 3 and 4 lasts approximately 10 to 30 minutes, depending on age, and sleep lightens to stage 2 before the initiation of the first REM episode, which occurs 90 to 120 minutes after sleep onset. NREM and REM sleep continue in this manner for 4 to 5 cycles per 8 hours. Each cycle is about 90 minutes, but the sleep stages in those cycles change across the night. The duration of each episode of NREM stage 3 and 4 decreases each cycle and the duration of each REM episode increases with each cycle. During the third and fourth NREM-REM cycles there is minimal δ wave activity, and REM periods are of 20 to 30 minutes' duration.

The observation that slow wave sleep diminishes progressively across NREM-REM cycles during the night led to the hypothesis that slow wave sleep/slow wave activity is precisely controlled, reflecting the operation of a sleep homeostat.[3] This hypothesis was established and supported with many studies using both visual scoring and various quantitative EEG methods such as spectral analysis. Quantitative EEG methods yield several indices of slow wave activity that prove to be more sensitive than visual scoring of slow wave sleep. Numerous studies that have deprived sleep, extended sleep, or added daytime naps have shown that slow wave sleep and slow wave activity increase and decrease in the predicted directions (ie, the index increases with increasing hours of wake and decreases with increasing hours of sleep), as would be hypothesized for a sleep homeostat. One important caveat is that all of these studies involved acute, not chronic, manipulations of sleep. Given this hypothesis and the extensive data supportive of the hypothesis, drugs that enhance slow wave sleep should have important functional and clinical significance.

DRUG EFFECTS ON SLEEP STAGES
Benzodiazepine Receptor Agonists

The major class of drugs indicated for the treatment of insomnia is the benzodiazepine receptor agonists (BzRAs). The class includes benzodiazepines and nonbenzodiazepines that act at the benzodiazepine receptor. Benzodiazepines are known to reduce stage 3 to 4 sleep.

For example, estazolam 2 mg in 35-year-old insomniacs reduced stage 3 to 4 sleep from 4% to 1%.[4] Temazepam 15 and 30 mg in 38-year-old insomniacs reduced stage 3 to 4 sleep from 8% to 5%.[5] Both drugs reduced stage 1 sleep from 11% and 16% to 9%. In elderly insomniacs (60–85 years), triazolam 0.125 mg had no effect on sleep stages; stage 1 was 22% and stage 3 to 4 was 5% on both placebo and active drug.[6] In each of the studies, total sleep time was increased and, where measured, self-reported sleep was improved. In the elderly study cited earlier, the improved sleep time was associated with an improvement in daytime sleepiness as measured by the multiple sleep latency test (MSLT). This improved MSLT was found with 22% stage 1 sleep the previous night in the elderly subjects. These benzodiazepine data highlight the importance of caution in interpreting the significance of sleep stage changes and the biology associated with them. For example, it is known that, in humans, stage 3 to 4 sleep is associated with the highest arousal threshold. However, although benzodiazepines decrease stage 3 to 4 sleep, they also increase arousal threshold.[7] Given the known action of these drugs on the cortex, one has to question whether these declines represent a drug effect on stage 3 to 4 sleep or on the ability of the cortex to produce high-amplitude slow waves, which is our surrogate measure of stage 3 to 4 sleep.

Alternatively, the nonbenzodiazepine BzRAs do not seem to consistently alter sleep stages.[8] In one study of healthy 21 to 35-year-old normals, zolpidem 0 to 20 mg did not affect stage 1 or stage 3 to 4.[9] The high dose reduced REM sleep. Zopiclone 0 to 15 mg in middle-aged insomniacs reduced stage 1 from 12% to 8%.[10] At the high dose, it reduced stage 3 to 4 (9% to 4%) and REM sleep (20% to 18%). The S-isomer, eszopiclone (0, 1, 2, 3, 3.5 mg), in healthy volunteers did not alter stage 3 to 4 or stage 1 sleep at any dose.[11] In these studies, all the BzRAs, both Bz and non-Bz, that were studied improved sleep time or efficiency, and, where assessed, improved self-reports of sleep. None of these drugs, at clinical doses, suppress REM sleep, although there are reports of increases in latency to REM sleep.

γ-Aminobutyric Acid Reuptake Inhibitor

Tiagabine, a selective γ-aminobutyric acid (GABA) reuptake inhibitor indicated for epilepsy, has been studied for its effects on sleep. In a study of the effects of tiagabine (0, 2, 4, 8 mg) on the sleep of older adults, the 4- and 8-mg doses increased slow wave sleep by approximately 15 and 40 minutes, respectively. It did not reduce sleep latency and had inconsistent effects on sleep time and self-ratings of sleep.[12] In another study of healthy elderly people, 5 mg tiagabine doubled the minutes of slow wave sleep, and also improved sleep efficiency, but not self-reported sleep quality.[13] Sleep efficiency was low, 78%, in the placebo group and time in bed was unrestricted, making it difficult to interpret these results. In a study of elderly insomniacs receiving 0, 2, 4, 6, and 8 mg, the 4- to 8-mg doses increased slow wave sleep, the 6- and 8-mg doses reduced stage 1 sleep and number of awakenings, but had no effect of sleep efficiency or self-reported sleep.[14] In middle-aged adults with insomnia tiagabine (0, 4, 6, 8, 10 mg) again increased slow wave sleep in a dose-related manner, but had no effects on sleep latency, wake after sleep onset, or total sleep time.[15] In another study of middle-aged insomniacs, tiagabine (0, 4, 8, 12, 16 mg) increased 3 to 4 sleep from 7% to 29%, but did not consistently improve sleep latency, wake after sleep onset, or sleep time.[16]

One study has attempted to assess the functional significance of slow wave sleep enhancement with tiagabine in healthy normals during sleep restriction, which is known to impair next-day function. Healthy volunteers were randomized to placebo or 8 mg tiagabine before sleep for 4 nights during which bedtime was restricted to 1 to 6 am.[17] Relative to placebo, tiagabine increased slow wave sleep by about 30 minutes and the sleep restriction–associated impairment of psychomotor vigilance performance was diminished by the drug. The amount of slow wave sleep during the restriction was positively correlated with average daily sleep latency on the MSLT, that is greater slow wave sleep was correlated with longer latencies on the MSLT (ie, less daytime sleepiness). However, many other outcome measures of daytime function in the study did not show this relation with stage 3 to 4 sleep. The study also has implications for the use of sleep restriction in insomnia therapy, in that the depth of sleep may be enhanced through increased stage 3 to 4 sleep (see later discussion).

γ-Aminobutyric Acid A Agonist

Gaboxadol is a selective extrasynaptic γ-amino-butyric acid A (GABA_A) agonist that was being developed as a hypnotic, but was abandoned in 2007 because of an inadequate therapeutic/safety ratio. An early study of healthy adults showed that 20 mg gaboxadol increased slow wave sleep time relative to placebo from 56 to 80 minutes.[18] Another study of healthy adults introduced a 4 to 6 pm nap, which typically reduces subsequent nocturnal slow wave sleep, and 20 mg garboxadol administered before the nocturnal sleep increased slow wave sleep relative to placebo from 54 to 78 minutes.[19] In 2 large studies of healthy, middle-aged, volunteers undergoing a 4-hour phase advance, which was used as a model of transient insomnia, doses of 0, 5, 10, and 15 mg were administered.[20,21] The 10- and 15-mg doses increased slow wave sleep and increased total sleep time, primarily by reducing wake after sleep onset. These doses also improved self-reports of sleep time. In healthy elderly people without sleep complaints, gaboxadol 15 mg increased stage 3 and 4 sleep and reduced stage 1 sleep.[22] It also improved sleep time and wake after sleep onset as well as self-reported sleep time and sleep quality. In 2 studies of middle-aged insomniacs at doses of 0, 10, 15, 20 mg, gaboxadol increased stage 3 and 4 sleep and, at the 15 and 20 mg doses, it also increased sleep time by primarily reducing wake time after sleep onset.[23,24] In elderly patients with insomnia, gaboxadol 10 mg increased stages 2, 3, and 4 and reduced wake after sleep onset, but had no effect on sleep latency.[25]

As with tiagabine, a study used the sleep restriction paradigm to investigate the capacity of gaboxadol to enhance slow wave sleep during sleep restriction and thereby reduce the performance-impairing effect of the restriction.[26] In this study of healthy volunteers, slow wave sleep was increased by 17 minutes relative to placebo and, although a positive correlation of slow wave sleep to MSLT was found, psychomotor vigilance was not improved relative to placebo. The failure to reverse the performance-impairing effect of sleep restriction may be caused by a lessoned effect of gaboxadol on slow wave sleep (17 vs 30 minutes' increase) compared with the tiagabine study.

GABA_B Agonist

γ-Hydroxybutyrate (GHB) and the sodium salt of GHB, sodium oxybate, have a long history of study for their sedative effects. GHB is present in the central nervous system, synthesized from GABA as its active metabolite. When administered orally in supraphysiologic doses, as GHB or sodium oxybate, it is believed to act specifically, but weakly, at the GABA_B receptor, hence the need for supraphysiologic doses.[27] In healthy people 23 to 63 years old, a single GHB 2.25-g dose administered 15 minutes before sleep increased slow wave sleep from 10.5% to 13.6%, but it did not increase total sleep time.[28] In healthy young men, 2.5, 3.0, and 3.5 g GHB increased the minutes of slow wave sleep in a dose-related manner and reduced initial sleep latency, but did not increase total sleep.[29] The slow wave sleep effects in these studies were limited to the first third of the night, hence the need for a second nightly dose when treating narcolepsy, its current US Food and Drug Administration indication.

In narcolepsy, early studies used low total doses (50–60 mg/kg) of GHB given before sleep and 3 to 4 hours later. In 20 patients with narcolepsy, GHB 50 mg/kg increased slow wave sleep and decreased stage 1 sleep.[30] It reduced the number of awakenings, but did not increase total sleep time and had no effect on the excessive sleepiness of the narcopletics as measured by the MSLT. In a study of 24 narcoleptics, GHB 60 mg/kg, in divided doses, increased slow wave sleep and reduced the number of awakenings, and it improved self-rated daytime sleepiness.[31]

Showing therapeutic potential to improve both sleep and daytime sleepiness, several larger multisite clinical trails of sodium oxybate, the sodium salt of GHB, were conducted. Sodium oxybate was administered to narcoleptics in a titrated dosing schedule of 4.5, 6, 7.5, and 9 g.[32] The 7.5- and 9-g doses increased stage 3 and 4 sleep in the second half of the night and δ power across the night. Accompanying the nocturnal changes were improvements in daytime alertness as measured by the maintenance of wakefulness test (MWT). In a larger multisite trial of sodium oxybate in narcoleptics, 4.5-, 6-, and 9-g doses were administered, stage 3 and 4 sleep was increased in a dose-related manner, and stage 1 sleep was reduced at the 6- and 9-g doses.[27,33] MWT scores were improved.

α-2-Δ Ligands

Several antiepileptic drugs with unique mechanisms of action have been explored for their sleep effects. These drugs do not bind at $GABA_A$, $GABA_B$, or Bz receptors, but rather at the α-2-δ subunits of voltage-gated calcium channels. Pregabalin, with a wide range of therapeutic indications, was evaluated for its effects on the sleep of healthy volunteers. Pregabalin 450 mg was compared with alprazolam 3 mg and placebo, all administered before sleep.[34] Relative to placebo, pregabalin increased stage 3 and 4 sleep, whereas alprazolam reduced stage 3 and 4 sleep. Pregabalin also reduced the number of awakenings, but it

did not increase sleep time in these normal volunteers. Both drugs improved ratings of sleep quality and ease of falling asleep. In patients with controlled epilepsy, but remaining self-reported sleep disturbance, pregabalin 300 mg taken twice daily (not specifically before sleep) had no effect on stage 3 and 4 sleep, but it did reduce the number of awakenings relative to placebo.[35]

Another α-2-δ–acting drug, gabapentin, has indications for epilepsy and neuropathic pain. In healthy volunteers, gabapentin was titrated to a 1800-mg daily dose, taken in divided doses in the morning, midday, and before sleep.[36] It increased slow wave sleep from 8% to 13%, but did not affect other sleep stages. No differences in self-reported sleep or daytime sleepiness were observed. The sleep of patients with localization-related epilepsy controlled with various single antiepileptic drugs (AED) was compared with that of patients discontinued from their AEDs.[37] Gabapentin 900 mg increased slow wave sleep (19%) relative to the control patients (11%), but it did not alter other sleep stages or increase sleep time. The effect of gabapentin 300 and 600 mg was studied in healthy middle-aged adults, whose sleep was disrupted with a presleep 118-mL dose of 40% alcohol.[38] The 600-mg dose, relative to placebo and alcohol, increased slow wave sleep, whereas both doses reduced stage 1 sleep and the number of awakenings and increased sleep efficiency.

Serotonergic Antagonists and Inverse Agonists

Serotonergic antagonists also increase stage 3 to 4 sleep, but do not consistently improve sleep time or insomnia-related symptoms. Ritanserin, a $5-HT_{2A/2C}$ receptor antagonist with an approximately 40-hour half-life, is one such drug. In healthy volunteers, ritanserin 5 mg, administered in the morning, increased the amount of subsequent nighttime slow wave sleep by almost 50%, but there was no relation of the increased slow wave activity to any daytime performance measures, or reports about the efficiency or quality of sleep.[39] It did not increase sleep time or decrease sleep latency. In a dose study of ritanserin 1, 3, 10, and 30 mg administered in the morning to healthy volunteers, ritanserin increased slow wave sleep duration in a dose-related manner relative to placebo.[40] Again, no effects on sleep time or self-rated sleep measures were observed. A study in healthy volunteers compared ritanserin 5 mg to 20 and 40 mg ketanserin, which has less affinity to $5-HT_{2C}$ receptors than ritanserin.[41] Both drugs were administered 90 minutes before sleep and ritanserin increased slow wave sleep relative to placebo, and the increase was larger than that of ketanserin. Ketanserin reduced number of awakenings and wake after sleep onset to a greater extent than ritanserin. Given the daytime administration of ritanserin, its effects on driving performance and subsequent nighttime sleep were compared with those of lorazepam.[42] Lorazepam 1.5 mg and ritanserin 5 mg, both given twice a day (11:00 and 17:00 hours), had differential effects on driving and sleep. Lorazepam impaired driving and increased daytime sleepiness as measured by the MSLT, whereas ritanserin had no effects on sleepiness and driving performance. Ritanserin increased nocturnal slow wave sleep, whereas lorazepam had no effects on stage 3 to 4 sleep.

Ritanserin has also been studied in poor sleepers and other patient groups. In a study of young healthy volunteers, self-described as poor sleepers, 5 mg ritanserin increased slow wave sleep and δ EEG power spectra and it also increased REM and total sleep times and self-rated sleep quality.[43] In middle-aged poor sleepers, ritanserin 5 mg, administered after dinner, doubled the amount of slow wave sleep and reduced the amount of stage 1 sleep.[44] It did not alter sleep time or rating of sleep quality. In middle-aged patients with dysthymic disorder, ritanserin 10 mg versus placebo taken at breakfast doubled the percentage of stage 3 and 4 sleep.[45] It also reduced the number of sleep stage shifts, but had no effects on sleep time or self-rated sleep. A study assessed the effects of ritanserin 5 and 10 mg on the sleep of patients with narcolepsy.[46] Both doses increased stage 3 and 4 sleep, and the 10-mg dose decreased stage1 sleep, but neither dose improved daytime sleepiness.

Several 5-HT$_{2A}$ inverse agonists have been assessed as potential treatments for insomnia. The drug SR46349B (eplivanserin), in a 1-mg dose administered 3 hours before bedtime to healthy adults, increased stage 3 and 4 sleep from 19% to 32% and increased δ power spectra, but did affect self-reported sleep quality.[47] In a dose-ranging study 1, 10, or 40 mg eplivanserin in healthy adults increased slow wave sleep time by about 30%, but not in a dose-related manner.[48] Relative to placebo, it improved sleep efficiency and reduced the number of awakenings.

A recent study of a selective 5-HT$_{2A}$ inverse agonist, nelotanserin, suggests potential slow wave sleep enhancement and sleep consolidation.[49] At doses of 10, 20, and 40 mg administered to healthy adults before an afternoon nap, slow wave sleep was increased in a dose-related manner with the increase being from 47 to 82 minutes at the 40-mg dose. Total sleep time and the other sleep stages were not affected, but the number of awakenings, sleep stage shifts, and microarousals were all reduced.

Summary

The Bz and non-Bz agonists all improve insomnia; the Bzs mildly, but consistently, reduce stage 3 to 4 sleep and the non-Bz agonists do not affect stage 3 and 4 sleep. Thus, clinically, these drugs improve insomnia, but some reduce stage 3 and 4 sleep. However, some of the serotonergic antagonists, inverse agonists, and GABA reuptake inhibitors increase stage 3 and 4 sleep, but do not consistently improve measures of insomnia. A GABA$_A$ agonist seems to both increase stage 3 and 4 sleep and improve various measures of insomnia, and a GABA$_B$ agonist increases stage 3 and 4 sleep, consolidates sleep by reducing sleep stage shifts and awakenings, and improves the daytime sleepiness associated with narcolepsy.

Thus, modulations of stage 3 to 4 sleep have no consistent relation to improving insomnia. GHB/sodium oxybate increases stage 3 to 4 sleep and improves daytime alertness in narcolepsy. Stage 1 sleep reductions are reported with some of the drug classes discussed earlier, but not consistently so. These inconsistencies raise the question as to whether the functional significance of drug-related sleep stage alterations relate to the specific nature of sleep stage deficiencies in a given sleep disorder.

SLEEP STAGE VARIATIONS IN SLEEP DISORDERS
Primary Insomnia

Many studies have attempted to document PSG differences in the sleep of people with insomnia compared with those without insomnia. Most studies have failed to find differences in measures of onset and maintenance (ie, sleep latency, wake after sleep onset) or in sleep stage distribution.[50–52] An early, and the most frequently referenced, study was that of Carskadon and colleagues[53] in 1976, in which 122 drug-free insomniacs did not differ in PSG sleep from noninsomniacs. Plots of the distribution of sleep efficiency in the two groups showed considerable overlap. Among those studies showing PSG differences, increased wake time after sleep onset and less stage 3 and 4 sleep in insomniacs relative to controls has been reported.[54,55] Studies using EEG spectral analyses have compared patients with primary insomnia to age-matched controls. Some studies have failed to find substantial differences in EEG power in the δ and θ bands,[56] whereas others have reported differences.[57] One consistent finding reported in several studies is an increase in β and γ EEG activity in patients with insomnia compared with age-matched controls.[57,58]

Given the inability to find consistent PSG deviations from normal controls, particularly in total sleep times, a distinction between insomniacs showing objective sleep disturbance and those with no objective sleep disturbance was incorporated in the diagnostic nomenclature. The International Classification of Sleep Disorders (ICSD) includes the diagnostic entity "sleep state misperception" to account for those reporting disturbed sleep, but showing normal PSGs. Many studies were for 1 to 2 nights, which may be an inadequate assessment, so a study of patients with sleep state misperception sampled their sleep for 2 nights on each of 3 occasions separated by 2 weeks.[59] This study found patients with sleep state misperception had increased stage 1 sleep relative to age-match controls (14% vs 11%). Spectral analyses of the sleep EEG of patients with sleep state misperception have found lower δ and greater α, σ and β activity than controls.[60] As mentioned earlier, it is not clear whether the observed changes in sleep stages, when observed, were inherent in the condition or secondary to pathophysiologic events such as apneas and hypopneas, which cause EEG arousals.

Sleep Apnea and Periodic Leg Movement Disorders

The characteristic effect of these primary sleep disorders is the fragmentation of sleep with brief EEG arousals (ie, 3–15 seconds) and/or awakenings that follow each apnea or leg movement event. The effect on sleep stages of these primary sleep disorders is an increase in stage 1 sleep to 50% to 60% in patients with severe obstructive sleep apnea syndrome (OSAS) or to 25% and more in patients with periodic leg movements.[61,62] Stage 3 to 4 sleep is reduced to 3% and less. Although controls were not included in these studies, the degree of stage 1 increase and stage 3 to 4 reduction, corrected for age, would be considered abnormal. The degree to which sleep is fragmented, as documented by brief EEG arousal indices and secondarily reflected in the sleep stage deviations, relates to objective assessments of daytime sleepiness and the daytime sleepiness complaints of these patients. Treatment of OSAS, whether by surgery or continuous positive airway pressure, reduces the number of brief arousals, normalizes the sleep

stage deviations, and improves the daytime sleepiness.[63] Similarly, treatment of periodic leg movements improves sleep continuity and the daytime symptoms.[64,65]

The functionally impairing and sleep disruptive effects of primary sleep disorders has been modeled in healthy normals by fragmenting sleep with auditory tones producing brief EEG arousals. In one such study, the sleep of healthy young adults was disrupted with brief arousals on average 14 times per hour of sleep, which clinically would be considered a mild to moderate arousal index.[66] The consequent effect on sleep stages was to increase stage 1 sleep from 10% to 19% and to reduce stage 3 and 4 sleep from 19% to 5%. This fragmentation of sleep produced mild daytime sleepiness, reducing the average sleep latency on the MSLT from 14 minutes to 9 minutes.

Narcolepsy

The classic tetrad of symptoms in narcolepsy is excessive daytime sleepiness, cataplexy, sleep paralysis, and sleep onset hallucinations, with many considering disturbed nocturnal sleep to be a fifth symptom. Studies have generally shown reduced sleep efficiencies in patients with narcolepsy compared with age-matched healthy controls and some have shown increased stage 1 sleep.[67] In drug-free narcoleptics, stage 1 sleep was increased (21% vs 14%), but percent stage 3 and 4 (10%) was the same in both groups.[67] In another small study, drug-free narcoleptics compared with age-match controls showed a greater percentage of stage 1 (17% vs 9%) and reduced (11% vs 15%) percentage of 3 and 4.[68] However, a larger study found no differences in any sleep stages between narcoleptics and controls.[69] A study that conducted EEG spectral analyses in narcoleptics found no differences from age-matched controls in visually scored stage 3 and 4 sleep, but did find diminished slow wave activity and power.[70]

Summary

Insomniacs do not show consistent disturbance of sleep stages but, when present, the most disturbance seen is a mild increase in stage 1 sleep (10%–15%). Functional daytime impairment occurs in patients with primary sleep disorders (ie, apnea, periodic leg movements) because of the fragmentation of sleep by brief EEG arousals, which is then also reflected in higher percentages of stage 1 sleep and reductions of stage 3 and 4 sleep. Sleep stages 3 and 4 of patients with narcolepsy are not consistently abnormal, whereas stage 1 seems increased in most studies of narcoleptics. The major pathologic sign of narcolepsy is sleep onset REM periods. Overall, the data from patients with various sleep disorders suggest that, in the absence of frequent EEG arousals and sleep fragmentation, which tend to increase stage 1 sleep and reduce stages 3 and 4, there are no systematic changes in sleep stage distribution. The final question then is: What are normal variations in sleep staging and what are the functional consequences of sleep stage manipulation in healthy normals?

SLEEP STAGE VARIATIONS IN NONPATIENTS
Age and Sex Variations

Beyond the sleep stage changes of the first decade of life, the major variation in sleep stages occurs with aging. NREM stages 3 and 4 decline with age from approximately 20% in young adults, to 10% in the fourth decade, and to 6% in the sixth decade in one study.[71] Computer analyses of the δ wave activity of stage 3 and 4 sleep suggest that the age-related decline can be attributed to a reduction in δ wave amplitude and not specifically in the number of δ waves.[72] Because sleep-disordered breathing (SDB), which fragments sleep thereby increasing stage 1 and reducing stages 3 and 4 sleep, increases with age, valid data on age-dependent variations in sleep stages have to include concurrent assessment of SDB events, which was done in the data cited earlier. In contrast, REM sleep time shows little variation across the life span after the first year.

The other major variation in sleep stages is related to sex. Sex differences in the sleep of elderly volunteers have been well described.[72] The most prominent and consistent sex-related finding has been a reduction in the percentage of visually scored stage 3 to 4 sleep in elderly men,[73] which has been extended using computer scoring of slow wave activity.[74] Whether this δ wave sleep difference reflects a sex-related anatomic difference that alters the electrophysiologic signal (eg, greater male skull thickness and increased dead space between the skull and cortex, thereby attenuating the signal), a differential prevalence of sleep pathologies that fragment and suppress δ wave activity (ie, a higher prevalence of SDB in men), or a homeostatic sleep process difference between men and women is not clear. Related to the earlier discussion of insomnia, although the decline in sleep wave sleep with age is more pronounced in men, the age-related increase in the prevalence of insomnia is more pronounced in women.

Recent small clinical studies of young to middle-aged adults (20–50 years) have confirmed the sex-related difference in δ wave sleep, using either visual or computer scoring.[74–79] Computer analyses of the sleep EEG in samples of young and middle-aged adults suggest that the δ wave difference between men and women is related to an anatomic difference that produces an electrophysiologic difference in signal amplitude. Power density differences in sleep EEG were found across a wide frequency range in NREM sleep (ie, were not limited to δ wave frequency bands), were found in the REM sleep EEG, and also were shown in the frequency of sleep spindles.[74–79] Men had smaller power densities and lower spindle frequency, likely because of their thicker skulls.

The studies discussed earlier had small samples of convenience. In a population-based sample of older persons (mean age 61 years), sex differences in sleep were reported.[80] Men had more wakefulness during sleep, more stage 1 sleep, and less stage 3 to 4 sleep than women. Given that SDB increases with age, the lighter sleep of the men in this population-based sample could be attributed to a higher prevalence of SDB. A recent study assessed sex differences in a younger (31–40 years old), large, community-based sample with concurrent assessment of SDB.[81] After correcting for SDB in these younger men, no stage 3 to 4 differences between men and women were found, but the men had a greater percentage of stage 1 sleep (13%).

Several studies have attempted to relate variations in sleep stages to measures of daytime function. Studies of night-to-night variations in REM sleep have shown positive correlations with memory function (ie, greater REM time is associated with better memory), although the REM-memory relation is controversial.[82] Beyond studies of a REM-memory relation, the functional significance of stage 3 and 4 sleep has received research attention. For example, in young men, slower reaction times were related to lesser amounts of visually scored stage 3 and 4 sleep.[83] However, most studies have been conducted in elderly people and have shown no relation between stages 3 and 4 sleep and measures of cognitive function.[84–87] Several more recent studies have used spectral EEG analyses to quantify δ activity.[88,89] On 1 or 2 of the half-dozen performance measures assessed, greater power in the 2 to 4 Hz frequency band was predictive of better performance. However, inclusion of 2 to 4 Hz frequency as δ, which is more typical of stage 1 than δ sleep, and unusually high percentages of visually scored stage 3 and 4 sleep (about 20% in those aged 50 and 60 years) raise questions about these studies.

Studies of Selective Sleep Stage Deprivation and Recovery

In an attempt to understand the functional and clinical relevance of variations in sleep stage distribution, selective sleep stage deprivation studies have been conducted. Although the most selective sleep stage deprivation studies have focused on REM sleep, a few early, selective δ sleep deprivation studies were conducted. The acute within-night response to loss of stage 3 to 4 sleep (ie, a rapid return to stage 3–4 sleep and increasingly higher arousal thresholds), makes stage 3 to 4 deprivation studies difficult to conduct.[90] In contrast, REM deprivation at least for a few days is easier to achieve.[91] These early studies found that, when stage 4 sleep was deprived by arousing the sleeping individual immediately on entry to stage 4 sleep, subsequent entries to stage 4 sleep increased within the night and on subsequent nights.[91,92] When uninterrupted sleep was permitted, a rebound in stage 4 sleep was observed.

Daytime performance has been tested after selective stage 4 or REM sleep deprivation, and decrements specific to sleep stage were not found after as many as 7 nights of the selective sleep stage deprivation.[91–93] In recent, long-term, partial sleep deprivation studies, restricting bedtime to 5 hours a night led to an increase in stage 3 to 4 sleep and daytime performance decrements. This stage 3 to 4 compensation disappears after 1 to 2 days, but the performance decrements associated with the sleep restriction continue to accumulate.[94] It was concluded from all of these approaches that the major predictor of performance decrement was total sleep time and not time spent in specific sleep stages.[95]

As mentioned earlier, when recovery sleep is allowed after sleep deprivation, a rebound in stage 3 and 4 sleep is observed. It has been shown repeatedly that visually scored stage 3 and 4 sleep, or slow wave activity measured by EEG spectral analysis, is increased during recovery sleep as a function of the number of hours of prior waking.[96] Without prior sleep deprivation within the night, the amount of δ activity declines during successive NREM-REM cycles. It is hypothesized, and generally accepted, that δ activity is reflective of a sleep regulatory process, termed process S.[96] But caution is needed because enhanced δ activity does not necessarily reflect the restorative processes of sleep. Post–sleep deprivation recovery of EEG δ activity does not relate to the recovery of daytime behavioral function in correlational studies. This hypothesis was tested by comparing restoration of daytime function after

selective deprivation of δ sleep during the recovery night following total sleep deprivation to a nondisturbed night of recovery sleep.[97] Recovery sleep restored performance, and there was no difference between recovery sleep with and without δ sleep. All of these sleep deprivation studies were acute and the sleep stage recovery associated with long-term sleep deprivation in humans is not well documented.

Studies of sleep stage variations in healthy volunteers have reported considerable changes in sleep stages as a function of age and sex. The major changes observed are an age-related reduction of stage 3 and 4 sleep that is more pronounced in men than women. There is also some evidence of an increase in stage 1 sleep with age in men. Selective sleep stage deprivation studies do not find a functional significance associated with the loss and recovery of specific sleep stages.

SUMMARY

Slow wave sleep changes as a function of age more rapidly in men than women, and stage 1 sleep increases slightly with age in men. After controlling for primary sleep disorders, which also increase with age, no functional or clinical significance is found with these changes. Similarly, in healthy normals, selective sleep stage deprivation studies have not found functional impairment associated with the loss and recovery of specific sleep stages. Large changes in sleep stages that are associated with functional impairment are found in some primary sleep disorders, but these changes are likely secondary to the fragmentation of sleep by brief arousals. The fragmentation is often associated with an increase in stage 1 sleep. To date, no consistent sleep stage changes, such as deficiencies of stage 3 to 4 sleep or increases of stage 1 sleep, have been reported in insomniacs.

Given the observation of these normal reductions in slow wave sleep and often increases in stage 1 sleep with age, and the absence of clear sleep stage changes in insomnia, the functional significance and clinical relevance of drug-related changes in stage 3 to 4 sleep remain to be shown. Studies showing that enhancement of slow wave sleep in healthy older adults is also associated with improved daytime function such as memory or vigilance will be an important step. Similarly, studies showing that the usual impairing effects of sleep time reductions can be reversed, such as the studies attempted with tiagabine and gaboxadol, will be of further importance. In patients with insomnia, the data for many of these agents suggest that, although sleep onset is not reduced, sleep maintenance may be improved, possibly through the reduced capacity for arousal associated with the enhanced stage 3 and 4 sleep.

REFERENCES

1. Roth T, Roehrs T. An overview of normal sleep and sleep disorders. Eur J Neurol 2000;7(S4):3–8.
2. Carakadon MA, Dement WC. Normal human sleep: an overview. In: Kryger MH, Roth T, Dement WC, editors. Principles and practice of sleep medicine. 4th edition. Philadelphia: Elsevier; 2005. p. 13–23.
3. Dijk DJ. Regulation and functional correlates of slow wave sleep. J Clin Sleep Med 2009;5:S6–15.
4. Lamphere J, Roehrs T, Zorick F, et al. Chronic hypnotic efficacy of estazolam. Drugs Exp Clin Res 1986;12:687–92.
5. Roehrs T, Vogel G, Vogel F, et al. Dose effects of temazepam tablets on sleep. Drugs Exp Clin Res 1986;12:693–9.
6. Roehrs T, Zorick F, Wittig R, et al. Efficacy of a reduced triazolam dose in elderly insomniacs. Neurobiol Aging 1985;6:293–6.
7. Roehrs T, Merlotti L, Rosenthal L, et al. Benzodiazepine associated reversal of the effects of experimental sleep fragmentation. Hum Psychopharm 1993;8:351–6.
8. Walsh J, Roehrs T, Decerck AC. Polysomnographic studies of the effects of zolpidem in patients with insomnia. In: Freeman H, Puech AJ, Roth T, editors. Zolpidem: an update of its pharmacological properties and therapeutic place in the management of insomnia. Paris: Elsevier; 1996. p. 129–39.
9. Merlotti L, Roehrs T, Koshorek G, et al. The dose effects of zolpidem on the sleep of healthy normals. J Clin Psychopharmacol 1989;1:9–14.
10. Lamphere JK, Roehrs TA, Zorick F, et al. The dose effects of zopiclone. Hum Psychopharm 1989;4: 41–6.
11. Rosenberg R, Caron J, Roth T, et al. An assessment of the efficacy and safety of eszopiclone in the treatment of transient insomnia in healthy adults. Sleep Med 2005;6:15–22.
12. Walsh JK, Randazzo AC, Frankowski S, et al. Dose-response effects of tiagabine on the sleep of older adults. Sleep 2005;28:673–6.
13. Mathias S, Wetter TC, Steiger A, et al. The GABA uptake inhibitor tiagabine promotes slow wave sleep in normal elderly subjects. Neurobiol Aging 2001;22: 247–53.
14. Roth T, Wright K, Walsh J. Effect of tiagabine on sleep in elderly subjects with primary insomnia: a randomized, double-blind, placebo-controlled study. Sleep 2006;29:335–41.
15. Walsh JK, Perlis M, Rosenthal M, et al. Tiagabine increases slow wave sleep in a dose-dependent fashion without affecting traditional efficacy

16. Walsh JK, Zammit G, Schweitzer PK, et al. Tiagabine enhances slow wave sleep and sleep maintenance in primary insomnia. Sleep Med 2006;7:155–61.
17. Walsh JK, Randazzo AC, Stone K, et al. Tiagabine is associated with sustained attention during sleep restriction: evidence for the value of slow-wave sleep enhancement? Sleep 2006;29:433–43.
18. Faulhaber J, Steiger A, Lancel M. The GABAA agonist THIP produces slow wave sleep and reduces spindling activity in NREM sleep in humans. Psychopharmacology 1997;130:285–91.
19. Winsky-Sommer R, Vyazovskiy VV, Homanics GE, et al. The EEG effects of THIP (Gaboxadol) on sleep and waking are mediated by the $GABA_A$-subunit-containing receptors. Eur J Neurosci 2007;25: 1893–9.
20. Walsh JK, Deacon S, Dijk DJ, et al. The selective extrasynaptic $GABA_A$ agonist, gaboxadol, improves traditional hypnotic efficacy measures and enhances slow wave activity in a model of transient insomnia. Sleep 2007;30:593–602.
21. Walsh JK, Mayleben D, Guico-Pabia C, et al. Efficacy of the selective extrasynaptic agonist, gaboxadol, in a model of transient insomnia: a randomized, controlled clinical trial. Sleep Med 2008;9:393–402.
22. Mathias S, Zihl J, Steiger A, et al. Effect of repeated gaboxadol administration on night sleep and next-day performance in healthy elderly subjects. Neuropsychopharmacology 2005;30:833–41.
23. Deacon S, Staner L, Staner C, et al. Effect of short-term treatment with gaboxadol on sleep maintenance and initiation in patient with primary insomnia. Sleep 2007;30:281–7.
24. Lundahl J, Staner L, Staner C, et al. Short-term treatment with gaboxadol improves sleep maintenance and enhances slow wave sleep in adult patients with primary insomnia. Psychopharmacology 2007; 195:139–46.
25. Lankford A, Corser BC, Zheng YP, et al. Effect of gaboxadol on sleep in adult and elderly patients with primary insomnia: results from two randomized, placebo-controlled, 30-night polysomnography studies. Sleep 2008;31:1359–70.
26. Walsh JK, Snyder E, Hall J, et al. Slow wave sleep enhancement with gaboxadol reduces daytime sleepiness during sleep restriction. Sleep 2008;31: 659–72.
27. Pardi D, Black J. γ-Hydroxybutyrate/sodium oxybate: neurobiology, and impact on sleep and wakefulness. CNS Drugs 2006;20:993–1018.
28. Lapierre O, Montplaisir J, Lamarre M, et al. The effect of gamma-hydroxybutyrate on nocturnal and diurnal sleep of normal subjects: further considerations on REM sleep-triggering mechanisms. Sleep 1990;13:24–30.

measures in adults with primary insomnia. J Clin Sleep Med 2006;2:35–41.

29. Van Cauter E, Plaat L, Schart MB, et al. Simultaneous stimulation of slow-wave sleep and growth hormone secretion by gamma-hydroxybutyrate in normal young men. J Clin Invest 1997;100:745–53.

30. Mamelak M, Black J, Montplaisir J, et al. A pilot study on the effects of sodium oxybate on sleep architecture and daytime alertness in narcolepsy. Sleep 2004;27:1327–34.

31. Scrima L, Hartman PG, Johnson FH, et al. The effects of γ-hydroxybutyrate on the sleep of narcolepsy patients: a double-blind study. Sleep 1990;3:479–90.

32. Lammer GJ, Arends J, Declerck AC, et al. Gamma-hydroxybutyrate and narcolepsy: a double-blind placebo-controlled study. Sleep 1993;16:216–20.

33. The Xyrem International Study Group. A double-blind placebo-controlled study demonstrates sodium oxybate is effective for the treatment of excessive daytime sleepiness in narcolepsy. J Clin Sleep Med 2005;1:391–7.

34. Hindmarch I, Dawson J, Stanley N. A double-blind study in healthy volunteers to assess the effects on sleep of pregabalin compared with alprazolam and placebo. Sleep 2005;28:187–93.

35. de Haas S, Otte A, de Weerd A, et al. Exploratory polysomnographic evaluation of pregabalin on sleep disturbance in patients with epilepsy. J Clin Sleep Med 2007;3:473–8.

36. Foldvary-Schaefer N, Sanchez I, Karafa M, et al. Gabapentin increases slow wave sleep in normal adults. Epilepsia 2002;43:1493–7.

37. Legros B, Bazil CW. Effects of antiepileptic drugs on sleep architecture: a pilot study. Sleep Med 2003;4:51–5.

38. Bazil CW, Battista J, Basner RC. Gabapentin improves sleep in the presence of alcohol. J Clin Sleep Med 2005;1:284–7.

39. Declerck AC, Wauquier A, Van Der Ham-Veltman PHM, et al. Increase in slow wave sleep in humans with the serotonin-S2 antagonist ritanserin. Curr Ther Res 1987;41:427–32.

40. Idzikowski C, Mills FJ, James RJ. A dose-response study examining the effects of ritanserin on human slow wave sleep. Br J Clin Pharmacol 1991;31:193–6.

41. Sharpley AL, Elliott JM, Attenburrow MJ, et al. Sleep wave sleep in humans: role of $5-HT_{2A}$ and $5-HT_{2C}$ receptors. Neuropharmacology 1994;33:467–71.

42. van Laar M, Volkerts E, Verbasten M. Subchronic effects of the GABA-agonist lorazepam and the $5-HT_{2A/2C}$ antagonist ritanserin on driving performance, slow wave sleep and daytime sleepiness in healthy volunteers. Psychopharmacology 2001;154:189–97.

43. Viola AU, Brandenberger G, Toussaint M, et al. Ritanserin, a serotonin-2 receptor antagonist, improves ultradian sleep rhythmicity in young poor sleepers. Clin Neurophysiol 2002;113:429–34.

44. Adam K, Oswald I. Effects of repeated ritanserin on middle-aged poor sleepers. Psychopharmacology 1989;99:219–21.

45. Paiva T, Arriaga F, Waugquer A, et al. Effects of ritanserin on sleep disturbances of dysthymic patients. Psychopharmacology 1988;96:395–9.

46. Mayer G. Ritanserin improves sleep quality in narcolepsy. Pharmacopsychiatry 2003;36:150–5.

47. Landolt HP, Meier V, Burgess HJ, et al. Serotonin-2 receptors and human sleep: effect of a selective antagonist on EEG power spectra. Neuropsychopharmacology 1999;21:455–66.

48. Hindmarch I, Cattelin F. Effect of two dose regimens of eplivanserin, a new sleep agent, on sleep and psychomotor performance of healthy subjects. Sleep 2008;31:A33.

49. Al-Shanna HA, Anderson C, Chuang E, et al. Nelotanserin, a novel selective human 5-hydroxytryptamine 2_A inverse agonist for the treatment of insomnia. J Pharmacol Exp Ther 2010;332:281–90.

50. Frankel BL, Coursey RD, Buchbinder R, et al. Recorded and reported sleep in chronic primary insomnia. Arch Gen Psychiatry 1976;33:615–23.

51. Edinger JD, Fins AI. The distribution and clinical significance of sleep time misperceptions among insomniacs. Sleep 1995;18:232–9.

52. Vanable PA, Aikens JE, Tadimenti L, et al. Sleep latency and duration estimates among sleep disorder patients: variability as a function of sleep disorder diagnosis, sleep history, and psychological characteristics. Sleep 2000;23:71–9.

53. Carskadon MA, Dement WC, Mitler MM, et al. Self-reports versus sleep laboratory findings in 122 drug-free subjects with complaints of primary insomnia. Am J Psychiatry 1976;133:1382–7.

54. Mendelson WB, James SP, Garnett D, et al. A psychophysiological study of insomnia. Psychiatry Res 1986;16:267–84.

55. Gillin JC, Duncan W, Pettigrew KD, et al. Successful separation of depressed, normal, and insomniac subjects by EEG sleep data. Arch Gen Psychiatry 1979;36:85–90.

56. Buysse DJ, Germain A, Hall M, et al. EEG spectral analysis in primary insomnia: NREM period effects and sex differences. Sleep 2008;31:1673–82.

57. Mercia H, Blois R, Gaillard JM. Spectral characteristics of sleep EEG in chronic insomnia. Eur J Neurosci 1998;10:1826–34.

58. Perlis ML, Smith MT, Andrews PJ, et al. Beta/gamma EEG activity in patients with primary and secondary insomnia and good sleeper controls. Sleep 2001;24:110–7.

59. Salin-Pascual RJ, Roehrs TA, Merlotti LA, et al. Long-term study of the sleep of insomnia patients with sleep-state misperception and other insomnia patients. Am J Psychiatry 1992;149:904–8.

60. Krystal AD, Edinger JD, Wohlgemuth WK, et al. NREM sleep EEG frequency correlates of sleep complaints in primary insomnia subtypes. Sleep 2002;25:626–36.

61. Conway WA, Zorick FJ, Sicklesteel JM, et al. Evaluation of the effectiveness of uvulopalatopharyngoplasty. Laryngoscope 1985;85:70–4.

62. Rosenthal L, Roehrs T, Sicklesteel J, et al. Periodic movements during sleep, sleep fragmentation, and sleep-wake complaints. Sleep 1984;7:326–30.

63. Zorick FJ, Roehrs T, Conway W, et al. Response to CPAP and UPPP in apnea. Henry Ford Hosp Med J 1990;38:223–6.

64. Brodeur C, Montplaisir J, Marinier R. Treatment of restless leg syndrome and periodic movements during sleep with L-dopa: a double-blind controlled study. Neurology 1988;35:1845–8.

65. Montplaisir J, Allen RP, Walters AS, et al. Restless legs syndrome and periodic limb movements during sleep. In: Kryger MH, Roth T, Dement WC, editors. Principles and practice of sleep medicine. 4th edition. Philadelphia: Elsevier Saunders; 2005. p. 839–52.

66. Roehrs T, Merlotti L, Petrucelli N, et al. Experimental sleep fragmentation. Sleep 1994;17:438–43.

67. Nykamp K, Rosenthal L, Helmus T, et al. Repeated nocturnal sleep latencies in narcoleptic, sleepy and alert subjects. Clin Neurophysiol 1999;110:1531–4.

68. Khatami R, Landolt HP, Achermann P, et al. Insufficient non-REM sleep intensity in narcolepsy-cataplexy. Sleep 2007;8:980–9.

69. Vernet C, Arnulf I. Narcolepsy with long sleep time: a specific entity? Sleep 2009;29:1229–35.

70. Mukai J, Uchida S, Miyazaki S, et al. Spectral analysis of all-night human sleep EEG in narcoleptic patients and normal subjects. J Sleep Res 2003;12:63–71.

71. Roth T, Roehrs T. Sleep organization and regulation. Neurology 2000;54:S2–7.

72. Bliwise DL. Normal aging. In: Kryger MH, Roth T, Dement WC, editors. Principles and practice of sleep medicine. 3rd edition. Philadelphia: Elsevier; 2000. p. 16–26.

73. Hoch CC, Dew MA, Reynolds CF III, et al. A longitudinal study of laboratory- and diary-based sleep measures in healthy "old old" and "young old" volunteers. Sleep 1994;17:489–96.

74. Reynolds CF, Monk TH, Hock CC, et al. Electroencephalographic sleep in the healthy "old old": a comparison with the "young old" in visually scored and automated measures. J Gerontol 1991;46:M39–46.

75. Dijk DJ, Beersma DGM, Bloem GM. Sex differences in the sleep EEG of young adults: visual scoring and spectral analysis. Sleep 1989;12:500–7.

76. Mourtazaev MS, Kemp B, Zwinderman AH, et al. Age and gender affect different characteristics of slow waves in the sleep EEG. Sleep 1989;18:557–64.

77. Armitage R. The distribution of EEG frequencies in REM and NREM sleep stages in healthy young adults. Sleep 1995;18:334–41.

78. Carrier J, Land S, Buysse DJ, et al. The effects of age and gender on sleep EEG power spectral density in the middle years of life (20–60 years old). Psychophysiology 2001;38:232–42.

79. Hupponen E, Mimanen SL, Varri A, et al. A study on gender and age differences in sleep spindles. Neuropsychobiology 2002;45:99–105.

80. Redline S, Kirchner L, Quan SF, et al. The effects of age, sex, ethnicity, and sleep architecture. Arch Intern Med 2004;164:406–18.

81. Roehrs T, Kapke A, Roth T, et al. Sex differences in the polysomnographic sleep of young adults: a community-based study. Sleep Med 2006;7:49–53.

82. Siegel JM. The REM sleep-review consolidation hypothesis. Science 2001;294:1058–63.

83. Jurado JL, Villegas G, Buela-Casal G. Normal human subjects with show reaction times and larger time estimations alter waking have diminished delta sleep. Electroencephalogr Clin Neurophysiol 1989;73:124–8.

84. Berry DTR, Webb WB. Sleep and cognitive functions in normal older adults. J Gerontol 1985;40:331–5.

85. Feinberg I, Koresko RL, Heller N. EEG sleep patterns as a function of normal and pathological aging in man. J Psychiatr Res 1967;5:107–44.

86. Prinz PN. Sleep patterns in healthy aged: relationship with intellectual function. J Gerontol 1977;32:179–86.

87. Spiegel R, Koberle S, Allen SR. Significance of slow wave sleep: considerations from a clinical viewpoint. Sleep 1986;9:66–79.

88. Crenshaw MC, Edinger JD. Slow-wave sleep and waking cognitive performance among older adults with and without insomnia complaints. Physiol Behav 1999;66:485–92.

89. Edinger JD, Glenn DM, Bastian LA, et al. Slow-wave sleep and waking cognitive performance II: findings among middle-aged adults with and without insomnia complaints. Physiol Behav 2000;70:127–34.

90. Gilliland MA, Bergmann BM, Rechtschaffen A. Sleep deprivation in the rat: VIII. High EEG amplitude sleep deprivation. Sleep 1989;12:53–9.

91. Agnew HW, Webb WB, Williams RL. Comparison of stage four and 1-REM sleep deprivation. Percept Mot Skills 1967;24:851–8.

92. Agnew HW, Webb WB, Williams RL. The effects of stage four sleep deprivation. Electroencephalogr Clin Neurophysiol 1964;17:68–70.

93. Johnson LC, Naitoh P, Moses JM. Interaction of REM deprivation and stage 4 deprivation with total sleep loss: experiment 2. Psychophysiology 1974;11:147–59.

94. Banks S, Dinges DF. Behavioral and physiological consequences of sleep restriction. J Clin Sleep Med 2007;3:519–28.

95. Johnson LC. Are stages of sleep related to waking behavior? Am Sci 1973;61:326–38.

96. Borbely AA, Achermann P. Sleep homeostasis and models of sleep regulation. In: Kryger MH, Roth T, Dement WC, editors. Principles and practice of sleep medicine. 4th edition. Philadelphia: Elsevier Saunders; 2005. p. 405–17.

97. Lubin A, Moses JM, Johnson LC. The recuperative effects of REM sleep and stage 4 sleep on human performance after complete sleep loss. Psychophysiology 1974;11:133–46.

Antidepressant and Antipsychotic Drugs

Andrew D. Krystal, MD, MS

- Antidepressant drugs • Antipsychotic drugs
- Pharmacologic effects • Sleep-wake effects

The antidepressant and antipsychotic drugs are a set of agents with a wide range of different pharmacologic effects. Many of these pharmacologic effects have an impact on sleep-wake function. This can involve promoting sleep, promoting wakefulness, altering the amount or timing of sleep stages across the night, and increasing the likelihood of restless legs syndrome (RLS) and/or periodic movements of sleep, which can disturb sleep. Depending on the time of day of administration, the pharmacokinetics of the drug, the dose of the drug, and the context, some of these effects may be therapeutic and some may be adverse. For example, when administered at bedtime to a patient with sleep difficulty, the sleep-promoting effects of an antipsychotic medication can be therapeutic. If that medication is administered in the morning or if the combination of dosage and half-life of the medication result in next-day effects, however, the sleep promotion associated with this medication can be problematic. Some of the effects on sleep-wake function of these medications, such as altering the amount or timing of sleep stages, are of uncertain clinical significance but have long been of interest in terms of research that pursues whether or not these changes might be linked to therapeutic effects, such as antidepressant effects, sleep restoration, and improvement in negative symptoms in schizophrenia.

This article reviews the pharmacology and associated sleep-wake effects of the antidepressant and antipsychotic medications. It discusses factors relevant to these effects, such as pharmacokinetic properties, dosing, and therapeutic target. Comprehensive review of the clinical trials related to the use of these agents for the treatment of sleep-wake disorders are not covered in this article but are included in articles in Part II of this volume (Table 1).

PHARMACOLOGIC MECHANISMS OF ANTIDEPRESSANTS AND ANTIPSYCHOTICS: EFFECTS ON SLEEP-WAKE FUNCTION
Promoting Sleep by Blocking the Activity of Wake-Promoting Neurotransmitters

Sleep promotion occurs with antidepressants and antipsychotics that block receptors that mediate the wake-promoting effects of several neurotransmitters, including the serotonin (5-hydroxytryptamine [HT]) type 2 receptor (5-HT2), histamine (H1) receptors, muscarinic acetylcholine (Ach) receptors, norepinephrine receptors, and dopamine (DA) receptors.[1–6] These effects can potentially improve sleep at night but also have the potential to cause daytime sedation.

5-HT2 antagonism
The 5-HT system and its effects on sleep are complex. There is some evidence in both human and animal studies that suggests, however, that agents that selectively block 5-HT2 receptors improve the ability to stay asleep.[7–10] The inconsistency of findings in such studies has led to the hypothesis that the sleep-promoting effects of 5-HT2 antagonism may depend on the ratio of effects on 5-HT2A and 5-HT2C receptor subtypes as well as other factors. These data, however, along with the tendency of antidepressant and antipsychotic medications that have 5-HT2 antagonist effects to enhance sleep, have led to the general belief that 5-HT2 antagonism may be associated with sleep enhancement.

Duke University School of Medicine, Duke University Medical Center, Box 3309, Trent Drive, Durham, NC 27710, USA
E-mail address: kryst001@mc.duke.edu

Sleep Med Clin 5 (2010) 571–589
doi:10.1016/j.jsmc.2010.08.010
1556-407X/10/$ — see front matter © 2010 Elsevier Inc. All rights reserved.

sleep.theclinics.com

Table 1
Pharmacologic mechanisms of sleep-wake effects of antidepressants and antipsychotics

Mechanism	Sleep Promotion	Wake Promotion	REM Suppression	Increases SWS	Promotes RLS/PLMS
H1 antagonism	√				
Ach antagonism	√		√		
5-HT2 antagonism	√			√	
α_1-Antagonism	√				
α_2-Antagonism		√			
D1/D2 antagonism	√				√
5-HT reuptake inhibition		√	√		√
NE reuptake inhibition		√			
DA reuptake inhibition		√			
MAO inhibition		√	√		√
5-HT1A agonism		√	√		

Abbreviations: NE, norepinephrine; SWS, slow-wave sleep.

Histamine antagonism

Histamine is one of the most important wake-promoting neurotransmitter systems in the brain. It mediates its effects by binding to the H1 receptor.[1] Agents that increase histamine's release and binding to H1 receptors enhance wakefulness.[11]

Many antidepressant and antipsychotic agents block these H1 receptors and, thereby, promote sleep.[12,13] Although there is ample experience with agents with H1 antagonism, few data exist on the sleep-wake effects of medications with H1 antagonism effects and minimal effects on other receptor systems. As a result, understanding of the sleep-wake effects of H1 antagonism remains limited. Recent studies have been performed with doxepin at dosages from 1–6 mg where it seems to be a selective H1 antagonist (discussed later).[14,15] The data suggest that H1 antagonism may have its greatest sleep-enhancing effects at the end of the night. In these studies, differences between doxepin and placebo were greatest in hours 7 to 8 of the night despite achieving peak blood level 1.5 to 4 hours after dosing.[14,15] These data suggest that the sleep enhancement of H1 antagonism is dissociated from blood level and may be more related to time of day. Further evidence to support this conclusion and to suggest that the sleep-enhancing effects may be affected by activity level as well is that doxepin (1–6 mg) was not associated with sedation when assessed after waking; just 1 hour after the peak, sleep-enhancing effect was observed.[14,15]

α_1-Adrenergic antagonism

The wake-promoting effects of norepinephrine in the central nervous system are well established and believed to be mediated at least in part by α_1 receptors.[1,16] This mechanism is believed to be responsible for some of the arousal achieved by stimulants, such as dextroamphetamine and methylphenidate.[16] On this basis, antidepressant and antipsychotic medications that block α_1 receptors are believed to have sleep-enhancing effects.[17,18]

Dopamine antagonism

Like norepinephrine, DA is also believed to be an important wake-promoting neurotransmitter.[1] There is evidence that some of the wake-promoting effects of the stimulants, dextroamphetamine and methylphenidate, are mediated through increasing dopaminergic activity at both D1 and D2 receptor subtypes.[16] Antipsychotic medications block these receptors and are believed to be associated with some degree of sleep-promoting effects as a result.[13]

Cholinergic antagonism

Ach is one of the most important neurotransmitters mediating arousal.[19] For example, cholinergic neurons form the core of the brainstem reticular activating system.[20] Some of the arousal effects of Ach seem to be mediated via muscarinic cholinergic receptors, which are blocked by any antidepressant and antipsychotic medications, resulting in a decrease in arousal and promotion of sleep.[21]

Promoting Wakefulness by Inhibiting the Reuptake or Metabolism of Wake-Promoting Neurotransmitters

Wake promotion may occur with antidepressants that block the reuptake or metabolism of neurotransmitters that bind to receptors that promote wakefulness, including the 5-HT type 1 (5-HT1) and 5-HT2 receptors, norepinephrine (α_1) receptors, and DA receptors.[1–6] This wake promotion may be therapeutic in many instances; however, there is also the potential for these effects to lead to sleep disturbance.

Norepinephrine reuptake inhibition

Several antidepressants block the reuptake of norepinephrine, including agents referred to as selective serotonin reuptake inhibitors (SSRIs)—fluoxetine, paroxetine, citalopram, and escitalopram; serotonin-norepinephrine reuptake inhibitors (SNRIs)—duloxetine, venlafaxine, and desvenlafaxine; tricyclic antidepressants (TCAs)—including amitriptyline, desipramine, doxepin, trimipramine, imipramine; and bupropion, a norepinephrine and DA reuptake inhibitor. Although it might be expected that SSRIs only block 5-HT reuptake and not norepinephrine, the data related to this issue suggest that SSRIs and SNRIs represent a continuum with respect to the capacity to block norepinephrine.[22] Some of these agents, such as escitalopram, have minimal norepinephrine reuptake inhibition at dosages typically used to treat depression, whereas others (paroxetine, duloxetine, and venlafaxine) have greater associated norepinephrine reuptake inhibition in antidepressant dosages.[23,24] Norepinephrine reuptake is expected to increase the amount of norepinephrine in the synapse, thereby increasing binding to α_1-adrenergic receptors and promoting wakefulness.[1,16]

5-HT reuptake inhibition

Inhibition of 5-HT reuptake occurs with SSRIs, SNRIs, TCAs, and the antidepressant, trazodone, and is expected to promote wakefulness by increasing the binding to 5-HT1 and 5-HT2 receptors.[25,26] As discussed above, increasing the binding to 5-HT2 receptors is expected to promote wakefulness and suppress non–rapid eye movement (REM) sleep.[7–9] By increasing binding to 5-HT1 receptors, an increase in wakefulness may occur in association with suppression of REM sleep.[27] Daytime sedation has also been associated with inhibition of 5-HT reuptake (SSRIs, SNRIs, and TCAs); however, it is unclear if this is a primary effect or a secondary effect of sleep disruption occurring in conjunction with 5-HT reuptake inhibition.[28–30]

Dopamine reuptake inhibition

Bupropion is the only antidepressant or antipsychotic agent that inhibits DA reuptake. DA reuptake inhibition is expected to have wake-promoting effects.[1,16] This view is based to a degree on the fact that several stimulants also inhibit DA reuptake; however, a similar clinical profile cannot be assumed for bupropion due to differences in potency and potential regional specificity of DA reuptake.[31,32]

Inhibition of monoamine oxidase

Monoamine oxidase is the enzyme that breaks down biogenic amines, including norepinephrine, 5-HT, epinephrine, melatonin, phenylethylamine, trace amines, and DA.[33] As a result, medications that inhibit this enzyme, monoamine oxidase inhibitors (MAOIs), increase the available amount of NE, 5-HT, epinephrine, and DA, and, much like agents that inhibit the reuptake of these neurotransmitters, MAOIs may have some degree of wake-promoting effects.[4,34,35] There are two forms of MAOIs, one of which is primarily involved in the metabolism of 5-HT, NE, epinephrine, melatonin, and DA, referred to as MAO type A, whereas the other, MAO type B, primarily metabolizes DA, phenylethylamine, and trace amines, and both have been associated with disturbances of sleep.[35] Daytime sedation is sometimes reported with MAOI, particularly with MAO type A inhibitors; however, it is unclear if this is due to the MAO inhibition or other of the many effects of these agents. It is unclear whether or not there are sleep-wake effects due to the inhibition of melatonin metabolism by MAO type A inhibitors.

Suppression of REM Sleep

Among antidepressant and antipsychotic agents, suppression of REM sleep seems to primarily derive from blockade of Ach receptors (occurs primarily with TCAs and several of the antipsychotic agents) and increasing 5-HT binding to 5-HT1A receptors, which occurs with TCAs, MAOIs, SSRIs, and SNRIs.[25,27,36,37] The significance of REM sleep suppression is unclear. Given the observation that REM latency is shortened in major depression and that depressed patients have an increase in the amount and intensity of REM compared with healthy controls, the fact that REM suppression occurs with nearly all antidepressant medications has led to the hypothesis that suppression of REM sleep is a mechanism by which antidepressants have a therapeutic effect on depression.[4,38–41] This remains controversial, however, because several agents that have consistently been demonstrated to have antidepressant effects seem to lack REM suppression (bupropion, mirtazapine, and nefazodone).[42] Patients with schizophrenia also have shortened REM latency and an increase in the amount of REM sleep and this has been linked to greater severity of delusions, hallucinations, and disorganization of thought and behavior.[42,43] There are no data available, however, related to the question of whether or not the pharmacologic suppression of REM sleep is associated with therapeutic effects in patients with schizophrenia.[42]

Increasing Slow Wave Sleep Time and Slow Wave Amplitude

An increase in the amount of slow wave sleep and in the amplitude of electroencephalogram (EEG) slow waves in sleep occurs with antidepressants and antipsychotics that block 5-HT2 receptors.[7–10,37,44–47] Although some debate exists regarding the extent to which this effect is associated with different subtypes of 5-HT2 receptors. There is also debate about the clinical significance of this effect. Because an increase in slow wave sleep and slow wave amplitude occurs in recovery sleep after sleep deprivation, some investigators have hypothesized that these slow wave effects might be associated with enhancing restoration from sleep.[48] Slow wave sleep also is diminished in depressed patients.[38] Whether or not increasing slow wave sleep and slow wave amplitude has any beneficial effect in depression remains unclear. There is also evidence for diminished slow wave sleep time and slow wave amplitude in non-REM sleep in schizophrenia and that these changes are associated with greater functional impairment and deficits in cognitive and social deficits.[42,43,49] As with major depression, however, it remains unknown whether or not increasing slow wave sleep time and slow wave activity has therapeutic effects in patients with schizophrenia.[42]

Promoting Restless Legs Syndrome and Periodic Limb Movements of Sleep

Several antidepressants and antipsychotics seem to have the potential to cause or exacerbate RLS and periodic limb movements of sleep (PLMS), which can be associated with difficulties with sleep onset, sleep maintenance complaints, and/or daytime sleepiness.[50] A deficiency in iron, as indicated by serum ferritin at the low end of normal or below, can exacerbate this problem.[51] The mechanisms by which some antidepressant and antipsychotic medications promote RLS and PLMS are incompletely understood; however, this seems to be associated with increasing 5-HT availability and DA receptor blockade.[38,42,52] On this basis, it is expected that SSRIs, SNRIs, TCAs, MAOIs, and

all of the antipsychotics have the potential to increase RLS and PLMS. A recent review article concluded, however, that of the antidepressants and antipsychotics, those most strongly associated with drug-induced RLS in the published literature are escitalopram, fluoxetine, mianserin, mirtazapine, and olanzapine, whereas those agents most strongly associated with PLMS are bupropion, citalopram, fluoxetine, paroxetine, sertraline, and venlafaxine.[50] Of these medications, the link of bupropion and PLMS is most controversial because some studies have not found any evidence of an association of PLMS and bupropion.[53]

IMPACT OF DOSE AND PHARMACOKINETICS ON SLEEP-WAKE EFFECTS OF ANTIDEPRESSANT AND ANTIPSYCHOTIC DRUGS

In addition to the pharmacologic considerations (discussed previously), whether or not sleep-wake effects occur with antidepressant and antipsychotic medications and what type of effects are observed depend on several other factors, including the dosage of the medication, the medication half-life, and the medication time to maximum plasma concentration (Tmax), an indicator of the speed of absorption. The data relevant to these issues for many antidepressant and antipsychotic medications appear in **Table 2**.

Dose

Increasing dose generally increases the likelihood that a medication having a pharmacologic effect has an associated clinical effect and also increases the duration of clinical effects. Changes in dosage may also alter the balance between different pharmacologic effects associated with a given medication. One example of the effects of dosage on clinical effects is the antidepressant, mirtazapine. Mirtazapine has several potent pharmacologic effects that promote sleep; however, it is also associated with antagonism of the α_2- adrenergic receptor, a presynaptic autoreceptor that inhibits norepinephrine release, and, as a result, blocking this receptor promotes wakefulness. It has been hypothesized that a decrease in sedation occurring with mirtazapine with increasing dosage is due to a relative increase in the importance of this α_2-antagonism at larger doses.[54] As discussed previously, doxepin is another example of dose-dependent effects. Doxepin's most potent pharmacologic effect is H1 antagonism, and, as a result, if the dosage is dropped to a low-enough level, it is possible to achieve a predominant antihistaminergic effect without the other effects that can occur with this medication, including 5-HT and norepinephrine reuptake inhibition, anticholinergic effects, and antiadrenergic and anticholinergic effects.[14,15] Recent studies suggest that at dosages from 1 to 6 mg (more than 10 times less than the usual antidepressant dosage), a unique profile of sleep-wake effects becomes apparent presumed to reflect this selective H1 antagonism, including a predominant sleep-enhancing effect in the last third of the night without significant morning impairment.[14,15]

Half-Life

Half-life plays an important role, along with dosage, in determining the duration of clinical effects. The longer the half-life, the longer the effects are likely to last, although the recent data with low-dose doxepin suggest that factors other than the blood level of medications can affect the nature of sleep-wake effects observed.[14,15] In this regard, medications that promote sleep that are dosed at bedtime and that have longer half-lives are more likely to be associated with sleep enhancement toward the end of the night and with daytime sedation. Similarly, those with wake-promoting effects dosed during the day that have longer half-lives are more likely to disrupt sleep.

Tmax

Tmax, the time until peak blood level, occurs reflects the rate of absorption of a given medication and primarily affects the speed with which sleep-wake effects may become evident. For some medications with very long half-lives that maintain clinically significant serum levels throughout the day, Tmax is likely to have a minimal effect. For medications given as a single dosage or those with shorter half-lives, however, the Tmax can have a substantial effect on the timing of sleep-wake effects. This is most likely to be apparent with sleep-promoting medications given at bedtime where, if absorption is very slow (Tmax is very long), significant blood levels may not be achieved in time to enhance sleep onset (eg, olanzapine, ziprasidone, and haloperidol).

THE SLEEP-WAKE EFFECTS OF ANTIDEPRESSANT MEDICATIONS

The specific properties of the antidepressant medications are reviewed. The following pharmacologically based categories of agents are discussed: (1) TCAs, (2) trazodone, (3) mirtazapine, (4) selective 5-HT reuptake inhibitors, (5) SNRIs, (6) bupropion, and (7) MAOIs. The typical dosage,

Tmax, half-life, pharmacologic effects, and sleep-wake effects of these agents appear in **Table 2**.

Tricyclic Antidepressants

Pharmacology

The TCAs are a group of related compounds that have in common a cyclic chemical structure. These medications differ in terms of the side-chains that come off of this cyclic structure. All of the TCAs are thought to achieve their antidepressant effects via inhibition of 5-HT and norepinephrine reuptake. As discussed previously, this may be associated with wake-promoting effects, suppression of non-REM sleep, suppression of REM sleep (5-HT reuptake inhibition), RLS, or PLMs (5-HT reuptake inhibition). Doxepin and amitriptyline are associated with a greater 5-HT than norepinephrine reuptake inhibition. Desipramine is associated with greater norepinephrine than 5-HT reuptake inhibition and, as a result, may have a wake-promoting effect. Trimipramine seems to have minimal effects on both norepinephrine and 5-HT reuptake. Other than norepinephrine and 5-HT reuptake inhibition, the most important effects of the TCAs are H1 antagonism, muscarinic anticholinergic effects, and α_1- and α_2-adrenergic antagonism. Doxepin is the TCA with the greatest relative H1 antagonism potency and trimipramine is also a potent H1 antagonist. As discussed previously, this likely plays a role in sleep enhancement, particularly in the latter part of the night. Amitriptyline is the most anticholinergic of the TCAs. The anticholinergic effects are also likely to promote sleep to a degree as well as suppress REM sleep. Amitriptyline, doxepin, and trimipramine are all associated with α_1- and α_2-adrenergic antagonism, which is thought to enhance sleep.

Metabolism of TCAs involves several liver cytochrome P450 isoenzymes, including CYP2C19, CYP2D6, CYP1A2, and CYP3A4.[55-58] As a result, blood levels of TCAs are affected by factors that alter the function of these isoenzymes, including polymorphisms in the population, age, grapefruit juice, and medications, such as the antidepressants fluoxetine and paroxetine, the stimulant methylphenidate, and many antipsychotic medications.

The half-life of the TCAs is all at least 10 hours. As a result, for those with sedating effects dosed at bedtime, there is significant potential for daytime sedation depending on the dosage. Agents that may have wake-promoting effects, such as desipramine, also have the potential to disrupt sleep at night when dosed in the morning. The Tmax of these agents varies from 1.5 to

Table 2
Key attributes of antidepressant and antipsychotic medications

Medication	Type	Dosage[a]	Tmax (h)	Half-life (h)	Mechanisms of Sleep Effects	Possible Sleep Effects
ANTIDEPRESSANTS						
Amitriptyline	Tricyclic	10–300 mg	2–5	10–100	Antagonism of NE, HA, Ach, 5-HTT, NET	↑ Sleep, ↓ REM, ↑ RLS/PLMS
Doxepin	Tricyclic	25–300 mg	1.5–4	10–50	Antagonism of NE, HA, Ach, 5-HTT, NET	↑ Sleep, ↓ REM, ↑ RLS/PLMS
Doxepin	Tricyclic	3–6 mg	1.5–4	10–50	Antagonism of HA	↑ Sleep
Trimipramine	Tricyclic	25–300 mg	2–8	15–40	Antagonism of NE, HA, Ach	↑ Sleep, ↑ RLS/PLMS
Trazodone	Phenylpiperazine	25–600 mg	1–2	7–15	Antagonism of 5-HT2, NE, HA, 5-HTT	↑ Sleep, ↓ REM, ↑ RLS/PLMS, ↑ SWS
Mirtazapine	Tetracyclic	7.5–45 mg	0.25–2	20–40	Antagonism of 5-HT2, HA	↑ Sleep, ↓ REM, ↑ RLS/PLMS
Fluoxetine	SSRI	10–80 mg	6–8	96–144	Antagonism of 5-HTT, NET	↓ Sleep, ↓ REM, ↑ RLS/PLMS
Paroxetine	SSRI	10–50 mg	6–10	21	Antagonism of 5-HTT, NET	↓ Sleep, ↓ REM, ↑ RLS/PLMS
Sertraline	SSRI	25–200 mg	8	24	Antagonism of 5-HTT, NET	↓ Sleep, ↓ REM ↑ RLS/PLMS
Citalopram	SSRI	20–60 mg	4	35	Antagonism of 5-HTT	↓ Sleep, ↓ REM, ↑ RLS/PLMS
Escitalopram	SSRI	10–20 mg	5	27–32	Antagonism of 5-HTT	↓ Sleep, ↓ REM, ↑ RLS/PLMS
Venlafaxine	SNRI	75–225 mg	2–5.5	5–11	Antagonism of 5-HTT, NET	↓ Sleep, ↓ REM, ↑ RLS/PLMS
Desvenlafaxine	SNRI	50–400 mg	0.5	11	Antagonism of 5-HTT, NET	↓ Sleep, ↓ REM, ↑ RLS/PLMS
Duloxetine	SNRI	40–60 mg	6	9–19	Antagonism of 5-HTT, NET	↓ Sleep, ↓ REM, ↑ RLS/PLMS
Bupropion XL	Aminoketone	150–450 mg	1.5	21	Antagonism of NET and DAT	↓ Sleep
Phenelzine	"Irreversible" MAOI	15–90 mg	2–4	2.5	MAO A and B inhibition	↓ Sleep, ↓ REM, ↑ RLS/PLMS

Isocarboxazid	"Irreversible" MAOI	10–40 mg	3–5	2.5	MAO A and B inhibition	↓ Sleep, ↓ REM, ↑ RLS/PLMS
Tranylcypromine	"Reversible" MAOI	30–60 mg	1–3	2.5	MAO A and B inhibition	↓ Sleep, ↓ REM, ↑ RLS/PLMS
Selegiline	"Reversible" MAOI	5–10 mg	0.7–1.5	10	MAO B Inhibition	↓ Sleep
Selegiline transdermal	"Reversible" MAOI	6–12 mg	Rapid	10	MAO B Inhibition	↓ Sleep
ANTIPSYCHOTICS						
Olanzapine	Thiobenzodiazepine	2.5–20 mg	4–6	20–54	Antagonism of HA, NE, Ach, 5-HT2, DA	↑ Sleep, ↑ SWS, ↑ RLS/PLMS
Quetiapine	Dibenzothiazepine derivative	25–300 mg	1–2	7	Antagonism of HA, NE, Ach, 5-HT2, DA	↑ Sleep, ↓ REM, ↑ RLS/PLMS
Risperidone	Benzisoxazole derivative	1–8 mg	1	3–20	Antagonism of DA, 5-HT, NE, HA	↑ Sleep, ↓ REM, ↑ RLS/PLMS, ↑ SWS
Ziprasidone	Benzothiazolyl piperazine derivative	20–160 mg	5	4–10	Antagonism of DA, 5-HT, NE, HA, 5-HTT, NET	↑ Sleep, ↓ REM, ↑ RLS/PLMS, ↑ SWS
Aripiprazole	Benzisoxazole derivative	10–30 mg	3–5	75	Partial DA, 5-HT1A agonist; antagonist of 5-HT2A, NE, HA	± Sleep, ? REM, ↑ RLS/PLMS, ? SWS
Clozapine	Dibenzodiazepine	12.5–500 mg	3	16	Antagonism of DA, Ach, 5-HT, NE, HA	↑ Sleep, ↑ RLS/PLMS, ↑ SWS
Thiothixene	Thioxanthene derivative	2–60 mg	2–4	34	Antagonism of DA, Ach, NE	↑ Sleep, ↓ REM, ↑ RLS/PLMS, ↑ SWS
Thioridazine	Piperidine phenothiazine	10–800 mg	2–4	10	Antagonism of DA, NE, Ach, 5-HT, HA	↑ Sleep, ? REM, ↑ RLS/PLMS, ? SWS
Chlorpromazine	Dimethylamine phenothiazine derivative	10–2000 mg	2–4	15–30	Antagonism of DA, Ach, 5-HT, NE, HA	↑ Sleep, ? REM, ↑ RLS/PLMS, ? SWS
Haloperidol	Butyrophenone	0.5–100 mg	4–6	12–36	Antagonism of DA, NE, HA	↑ Sleep, ↓ REM, ↑ RLS/PLMS, ↑ SWS

Abbreviations: HA, histamine; NE, norepinephrine; NET, norepinephrine transporter; SWS, slow-wave sleep; 5-HTT, serotonin transporter.

[a] Refers to daily dosage.

Data from Refs. 2,53,98,99,101,103,107,108,111,112,115–117,125–153

8 hours (see **Table 2**). On this basis, effects on sleep onset may not be observed from single doses taken at bedtime of some of the TCAs.

Studies of sleep-wake effects

Studies of the effects of TCAs on sleep include trials of their use as antidepressants and a few studies in patients with primary insomnia. Studies of the treatment of depression have documented the sleep-onset and maintenance effects of some TCAs, including amitriptyline, doxepin, and trimipramine,[12,40,59–62] and that desipramine and nortriptyline have minimal sleep-enhancing effects.[40,63] Studies in primary insomnia patients document improvement in sleep quality and sleep efficiency (total sleep time divided by time in bed) but not sleep-onset latency with trimipramine at dosages from 50 to 200 mg.[64,65] Sleep onset, maintenance, and quality effects versus placebo have been documented in studies of doxepin (dosed at 25 to 50 mg).[64,66–68] As discussed previously, doxepin has also been studied (in dosages from 1 to 6 mg) in primary insomnia patients in whom it had selective H1 antagonism effects and was found to have sleep maintenance efficacy, particularly in the last third of the night, and also sleep-onset efficacy, although the latter effect was less consistently observed.[14,15,69]

In terms of effects of TCAs on sleep stages, doxepin and amitriptyline have been found to decrease the percentage of REM sleep and increase the latency to the onset of REM sleep, whereas no consistent effect on REM has been found for trimipramine.[40,59–61,65,70,71]

Although TCAs are reported to have the potential to cause or exacerbate PLMs and RLS, there is little systematic documentation of this. A recent review did not find any TCAs among those agents most strongly associated with RLS and PLMS.[50]

Trazodone

Pharmacology

Trazodone has a tetracyclic structure and its primary pharmacologic effects include antagonism of 5-HT1A, 5-HT2, α_1-adrenergic, and H1 receptors. Trazodone is also a weak inhibitor of 5-HT reuptake.[6,72] The antagonism of 5-HT1A, 5-HT2, α_1-, and H1 receptors is thought to contribute to sleep-enhancing effects of this agent. The 5-HT2 antagonism also is expected to lead to an increase in slow wave sleep/EEG slow wave activity. There is also the potential for 5-HT2C partial agonism to occur with trazodone therapy deriving from its active metabolite, methyl-chlorophenylpiperazine (mCPP), which can lead to wake-promoting effects.[73–75] The degree of mCPP effect is variable because many factors affect the key routes of metabolism of trazodone and mCPP, including genetic polymorphisms, which occur commonly in the population.[73,74] The primary metabolic pathways of trazodone are CYP3A4 and CYP2D6.[2]

Trazodone is typically dosed in a range from 200 to 600 mg for the treatment of major depression and is dosed from 25 to 150 mg for the off-label treatment of insomnia.[2] It has a Tmax of 1 to 2 hours and a half-life of 7 to 15 hours.[2] As a result, it has the potential to lead to sleep-onset and maintenance effects and daytime sedation when dosed just before bedtime.

Studies of sleep-wake effects

Despite the fact that trazodone is one of the most frequently administered insomnia therapies, there has been little systematic research on its sleep-wake effects. A few studies on the effects of trazodone on the sleep of healthy control subjects have been performed and found efficacy of improvement in sleep time and sleep maintenance.[76] The majority of evidence that trazodone enhances sleep derives from studies of its use in the treatment of major depression.[77–79] Several placebo-controlled studies of the use of trazodone as adjunctive treatment to antidepressant medications also document sleep-enhancing effects with trazodone.[80,81] A placebo-controlled study of trazodone (50 mg) in primary insomnia patients identified that several sleep parameters improved with trazodone therapy but the effect was only significant versus placebo in the first week of this 2-week study.[82] A pilot placebo-controlled trial in abstinent alcoholics with insomnia was also performed and identified therapeutic effects on sleep maintenance with trazodone.[83]

Trazodone's effects on sleep stages seem limited primarily to an increase in slow wave sleep and an increase in EEG delta activity during non-REM sleep.[44,76,77,79,81,84]

In terms of RLS/PLMS, trazodone is not among the medications that are those most commonly associated with drug-induced sleep-related movement difficulties.[50]

Mirtazapine

Pharmacology

The primary pharmacologic effects of mirtazapine are antagonism of 5-HT2, 5-HT3, α_1- and α_2-adrenergic, and H1 receptors.[85] These effects are expected to enhance sleep except for the α_2-antagonism, which increases norepinephrine release and, on this basis, can promote wakefulness.[86]

Mirtazapine is dosed from 7.5 to 45 mg. It has a Tmax of 0.25 to 2 hours and has a half-life of 20 to 40 hours.[2,85] On this basis, possible effects include sleep-onset effects, sleep maintenance effects, and daytime sedation when dosed at bedtime. The primary metabolism of mirtazapine occurs via CYP2D6, CYP3A4, and CYP1A2.[2]

Studies of sleep-wake effects

There are no published placebo-controlled trials of the mirtazapine treatment of insomnia. Evidence that mirtazapine has sleep-enhancing effects include a double-blind trial comparing this agent with fluoxetine in depressed patients and open-label studies in healthy volunteers.[45,87,88]

Small polysomnographic (PSG) studies of mirtazapine have been performed in healthy volunteers and depressed patients and suggest that this agent improves sleep onset, sleep maintenance, and total sleep time.[45,89] Mirtazapine led to an increased amount of slow wave sleep in one of two of these studies and did not affect REM sleep.

Mirtazapine has been reported to be among the agents most associated with drug-induced RLS.[50]

Selective Serotonin Reuptake Inhibitors

Pharmacology

As the name suggests, the primary pharmacologic effect of the SSRIs is to inhibit 5-HT reuptake. As a result, these agents are expected to have the potential to disturb sleep, suppress REM sleep, and cause or exacerbate RLS and PLMS. They also have varying degrees of norepinephrine reuptake inhibition, which also are expected to be associated with the potential for sleep disruption.[22-24]

Half-life of the SSRIs varies from 21 to 144 hours, suggesting that they have the potential to disturb sleep and to cause or exacerbate RLS and PLMs when dosed in the morning.

The SSRIs vary in terms of the primary liver cytochromes involved in their metabolism. Fluoxetine is primarily metabolized by CYP2D6 and CYP2C9, fluvoxamine is primarily metabolized by CYP1A2 and CYP2D6, paroxetine is primarily metabolized by CYP2D6, and citalopram is metabolized primarily via CYP2C19.

Studies of sleep-wake effects

There are few placebo-controlled studies that focused on delineating the sleep-wake effects of SSRIs. One placebo-controlled study in older insomnia patients was performed with paroxetine and reported a beneficial effect in terms of ratings of sleep quality, daytime alertness, and mood; however, the investigators concluded that paroxetine was not effective because they observed no effect versus placebo on sleep efficiency or categorical response rate.[90] SSRIs might have therapeutic effects on sleep via improving mood. Given the complexity of central 5-HT function,

however, it is possible that SSRIs might have a direct sleep promotion effect, at least in some individuals. As discussed previously, sedation is not infrequently observed with SSRIs, although it is unclear if this is a sleep promotion effect or consequence of disturbed sleep.[28-30] In this regard, the incidence of insomnia as an adverse event in trials of SSRIs in depressed patients is in the range of 7% to 22% as compared with 4% to 11% for placebo.[42] At the same time, the frequency of somnolence as an adverse event is in the range of 4% to 24% for SSRIs compared with 4% to 11% in placebo subjects.[42] Thus, SSRIs seem to be associated with the potential for both sleep disturbance and sleep promotion. It remains unknown what determines when sleep disturbance, sleep enhancement, or neither occurs or if they are related to each other. A factor that might contribute to either sleep disturbance or the experience of daytime somnolence is PLMS and RLS, which may be associated with SSRIs. SSRIs seem to be among the agents most strongly associated with drug-induced RLS and PLMS.[50,53]

Serotonin-Norepinephrine Reuptake Inhibitors

Pharmacology

The primary pharmacologic effects of the SNRIs is a dose-dependent inhibition of 5-HT and norepinephrine reuptake. On this basis, these agents are expected to have the potential to disturb sleep, suppress REM sleep, and cause or exacerbate RLS and PLMS. Compared with SSRIs, the SNRIs are expected to have greater associated wake promotion owing to their greater inhibition of norepinephrine reuptake. The SNRIs consist of three medications: venlafaxine, desvenlafaxine, and duloxetine.

The half-life of the SNRIs varies from 5 to 19 hours, suggesting that they have the potential to disturb sleep and to cause or exacerbate RLS and PLMs when dosed in the morning.

The SNRIs are primarily metabolized by CYP2D6 and their elimination is affected by factors that affect this isoenzyme.

Studies of sleep-wake effects

Few placebo-controlled studies have been performed that focused on delineating the sleep-wake effects of SNRIs. One placebo-controlled study of the PSG effects of duloxetine was performed in 24 healthy controls.[91] In this study, duloxetine was found to decrease the amount of REM sleep and increase the latency to the onset of REM sleep. The effects of duloxetine on sleep onset and maintenance were dependent on the dosing regimen. A regimen of 60 mg twice per day of duloxetine led to a diminished capacity to stay asleep compared with placebo, whereas a regimen of 80 mg taken each morning improved the ability to fall asleep and maintain sleep versus placebo.

A placebo-controlled trial of the sleep effects of venlafaxine dosed up to a maximum of 225 mg per day was also performed in depressed patients.[92] Compared with placebo, venlafaxine disturbed sleep in terms of a decrease in total sleep time and increase in wake time and also suppressed REM sleep in terms of an increase in REM latency and a decrease in total duration of REM sleep.

As with SSRIs, data exist on the rate at which insomnia and sedation were reported as adverse effects in trials of SNRIs performed in depressed patients. For venlafaxine, the rate of insomnia reported as a side effect was approximately 4% to 23% versus 2% to 10% with placebo and somnolence was reported by 5% to 23% versus 5% to 10% with placebo.[42] For duloxetine-treated patients, insomnia was reported by 8% to 16% of subjects versus 6% to 10% with placebo whereas somnolence was reported by 11% to 21% of subjects receiving duloxetine as compared with 3% to 8% of placebo-treated subjects. Although these data seem to suggest a comparable rate of insomnia and sedation as seen with SSRIs, studies systematically assessing sleep and wake function are needed to characterize the relative wake and sleep-promoting effects of the SNRIs and how these compare with SSRIs. One factor to consider is dosage because there may be greater noradrenergic reuptake inhibition with greater dosages of the SNRIs and a greater prevalence of insomnia because an adverse effect has been reported with higher dosages of venlafaxine.[42]

In terms of effects on PLMS and RLS, there is less clinical experience with the SNRIs than the SSRIs; however, the SNRI that has been available for the longest period of time in the United States, venlafaxine, is one of the agents most frequently associated with PLMS.[50] Presumably, this reflects the 5-HT reuptake inhibition of this agent.

Bupropion

Pharmacology
Bupropion's principal pharmacologic effects are inhibition of norepinephrine and DA reuptake. As a result, this medication is expected to promote wakefulness. No substantive effects on sleep stages or RLS/PLMS are expected from this pharmacologic profile.

The half-life of bupropion is approximately 21 hours and it is most commonly prescribed in the United States in an extended-release formulation. On this basis, there is the potential for the disturbance of nighttime sleep with morning dosing.

Primary metabolism of bupropion occurs via CYP2B6.

Studies of sleep-wake effects
Data on the sleep-wake effects of bupropion primarily derive from adverse events rates in placebo-controlled depression trials with this agent. These data suggest a rate of insomnia that is comparable to that of SSRIs and SNRIs with a lower rate of somnolence. Insomnia has been reported as an adverse event in 5% to 20% of bupropion-treated patients as compared with 2% to 8% of patients treated with placebo.[42] The somnolence rate with bupropion was 1% to 7% versus 2% to 7% among placebo-treated patients suggested minimal potential for sleep enhancement.[42]

There have also been several studies examining the PSG effects of bupropion in depressed patients.[53,92–97] Taken together, these studies suggest that bupropion has no consistent effect on sleep stage distribution and does not seem to suppress REM sleep.[42]

A few studies have been performed examining the effects of bupropion on PLMS. These studies suggest that bupropion does not increase PLMS; however, a recent review concluded that bupropion is among those agents with a strong association with drug-induced PLMS.[42,50]

Monoamine Oxidase Inhibitors

Pharmacology
Monoamine oxidase is involved in breaking down several neurotransmitters that have sleep-wake effects. As described previously, there are two types of monoamine oxidase, types A and B. Those that inhibit type A, including phenelzine, isocarboxazid, and tranylcypromine (see **Table 2**), increase the availability of 5-HT, NE, epinephrine, melatonin, and DA, and are expected to be associated with wake promotion, REM suppression, and the potential for increasing RLS/PLMS. The monoamine oxaidase type B inhibitors primarily increase the availability of DA, phenylethylamine, and trace amines and are expected to be primarily associated with wake promotion. The MAOIs also can have anticholinergic effects that are expected to promote sleep and suppress REM activity and many also block adrenergic receptors and have antihistaminergic effects that may promote sleep.

The Tmax of MAOIs varies from 0.5 to 5 hours and their half-life is 2.5 to 10 hours. Those with shorter half-lives, such as phenelzine, isocarboxazid, and tranylcypromine, are less likely to disturb sleep if dosed in the morning than selegeline, which has a 10-hours half-life.

In terms of the metabolism of MAOIs, phenelzine is inactivated hepatically by acetylation. The metabolism of tranylcypromine occurs via ring-hydroxylation and N-acetylation. The metabolism of selegiline primarily occurs via liver cytochromes, CYP2B6 and CYP3A4, with CYP2A6 playing a minor role.

Studies of sleep-wake effects

Few controlled trials document the sleep-wake effects of MAOIs. Disturbance of sleep has been observed with phenelzine, tranylcypromine, and isocarboxazid, and suppression of REM sleep has been reported to occur with phenelzine and tranylcypromine.[4]

THE SLEEP-WAKE EFFECTS OF ANTIPSYCHOTIC MEDICATIONS

In this section the properties of the antipsychotic medications are reviewed. The antipsychotic effects of these medications are primarily believed to be mediated by antagonism of DA receptors.[98–100] This section discusses these agents using as a framework the two traditional categories: typical antipsychotics, an older group of agents that do not block 5-HT receptors, and atypical antipsychotics, which do block 5-HT receptors in addition to having antidopaminergic effects.[99,101,102] The typical dosage, Tmax, half-life, pharmacologic effects, and sleep-wake effects of these agents appear in **Table 2**.

Typical Antipsychotics

Pharmacology

In addition to antagonism of DA receptors, typical antipsychotics may also have anticholinergic, antihistaminergic, and antiadrenergic effects. All of these effects are expected to be sleep enhancing. Of the atypical antipsychotics, those with the greatest antihistaminergic effects relative to their other pharmacologic effects include chlorpromazine and thioridazine.[103–105] These agents, although classified as typical antipsychotics, also have some degree of 5-HT2 antagonism and are expected to be among the most sedating typical antipsychotics owing to this 5-HT2 antagonism and strong H1-blocking effects. Given their 5-HT2 antagonism they are also expected to increase the amount of slow wave sleep and increase slow wave activity. Chlorpromazine and thioridazine also have high anticholinergic activity, which has the potential to lead to a suppression of REM sleep. Those agents that are most potent for blocking DA receptors, such as haloperidol, pimozide, and thiothixene, and have greater potential for triggering leg restlessness and PLMS, which

can interfere with the ability to fall or stay asleep.[51,106] These higher-potency DA antagonists also have anticholinergic effects, which carry with them potential suppression of REM sleep.

The Tmax of thiothixene, thioridazine, and chlorpromazine is approximately 2 to 4 hours (see **Table 2**), suggesting that, when delivered as a single bedtime dose, a sleep-onset effect is less likely with these agents than with agents with shorter Tmax. The likelihood of an effect on sleep onset is even less with haloperidol because it has a Tmax of 4 to 6 hours. Because the half-life of these agents is 10 to 36 hours, there is the potential for sleep maintenance effects and daytime sedation with bedtime dosing and long-lasting daytime sedation when administered in the morning.

The primary metabolism of the typical antipsychotics occurs via the liver cytochromes, CYP1A2 (haloperidol), CYP2D6 (haloperidol, thioridazine, and chlorpromazine), and CYP3A4 (haloperidol and pimozide).

The typical antipsychotics vary in their side-effect profiles as a function of the potency of DA antagonism to blockade of other receptor subtypes. Those with highest DA antagonist potency, including haloperidol, pimozide, and thiothixene, are the most strongly associated with a set of movement-related adverse effects, referred to as extrapyramidal side effects, including parkinsonian symptoms and tardive dyskinesia.[103] With greater DA antagonist potency, these agents can achieve an antipsychotic effect with lower levels of other types of pharmacologic effects, such as anthihistaminic, antiadrenergic, and antihicholinergic effects, although these side effects may still be experienced by some individuals treated with these higher-potency agents and are dose dependent.

Studies of sleep-wake effects

There are few data derived from studies focusing on the sleep-wake effects of typical antipsychotics. In one open-label study, the PSG effects of clinical dosing of thiothixene and haloperidol were compared in 14 medication-free schizophrenia patients.[107] Compared with baseline, both agents led to improvement in sleep-onset latency, wake time after sleep onset, and total sleep time. An increase in REM latency and a small increase in slow wave sleep time were observed with both medications, although no other effects on REM or slow wave sleep were observed. A similar study comparing PSG sleep indices in those treated with haloperidol and the atypical antipsychotic, risperidone, found that risperidone led to a greater increase in slow wave sleep.[108]

In terms of the frequency with which sleep-related effects are reported as adverse effects in placebo-controlled studies of typical antipsychotics, chlorpromazine and thioridazine are associated with the highest rate of reported somnolence (33%–57%), whereas 23% of haloperidol-treated patients had somnolence.[13] Insomnia is reported in approximately a quarter of patients treated with haloperidol and thioridazine.[13] It seems likely that this insomnia is due, at least in part, to RLS or PLMS being triggered by these medications. In this regard, PSG evidence of an increase in PLMS frequency has been reported with haloperidol.[109,110] It is also possible that PLMS is responsible for the somnolence reported with at least some of the typical antipsychotics.

Atypical Antipsychotics

Pharmacology

The atypical antipsychotics differ from the typical antipsychotics in terms of having 5-HT2 antagonism in addition to antagonism of DA receptors. On this basis, it might be expected that these agents are associated with greater sleep enhancement, greater increase in slow wave sleep, greater increase in slow wave activity, and perhaps greater weight gain associated with them than typical antipsychotics. Olanzapine, resiperidone, clozapine, and ziprasidone are the most potent 5-HT2 antagonists of the atypical antipsychotics.[13] In addition to the 5-HT2 and DA antagonist effects, atypical antipsychotics also have varying degrees of anticholinergic, antihistaminergic, and antiadrenergic effects, all of which are expected to enhance sleep to some degree. Of the atypical agents, olanzapine and clozapine seem to have the greatest antihistaminergic and anticholinergic effects[111] whereas resperidone is a potent α_1-adrenergic antagonist.[112] Quetiapine is a low-potency DA antagonist, and, as a result, it is administered in higher dosages leading to more significant clinical antihistaminergic and adrenergic effects than other atypical antipsychotics, which are more potent atagonists at these receptors.[101] Ziprasidone and aripiprazole are somewhat unique among the atypical antipsychotics because they are 5-HT1A agonists that are expected to be associated with wake promotion and suppression of REM sleep.[13] Aripiprazole is potent as a dopaminergic antagonist and has minor effects on adrenergic and histaminergic receptors at typical clinical dosages.[113,114] Overall, on the basis of antihistaminergic and antiadrenergic effects, the atypical antipsychotics with the greatest sleep enhancement are olanzapine, clozapine, and quetiapine; however, in terms of 5-HT2 antagonist effects, olanzapine, risperidone, ziprasidone, and clozapine are expected to enhance sleep to the greatest degree.[13] The greatest degree of REM suppression is expected with ziprasidone and arirprazole on the basis of their 5-HT1A agonist effects and with olanzapine and clozapine due to the associated anticholinergic effects.[13]

From a pharmacokinetic point of view, quetiapine and risperidone, which have Tmax of 1 to 2 hours, are most likely to have effects on sleep onset as a single dose at bedtime (see **Table 2**), whereas this is least likely with ziprasidone and olanzapine, which have Tmax in the range of 4 to 6 hours.[13] Quetiapine with an elimination half-life of 7 hours is least likely to be associated with daytime sedation with nighttime dosing and is affected by factors that alter the CYP3A4 and CYP2D6 liver enzymes.[13] The elimination of risperidone is also dependent on liver cytochromes, CYP2D6 and CYP3A4; however, its half-life is substantially more variable, suggesting that a wide range of variation in duration of sedation across the night and during the daytime is likely to be seen with this agent.[13] Ziprasidone metabolized primarily by CYP3A4 and to a lesser degree by CYP1A2 has a short half-life of 4 to 10 hours and, therefore, has a low likelihood of daytime effects when dosed at bedtime. Olanzapine has an elimination half-life that is affected by factors that alter CYP1A2 and CYP2D6, and, because the Tmax is approximately 25 to 50 hours, this agent is likely to be associated with daytime effects.[13] Aripiprazole and clozapine both have half-lives that exceed 15 hours and, as a result, have the potential for long-lasting effects.

Studies of sleep-wake effects

Several PSG trials of the sleep-wake effects of atypical antipsychotics have been performed in healthy volunteers and in those with mood disorders or schizoprhenia. Two of these were placebo-controlled crossover studies comparing sleep on an undisturbed night and a night where subjects were exposed to noise. In one of these studies (N = 14), quetiapine (dosed at 25 and 100 mg) was associated with significant effects on sleep-onset latency, total sleep time, sleep efficiency, and sleep quality and led to suppression of REM sleep.[115] In the other study, ziprasidone (dosed at 40 mg) was associated with significant effects on total sleep time, sleep efficiency, and number of awakenings as well as reported sleep quality.[116] In this study, ziprasidone was also found to significantly decrease the percentage of REM sleep and REM density and increase REM latency and slow wave sleep time.[116] Small PSG studies of olanzapine in healthy controls and in patients with mood disorders and schizophrenia suggest that this agent improves sleep latency, wake time after sleep onset, sleep efficiency, and sleep quality and increases slow wave sleep time.[117–123] Quetiapine (dosed from 25 to 75 mg) has also been studied in an open-label study in patients with primary insomnia and was reported to improve self-reported sleep-onset latency, sleep efficiency, and total sleep time.[124] Open-label PSG studies of the treatment of patients with schizophrenia with olanzapine (10 mg) have been performed and confirm that this agent decreases the number of awakenings, increases total sleep time, and increases the percentage of slow wave sleep.[117,125] Two small studies of clozapine in medication-free schizophrenia patients have been performed, indicating that this agent decreases wake time and awakenings, improves sleep time, and increases slow wave sleep time.[126,127] A PSG study of the effects of risperidone (0.5–1 mg) in few depressed patients was also performed and indicated that this medication decreased wake time after sleep onset and decreased the amount of REM sleep.[128] In a study comparing clinical treatment with haloperidol and risperidone, risperidone led to significantly greater slow wave sleep time.[108]

Adverse effects data suggest that the highest rates of sedation among the atypical antipsychotics occur with clozapine (52%), followed by risperidone (30%) and olanzapine (29%).[13] The agent with the lowest rate of somnolence as an adverse effect in placebo-controlled trials was aripiprazole, which is associated with somnolence in approximately 12% of cases.[13] Quetiapine and ziprasidone both are associated with somnolence as an adverse event in 16% of subjects.[13] In interpreting these data, the rate of sedation as an adverse effect reflects both the sleep enhancement of the medication as well as its pharmacokinetic properties.

Insomnia reported as an adverse effect was most common with aripiprazole, reported by 24% of subjects.[13] Risperidone and olanzapine are associated with insomnia as an adverse event in 17% to 18% of subjects, whereas quetiapine and ziprasidone have been associated with a 9% rate of insomnia.[13] As discussed previously, it is impossible to determine the extent to which RLS/PLMS might be contributing to the rates of insomnia or daytime sedation observed. Few studies have looked at the association of RLS/PLMS with atypical antipsychotic medications. The few that have studied this relationship, however, have reported an association of PLMS with olanzapine and risperidone among the atypical antipsychotics,[109,110] suggesting that at least some of the insomnia reported with these agents may have been PLMS related.

SUMMARY

This article has reviewed the pharmacology and associated sleep-wake effects of the antidepressant and antipsychotic medications. Although the available data on the sleep-wake effects of these medications are limited, the data that exist suggest a clear correspondence between the pharmacology of these agents and their varying effects on sleep-wake function. In this regard, antidepressants tend to be associated with inhibition of the reuptake of 5-HT or norepinephrine (and DA in the case of bupropion) or have 5-HT2 antagonism. The 5-HT reuptake inhibition seems associated with a tendency toward wake promotion, suppression of REM sleep, and triggering of RLS/PLMS. Sedation and some of the sleep disturbance seen with 5-HT reuptake inhibitors may be a direct pharmacologic effect or secondary to eliciting RLS/PLMS. The norepinephrine reuptake inhibition seems primarily associated with wake promotion whereas 5-HT2 antagonism may be associated with a tendency toward sleep promotion, slow wave sleep enhancement, and possibly weight gain/insulin resistance. The antipsychotics may also be antagonists of 5-HT2 receptors, in particular the atypical antipsychotics, although their antipsychotic effect seems to derive from DA antagonism, which seems to increase the risks of RLS/PLMS and may be sleep promoting. The other sleep-wake effects of the antidepressants and antipsychotics derive from pharmacologic effects not related to their antidepressant or antipsychotic mechanisms, including cholinergic antagonism (sleep promotion and suppression of REM sleep), histaminergic antagonism (sleep promotion and possibly increase in appetite), adrenergic antagonism (sleep promotion and orthostatic hypotension), and 5-HT1A agonist effects (wake promotion and suppression of REM sleep). This article also discusses how pharmacokinetic and dosing factors play a key role in determining the varied sleep-wake effects of these medications. It is hoped that this review of these principles provides a basis for understanding the sleep-wake effects of antipsychotic and antidepressant medications that is useful both for research and for clinical practice.

REFERENCES

1. Saper CB, Scammell TE, Lu J. Hypothalamic regulation of sleep and circadian rhythms. Nature 2005; 437:1257–63.
2. Krystal A. A compendium of placebo-controlled trials of the risks/benefits of pharmacologic treatments for insomnia: the empirical basis for U.S.

clinical practice. Sleep Med Rev 2009;13(4): 265–74.

3. Stahl SM. Essential Psychopharmacology. 2nd edition. New York: Cambridge University Press; 2000.

4. Mayers AG, Baldwin DA. Antidepressants and their effect on sleep. Hum Psychopharmacol 2005; 20(8):533–59.

5. Richelson E. Interactions of antidepressants with neurotransmitter transporters and receptors and their clinical relevance. J Clin Psychiatry 2003; 64(Suppl 13):5–12.

6. Baldessarini R. Drug therapy of depression and anxiety disorders. In: Brunton LL, Lazo JS, Parker KL, editors. Goodman and Gilman's: the pharmacological basis of therapeutics. 11th edition. New York: McGraw-Hill; 2006. p. 429–60.

7. Adam K, Oswald I. Effects of repeated ritanserin on middle-aged poor sleepers. Psychopharmacology (Berl) 1989;99(2):219–21.

8. Landolt HP, Meier V, Burgess HJ, et al. Serotonin-2 receptors and human sleep: effect of a selective antagonist on EEG power spectra. Neuropsychopharmacology 1999;21(3):455–66.

9. Morairty SR, Hedley L, Flores J, et al. Selective 5HT2A and 5HT6 receptor antagonists promote sleep in rats. Sleep 2008;31(1):34–44.

10. Rosenberg R, Seiden DJ, Hull SG, et al. APD125, a selective serotonin 5-HT(2A) receptor inverse agonist, significantly improves sleep maintenance in primary insomnia. Sleep 2008; 31(12):1663–71.

11. Lin JS, Dauvilliers Y, Arnulf I, et al. An inverse agonist of the histamine H(3) receptor improves wakefulness in narcolepsy: studies in orexin-/- mice and patients. Neurobiol Dis 2008;30:74–83.

12. Richelson E, Nelson A. Antagonism by antidepressants of neurotransmitter receptors of normal human brain in vitro. J Pharmacol Exp Ther 1984; 230(1):94–102.

13. Krystal AD, Goforth H, Roth T. Effects of antipsychotic medications on sleep in schizophrenia. Int Clin Psychopharmacol 2008;23:150–60.

14. Roth T, Rogowski R, Hull S, et al. Efficacy and safety of doxepin 1, 3 and 6 mg in adults with primary insomnia. Sleep 2007;30:1555–61.

15. Krystal AD, Durrence H, Scharf M, et al. Long-term efficacy and safety of doxepin 1 mg and 3 mg in a 12-week sleep laboratory and outpatient trial of elderly subjects with chronic primary insomnia. Sleep, in press.

16. Berridge CW. Neural substrates of psychostimulant-induced arousal. Neuropsychopharmacology 2006; 31(11):2332–40.

17. Hilakivi I, Leppavuori A, Putkonen PT. Prazosin increases paradoxical sleep. Eur J Pharmacol 1980;65:417–20.

18. Hilakivi I, Leppavuori A. Effects of methoxamine, and alpha-1 adrenoceptor agonist, and prazosin, an alpha-1 antagonist, on the stages of the sleep–waking cycle in the cat. Acta Physiol Scand 1984;120:363–72.

19. Lydic R, Baghdoyan HA. Acetylcholine modulates sleep and wakefulness: a synaptic perspective. In: Monti JM, Pandi-Perumal SR, Sinton CM, editors. Neurochemistry of sleep and wakefulness. Cambridge (UK): Cambridge University Press; 2008. p. 109–43.

20. Kanai T, Szerb JC. Mesencephalic reticular activating system and cortical acetylcholine output. Nature 1965;205:80–2.

21. Imeri L, Bianchi S, Angeli P, et al. Selective blockade of different brain stem muscarinic receptor subtypes: effects on the sleep-wake cycle. Brain Res 1994;636:68–72.

22. Nemeroff CB, Owens MJ. Pharmacologic differences among the SSRIs: focus on monoamine transporters and the HPA axis. CNS Spectr 2004; 9(6 Suppl 4):23–31.

23. Nutt DJ. The neuropharmacology of serotonin and noradrenaline in depression. Int Clin Psychopharmacol 2002;17(Suppl 1):S1–12.

24. Owens MJ, Knight DL, Nemeroff CB. Second-generation SSRIs: human monoamine transporter binding profile of escitalopram and R-fluoxetine. Biol Psychiatry 2001;50(5):345–50.

25. Leonard BE. Serotonin receptors and their function in sleep, anxiety disorders and depression. Psychother Psychosom 1996;65:66–75.

26. Wilson SJ, Bailey JE, Rich AS, et al. The use of sleep measures to compare a new 5HT1A agonist with buspirone in humans. Psychopharmacology 2005;19:609–13.

27. Leppävuori A. The effects of an alpha-adrenergic agonist or antagonist on sleep during blockade of catecholamine synthesis in the cat. Brain Res 1980;193(1):117–28.

28. Hu XH, Scott AB, Hunkeler EM, et al. Incidence and duration of side effects and those rated as bothersome with selective serotonin reuptake inhibitor treatment for depression: patient report versus physician estimate. J Clin Psychiatry 2004;65: 959–65.

29. Fava M, Rush AJ, Thase ME, et al. 15 years of clinical experience with bupropion HCl: from bupropion to bupropion SR to bupropion XL. Prim Care Companion J Clin Psychiatry 2005;7(3):106–13.

30. Sharpley AL, Williamson DJ, Attenburrow ME, et al. The effects of paroxetine and nefazodone on sleep: a placebo controlled trial. Psychopharmacology 1996;126:50–4.

31. Stahl SM, Pradko JF, Haight BR, et al. A review of the neuropharmacology of bupropion, a dual norepinephrine and dopamine reuptake inhibitor.

Prim Care Companion J Clin Psychiatry 2004;6: 159–66.

32. Mehta NB. The chemistry of bupropion. J Clin Psychiatry 1983;44(5 Pt 2):56–9.

33. Bolasco A, Carradori S, Fioravanti R. Focusing on new monoamine oxidase inhibitors. Expert Opin Ther Pat 2010;20(7):909–39.

34. Murphy DL, Sunderland T, Cohen RM. Monoamine oxidase-inhibiting antidepressants. A Clinical update. Psychiatr Clin North Am 1984;7:546–62.

35. Quitkin F, Rifkin A, Klein DF. Monoamine oxidase inhibitors. A review of antidepressant effectiveness. Arch Gen Psychiatry 1979;36(7):749–60.

36. Poland RE, McCracken JT, Lutchmansingh P, et al. Differential response of rapid eye movement sleep to cholinergic blockade by scopolamine in currently depressed, remitted, and normal control subjects. Biol Psychiatry 1997;41(9):929–38.

37. Maes M, Westenberg H, Vandoolaeghe E, et al. Effects of trazodone and fluoxetine in the treatment of major depression: therapeutic pharmacokinetic and pharmacodynamic interactions through formation of meta-chlorophenylpiperazine. J Clin Psychopharmacol 1997;17(5):358–64.

38. Benca RM, Obermeyer WH, Thisted RA, et al. Sleep and psychiatric disorders. A meta-analysis. Arch Gen Psychiatry 1992;49:651–68.

39. Gillin JC, Wyatt RJ, Fram D, et al. The relationship between changes in REM sleep and clinical improvement in depressed patients treated with amitriptyline. Psychopharmacology (Berl) 1978; 59:267–72.

40. Kupfer DJ, Spiker DG, Coble PA, et al. Sleep and treatment prediction in endogenous depression. Am J Psychiatry 1981;138:429–34.

41. Thase ME. Depression and sleep: pathophysiology and treatment. Dialogues Clin Neurosci 2006;8: 217–26.

42. Krystal AD, Thase ME, Tucker VL, et al. Bupropion HCL and sleep in patients with depression. Clin Psychol Rev 2007;3:123–8 Curr Psychiatry Rev.

43. Poulin J, Daoust AM, Forest G, et al. Sleep architecture and its clinical correlates in first episode and neuroleptic-naive patients with schizophrenia. Schizophr Res 2003;62:147–53.

44. Ware JC, Pittard JT. Increased deep sleep after trazodone use: a double-blind placebo-controlled study in healthy young adults. J Clin Psychiatry 1990;51 Suppl:18–22.

45. Winokur A, Sateia MJ, Hayes JB, et al. Acute effects of mirtazapine on sleep continuity and sleep architecture in depressed patients: a pilot study. Biol Psychiatry 2000;48(1):75–8.

46. Aslan S, Isik E, Cosar B. The effects of mirtazapine on sleep: a placebo controlled, double-blind study in young healthy volunteers. Sleep 2002;25(6): 677–9.

47. Schittecatte M, Dumont F, Machowski R, et al. Effects of mirtazapine on sleep polygraphic variables in major depression. Neuropsychobiology 2002;46(4):197–201.

48. Walsh JK. Enhancement of slow wave sleep: implications for insomnia. J Clin Sleep Med 2009;5(Suppl 2):S27–32.

49. Goder R, Boigs M, Braun S, et al. Impairment of visuospatial memory is associated with decreased slow wave sleep in schizophrenia. J Psychiatr Res 2004;38:591–9.

50. Hoque R, Chesson AL Jr. Pharmacologically induced/exacerbated restless legs syndrome, periodic limb movements of sleep, and REM behavior disorder/REM sleep without atonia: literature review, qualitative scoring, and comparative analysis. J Clin Sleep Med 2010;6(1):79–83.

51. Hornyak M, Feige B, Riemann D, et al. Periodic leg movements in sleep and periodic limb movement disorder: prevalence, clinical significance and treatment. Sleep Med Rev 2006;10: 169–77.

52. Winkelman JW, James L. Serotonergic antidepressants are associated with REM sleep without atonia. Sleep 2004;27:317–21.

53. Yang C, White DP, Winkelman JW. Antidepressants and periodic leg movements of sleep. Biol Psychiatry 2005;58:510–4.

54. Hughes AM, Lynch P, Rhodes J, et al. Electroencephalographic and psychomotor effects of chlorpromazine and risperidone relative to placebo in normal healthy volunteers. Br J Clin Pharmacol 1999;48(3):323–30.

55. Gillin JC, Duncan W, Pettigrew KD, et al. Successful separation of depressed, normal, and insomniac subjects by EEG sleep data. Arch Gen Psychiatry 1979;36:85–90.

56. Kupfer DJ, Ulrich RF, Coble PA, et al. Elextroencephalographic sleep of younger depressives. Comparison with normals. Arch Gen Psychiatry 1985;42:806–10.

57. Berger M, Doerr P, Lund R, et al. Neuroendocrinological and neurophysiological studies in major depressive disorders: are there biological markers of the endogenous subtype? Biol Psychiatry 1982; 17:1217–42.

58. Reynolds CF 3rd, Frank E, Houck PR, et al. Which elderly patients with remitted depression remain well with continued interpersonal psychotherapy after discontinuation of antidepressant medication? Am J Psychiatry 1997;154:958–62.

59. Nierenberg AA, Wright EC. Evolution of remission as the new standard in the treatment of depression. J Clin Psychiatry 1999;60(Suppl 22):7–11.

60. Richelson E. Synaptic effects of antidepressants. J Clin Psychopharmacol 1996;16(3 Suppl 2): 1S–9S.

61. Saller CF, Salama AI. Seroquel: biochemical profile of a potential atypical antipsychotic. Psychopharmacology 1993;112:285–92.
62. Tandon R. Neuropharmacological basis of clozapine's unique profile. Arch Gen Psychiatry 1993; 50:158–9.
63. Seeger TF, Seymour PA, Schmidt AW, et al. Ziprasidone: a new antipsychotic with combined dopamine and serotonin receptor antagonist activity. J Pharmacol Exp Ther 1995;275:101–13.
64. Beasley CM Jr, Tollefson G, Tran P, et al. Olanzapine versus placebo and haloperidol: acute phase results of the North American double-blind olanzapine trial. Neuropsychopharmacology 1996;14: 111–23.
65. Bymaster FP, Calligaro DO, Falcone JF, et al. Radioreceptor binding profile of the atypical antipsychotic olanzapine. Neuropsychopharmacology 1996;14:87–96.
66. Schotte A, Janssen PF, Gommeren W, et al. Risperidone compared with new and reference antipsychotic drugs: in vitro and in vivo receptor binding. Psychopharmacology 1996;124:57–73.
67. Sekine Y, Rikihisa T, Ogata H, et al. Correlations between in vitro affinity of antipsychotics to various central neurotransmitter receptors and clinical incidence of their adverse drug reactions. Eur J Clin Pharmacol 1999;55:583–7.
68. Farah A. Atypicality of atypical antipsychotics. Prim Care Companion J Clin Psychiatry 2005;7:268–74.
69. Newman-Tancredi A, Assie MB, Leduc N, et al. Novel antipsychotics activate recombinant human and native rat serotonin 5-HT1A receptors: affinity, efficacy and potential implications for treatment of schizophrenia. Int J Neuropsychopharmacol 2005;8:341–56.
70. Allison DB, Mentore JL, Heo M, et al. Antipsychotic-induced weight gain: a comprehensive research synthesis. Am J Psychiatry 1999;156:1686–96.
71. Bagnall A, Kleijnen J, Leitner M, et al. Ziprasidone for schizophrenia and severe mental illness. Cochrane Database Syst Rev 2000;4:CD001945.
72. Sultana A, Reilly J, Fenton M. Thioridazine for schizophrenia. Cochrane Database Syst Rev 2000;2:CD001944.
73. Thornley B, Rathbone J, Adams CE, et al. Chlorpromazine versus placebo for schizophrenia. Cochrane Database Syst Rev 2003;2:CD000284.
74. Srisurapanont M, Maneeton B, Maneeton N. Quetiapine for schizophrenia. Cochrane Database Syst Rev 2004;2:CD000967.
75. Duggan L, Fenton M, Rathbone J, et al. Olanzapine for schizophrenia. Cochrane Database Syst Rev 2005;2:CD001359.
76. El-Sayeh HG, Morganti C. Aripiprazole for schizophrenia. Cochrane Database Syst Rev 2006;2: CD004578.
77. Jayaram MB, Hosalli P, Stroup S. Risperidone versus olanzapine for schizophrenia. Cochrane Database Syst Rev 2006;2:CD005237.
78. Joy CB, Adams CE, Lawrie SM. Haloperidol versus placebo for schizophrenia. Cochrane Database Syst Rev 2006;4:CD003082.81.
79. Forsman A, Ohman R. Studies on serum protein binding of haloperidol. Curr Ther Res Clin Exp 1977;21:245–55.
80. He H, Richardson JS. A pharmacological, pharmacokinetic and clinical overview of risperidone, a new antipsychotic that blocks serotonin 5-HT2 and dopamine D2 receptors. Int Clin Psychopharmacol 1995;10:19–30.
81. Ereshefsky L. Pharmacokinetics and drug interactions: update for new antipsychotics. J Clin Psychiatry 1996;57(Suppl 11):12–5.
82. Hinze-Selch D, Mullington J, Orth A, et al. Effects of clozapine on sleep: a longitudinal study. Biol Psychiatry 1997;42:260–6.
83. Prakash C, Kamel A, Gummerus J, et al. Metabolism and excretion of a new antipsychotic drug, ziprasidone, in humans. Drug Metab Dispos 1997; 25:863–72.
84. Maixner S, Tandon R, Eiser A, et al. Effects of antipsychotic treatment on polysomnographic measures in schizophrenia: a replication and extension. Am J Psychiatry 1998;155:1600–2.
85. Salin-Pascual RJ, Herrera-Estrella M, Galicia-Polo L, et al. Olanzapine acute administration in schizophrenic patients increases delta sleep and sleep efficiency. Biol Psychiatry 1999;46(1):141–3.
86. Salin-Pascual RJ, Herrera-Estrella M, Galicia-Polo L, et al. Low delta sleep predicted a good clinical response to olanzapine administration in schizophrenic patients. Rev Invest Clin 2004;56: 345–50.
87. Lee JH, Woo JI, Meltzer HY. Effects of clozapine on sleep measures and sleep-associated changes in growth hormone and cortisol in patients with schizophrenia. Psychiatry Res 2001;103:157–66.
88. Yamashita H, Morinobu S, Yamawaki S, et al. Effect of risperidone on sleep in schizophrenia: a comparison with haloperidol. Psychiatry Res 2002;109: 137–42.
89. Sharpley AL, Bhagwagar Z, Hafizi S, et al. Risperidone augmentation decreases rapid eye movement sleep and decreases wake in treatment-resistant depressed patients. J Clin Psychiatry 2003;64:192–6.
90. Cohrs S, Rodenbeck A, Guan Z, et al. Sleep-promoting properties of quetiapine in healthy subjects. Psychopharmacology 2004;174:421–9.
91. Cohrs S, Meier A, Neumann AC, et al. Improved sleep continuity and increased slow wave sleep and REM latency during ziprasidone treatment: a randomized, controlled, crossover trial of 12

healthy male subjects. J Clin Psychiatry 2005;66: 989–96.

92. Tassaneeyakul W, Kittiwattanagul K, Vannaprasaht S, et al. Steady-state bioequivalence study of clozapine tablet in schizophrenic patients. J Pharm Pharm Sci 2005;8:47–53.

93. Markowitz JS, DeVane CL, Malcolm RJ, et al. Pharmacokinetics of olanzapine after single-dose oral administration of standard tablet versus normal and sublingual administration of an orally disintegrating tablet in normal volunteers. J Clin Pharmacol 2006;46:164–71.

94. Flores BH, Schatzberg AF. Mitazapine. In: Schatzberg A, Nemeroff C, editors. The American psychiatric publishing textbook of psychopharmacology. Washington, DC: American Psychiatric Publishing, Inc; 2004. p. 341–7.

95. Baldessarini RJ. Drugs and the treatment of anxiety disorders: depression and anxiety disorders. In: Hardman JG, Limbird LE, editors. Goldman and Gilman's: the pharmacologic basis of therapeutics. New York: McGraw-Hill; 2001. p. 447–83.

96. Rudorfer MV, Potter WZ. Metabolism of tricyclic antidepressants. Cell Mol Neurobiol 1999;19(3):373–409.

97. Rudorfer MV, Potter WZ. Pharmacokinetics of antidepressants. In: Meltzer HY, editor. Psychopharmacology: the third generation of progress. New York: Raven Press; 1987. p. 1353–63.

98. Ziegler V, Biggs JT, Ardekani AB, et al. Contribution to the pharmacokinetics f amitriptyline. J Clin Pharmacol 1978;18(10):462–7.

99. Shipley JE, Kupfer DJ, Griffin SJ, et al. Comparison of effects of desipramine and amitriptyline on EEG sleep of depressed patients. Psychopharmacology 1985;85:14–22.

100. Dunleavy DL, Brezinova V, Oswald I, et al. Changes during weeks in effects of tricyclic drugs on the human sleep brain. Br J Psychiatry 1972;120:663–72.

101. Roth T, Zorick F, Wittig R, et al. The effects of doxepin HCl on sleep and depression. J Clin Psychiatry 1982;43:366–8.

102. Feuillade P, Pringuey D, Belugou JL, et al. Trimipramine: acute and lasting effects on sleep in healthy and major depressive subjects. J Affect Disord 1992;24:135–45.

103. Ware JC, Brown FW, Moorad PJ, et al. Effects on sleep: a double-blind study comparing trimipramine to imipramine in depressed insomniac patients. Sleep 1989;12:537–49.

104. Riemann D, Voderholzer U, Cohrs S, et al. Trimipramine in primary insomnia: results of a polysomnographic double-blind controlled study. Pharmacopsychiatry 2002;35(5):165–74.

105. Hohagen F, Montero RF, Weiss E. Treatment of primary insomnia with trimipramine: an alternative to benzodiazepine hypnotics? Eur Arch Psychiatry Clin Neurosci 1994;244(2):65–72.

106. Rodenbeck A, Cohrs S, Jordan W, et al. The sleep-improving effects of doxepin are paralleled by a normalized plasma cortisol secretion in primary insomnia. Psychopharmacology (Berl) 2003;170: 423–8.

107. Hajak G, Rodenbeck A, Adler L, et al. Nocturnal melatonin secretion and sleep after doxepin administration in chronic primary insomnia. Pharmacopsychiatry 1996;29(5):187–92.

108. Hajak G, Rodenbeck. A, Voderholzer U, et al. Doxepin in the treatment of primary insomnia: a placebo-controlled, double-blind, polysomnographic study. J Clin Psychopharmacol 2001; 62(6):453–63.

109. Scharf M, Rogowski R, Hull S, et al. Efficacy and safety of doxepin 1 mg, 3 mg, and 6 mg in elderly patients with primary insomnia: a randomized double-blind, placebo-controlled crossover study. J Clin Psychiatry 2008;69(10):1557–64.

110. Buysse DJ, Reynolds CF, Hoch CC, et al. Longitudinal effects of nortriptyline on EEG sleep and the likelihood of recurrence in elderly depressed patients. Neuropsychopharmacology 1996;14(4):243–52.

111. Hartmann E, Cravens J. The effects of long term administration of psychotropic drugs on human sleep: III. The effects of amitriptyline. Psychopharmacology 1973;33:185–202.

112. Golden RN, Dawkins K, Nicholas L. Trazadone and nefazodone. In: Schatzberg A, Nemeroff C, editors. The American psychiatric textbook of psychopharmacology. Washington, DC: American Psychiatric Textbook, Inc; 2004. p. 315–25.

113. Caccia S, Ballabio M, Fanelli R, et al. Determination of plasma and brain concentrations of trazodone and its metabolite, 1-m-chlorophenylpiperazine, by gas-liquid chromatography. J Chromatogr 1981;5(210):311–8.

114. Greenblatt DJ, Friedman H, Burstein ES, et al. Trazodone kinetics: effects of age, gender and obesity. Clin Pharmacol Ther 1987;42:193–200.

115. Warner M, Peabody CA, Whiteford HA, et al. Trazodone and priapism. J Clin Psychiatry 1987;48(6):244–5.

116. Montgomery I, Oswald I, Morgan K, et al. Trazodone enhances sleep in subjective quality but not in objective duration. Br J Clin Pharmacol 1983; 16:139–44.

117. Saletu-Zyhlarz G, Abu-Bakr M, Anderer P, et al. Insomnia in depression: differences in objective and subjective sleep awakening quality to normal controls and accute effects of trazodone. Prog Neuropsychopharmacol Biol Psychiatry 2002;26:249–60.

118. Scharf MB, Sachais BA. Sleep laboratory evaluation of the effects and efficacy of trazodone in depressed insomniac patients. J Clin Psychiatry 1990;51:13–7.

119. Mouret J, Lemoine P, Minuit MP, et al. Effects of trazodone on the sleep of depressed subjects –

a polygraphic study. Psychopharmacology 1988; 95:37–43.

120. Nierenberg AA, Adler LA, Peselow E. Trazodone for antidepressant-associated insomnia. Am J Psychiatry 1994;151:1069–72.

121. Kaynak H, Kaynak D, Gozukirmizi E, et al. The effects of trazodone on sleep in patients treated with stimulant antidepressants. Sleep Med 2004; 5(1):15–20.

122. Walsh JK, Erman M, Erwin CW. Subjective hypnotic efficacy of trazodone and zolpidem in DSM-III-R primary insomnia. Hum Psychopharmacol 1998; 13:191–8.

123. Le Bon O, Murphy JR, Staner L, et al. Double-blind, placebo-controlled study of the efficacy of trazodone in alcohol post-withdrawal syndrome: polysomnographic and clinical evaluations. J Clin Psychopharmacol 2003;23(4):377–83.

124. Parrino L, Spaggiari MC, Boselli M, et al. Clinical and polysomnographic effects of trazodone CR in chronic insomnia associated with dysthymia. Psychopharmacology 1994;116:389–95.

125. DeBoer T. The pharmacologic profile of mirtazapine. J Clin Psychopharmacol 1996;57(Suppl 4): 19–25.

126. Fawcett J, Barkin RL. Review of the results from clinical studies on the efficacy, safety and tolerability of mirtazapine for the treatment of patients with major depression. J Affect Disord 1998; 51(3):267–85.

127. Winokur A, DeMartinis NA 3rd, McNally DP, et al. Comparative effects of mirtazapine and fluoxetine on sleep physiology measures in patients with major depression and insomnia. J Clin Psychiatry 2003;64(10):1224–9.

128. Sørensen M, Jørgensen J, Viby-Mogensen J, et al. A double-blind group comparative study using the new anti-depressant Org 3770, placebo and diazepam in patients with expected insomnia and anxiety before elective gynaecological surgery. Acta Psychiatr Scand 1985;71(4):331–46.

129. Ruigt GS, Kemp B, Groenhout CM, et al. Effect of the antidepressant Org 3770 on human sleep. Eur J Clin Pharmacol 1990;38:551–4.

130. Reynolds CF 3rd, Buysse DJ, Miller MD, et al. Paroxetine treatment of primary insomnia in older adults. Am J Geriatr Psychiatry 2006;14(9):803–7.

131. Chalon S, Pereira A, Lainey E, et al. Comparative effects of duloxetine and desipramine on sleep EEG in healthy subjects. Psychopharmacology (Berl) 2005;177(4):357–65.

132. Luthringer R, Toussaint M, Schaltenbrand N, et al. A double-blind, placebo-controlled evaluation of the effects of orally administered venlafaxine on sleep in inpatients with major depression. Psychopharmacol Bull 1996;32(4):637–46.

133. Nofzinger EA, Reynolds CF, Thase ME, et al. REM sleep enhancement by bupropion in depressed men. Am J Psychiatry 1995;152:274–6.

134. Nofzinger EA, Fasiczka MA, Berman S, et al. Bupropion SR reduces periodic limb movements associated with arousals from sleep in depressed patients with periodic limb movement disorder. J Clin Psychiatry 2000;61:858–62.

135. Ott GE, Rai U, Nuccio I, et al. Effect of bupropion SR on REM sleep: relationship to antidepressant response. Psychopharmacology 2002;165:29–36.

136. Ott GE, Rao U, Lin KM, et al. Effect of treatment with bupropion on EEG sleep: relationship to antidepressant response. Int J Neuropsychopharmacol 2001;7:275–81.

137. Evans L, Golshan S, Kelsoe J, et al. Effects of rapid tryptophan depletion on sleep electroencephalogram and mood in subjects with partially remitted depression on bupropion. Neuropsychopharmacology 2002;27:1016–26.

138. Miyamoto S, Duncan GE, Marx CE, et al. Treatments for schizophrenia: a critical review of pharmacology and mechanisms of action of antipsychotic drugs. Mol Psychiatry 2005;10:79–104.

139. Collaborative Working Group on Clinical Trial Evaluations. Adverse effects of the atypical antipsychotics paper. J Clin Psychiatry 1988; 59(Suppl 12):17–22.

140. Clark ML, Huber WK, Hill D, et al. Pimozide in chronic schizophrenic outpatients. Dis Nerv Syst 1975;36:137–41.

141. Sultana A, McMonagle T. Pimozide for schizophrenia or related psychoses. Cochrane Database Syst Rev 2000;3:CD001949.

142. Farde L. Selective D1- and D2-dopamine receptor blockade both induces akathisia in humans: a PET study with [11C]SCH 23390 and [11C]raclopride. Psychopharmacology 1992;107:23–9.

143. Wetter TC, Brunner J, Bronisch T. Restless legs syndrome probably induced by risperidone treatment. Pharmacopsychiatry 2002;35:109–11.

144. Kraus T, Schuld A, Pollmacher T. Periodic leg movements in sleep and restless legs syndrome probably caused by olanzapine. J Clin Psychopharmacol 1999;19:478–9.

145. Urban JD, Vargas GA, von Zastrow M, et al. Aripiprazole has functionally selective actions at dopamine D2 receptor-mediated signaling pathways. Neuropsychopharmacology 2007;32:67–77.

146. Gentile S. Long-term treatment with atypical antipsychotics and the risk of weight gain: a literature analysis. Drug Saf 2006;29:303–19.

147. Sharpley AL, Vassallo CM, Cowen PJ. Olanzapine increases slow-wave sleep: evidence for blockade of central 5-HT2C receptors in vivo. Biol Psychiatry 2000;47(5):468–70.

148. Lindberg N, Virkkunen M, Tani P, et al. Effect of a single-dose of olanzapine on sleep in healthy females and males. Int Clin Psychopharmacol 2002;17(4):177—84.
149. Sharpley AL, Vassallo CM, Pooley EC. Allelic variation in the 5-HT2C receptor (HT2RC) and the increase in slow wave sleep produced by olanzapine. Psychopathology 2001;153:271—2.
150. Gimenez S, Clos S, Romero S, et al. Effects of olanzapine, risperidone and haloperidol on sleep after a single oral morning dose in healthy volunteers. Psychopharmacology 2007;190(4):507—16.
151. Sharpley AL, Attenburrow ME, Hafizi S, et al. Olanzapine increases slow wave sleep and sleep continuity in SSRI-resistant depressed patients. J Clin Psychiatry 2005;66(4):450—4.
152. Moreno RA, Hanna MM, Tavares SM, et al. A double-blind comparison of the effect of the antipsychotics haloperidol and olanzapine on sleep in mania. Braz J Med Biol Res 2007;40(3): 357—66.
153. Wiegand MH, Landry F, Bruckner T, et al. Quetiapine in primary insomnia: a pilot study. Psychopharmacology 2008;196(2):337—8.

Stimulants in Excessive Daytime Sleepiness

Noriaki Sakai, DVM, PhD[a], Sachiko Chikahisa, PhD[a,b],
Seiji Nishino, MD, PhD[a,*]

KEYWORDS

- Amphetamine • Methamphetamine • Methylphenidate
- Modafinil • EDS • Narcolepsy

The term central nervous system (CNS) stimulant is a loosely defined but widely used scientific term. In *Drugs and the Brain* by S. Snyder, stimulants are defined as "drugs that have an alerting effect; they improve the mood and quicken the intellect."[1] In the *Handbook of Sleep Disorders* by J.D. Parkes, CNS stimulation implies "an increase in neuronal activity due to enhanced excitability, with a change in the normal balance between excitatory and inhibitory influences. This may result from blockage of inhibition, enhancement of excitation, or both."[2] In this review the generic term CNS stimulants is used for all wake-promoting compounds potentially used in the treatment of excessive daytime sleepiness (EDS). CNS stimulants are generally effective on EDS independent of the underlying cause. However, they should be used carefully because of their potential for misuse and abuse.

Several CNS stimulants are currently used in sleep medicine, including amphetaminelike compounds (L- and D-amphetamine and methamphetamine, L- and D-methylphenidate, pemoline), mazindol, modafinil, some antidepressants with stimulant properties (eg, bupropion), and caffeine. Most of these drugs promote wakefulness primarily through inhibition of dopamine (DA) reuptake/transport and in some cases through increased DA release. Inhibition of adrenergic uptake also likely has some stimulant effects. In the past decade, monoamine transporters (for DA, norepinephrine [NE], and serotonin [5-HT]) have been cloned and their molecular mechanisms have been elucidated. Biogenic monoamine transporters are located at nerve terminals, and play an important role in terminating transmitter action and maintaining transmitter homeostasis.

Genetically engineered mice lacking DA, NE, or 5-HT transporters (knockout [KO] mice) have also become available. In parallel with these advances, potent and selective ligands for these transporters have been developed. The results of pharmacologic studies using these new ligands in canine narcolepsy and KO mice models confirm the importance of the DA transporter (DAT) for the mechanism of action of amphetamines and amphetaminelike compounds (as well as mazinzol and bupropion) on wakefulness. However, the various stimulants also have differential effects on DA storage (via vesicular monoamine transporter [VMAT] inhibition) or DA release, and in most cases have negligible effects on other monoaminergic systems.

Modafinil is a more recent compound, which rapidly became a first-line treatment of EDS in narcolepsy. The mechanisms of action of modafinil

This work is partially supported by an NIH grant, R01MH072525.
The authors have nothing to disclose.
a Sleep and Circadian Neurobiology Laboratory, Stanford University School of Medicine, 1201 Welch Road, MSLS, P213, Palo Alto, CA 94304-5489, USA
b Department of Integrative Physiology, Institute of Health Biosciences, The University of Tokushima Graduate School, 3-18-18 Kuramoto-cho, Tokushima 770-8503, Japan
* Corresponding author.
E-mail address: nishino@stanford.edu

Sleep Med Clin 5 (2010) 591–607
doi:10.1016/j.jsmc.2010.08.009

have been controversial, but are now increasingly suggested to be primarily mediated by DA reuptake inhibition.

Other wake-promoting mechanisms include adenosine receptor antagonism, such as those found in caffeine. More recently, novel classes of wake-promoting therapeutics including glutamatergic and histaminergic modulators are being developed and preclinical and clinical evaluation are in progress.

This article reviews the neurochemical, neurophysiologic, and neuropharmacologic properties of the CNS stimulants most commonly used in sleep medicine, which gives a perspective on future stimulant treatments.

AMPHETAMINES AND AMPHETAMINELIKE COMPOUNDS
Historical Perspective

Amphetamine was first synthesized by Alles in 1897. The stimulant effects of amphetamine were recognized in 1929, and it was rapidly shown to be a safer and cheaper alternative to ephedrine as a stimulant. In World War II, amphetamine was extensively supplied to paratroopers and commandos to promote alertness and reduce fatigue.

The indications for amphetaminelike stimulants are limited, primarily including the treatment of narcolepsy and attention-deficit/hyperactivity disorder (ADHD). Narcolepsy was probably the first condition for which amphetamine was used clinically. It revolutionized therapy for this condition, although it was not curative. In 1959, Yoss and Daly[3] introduced methylphenidate, the piperazine derivative of amphetamine.

Many case series suggest the effectiveness of stimulants in treatment-resistant depression, although no controlled trials have been performed. Part of the beneficial effects of amphetamine on depression may be caused by a reduction of fatigue and apathy, rather than a genuine antidepressant effect. Combined therapy with stimulants, monoamine oxidase inhibitors (MAOIs) , and tricyclics is generally not advised because of significant hypertension or hyperthermia noted in certain cases. In patients with narcolepsy-cataplexy, the combination of amphetamines with low (anticataplectic) doses of tricyclics is often prescribed without any problem.

The effectiveness of amphetamine for antisocial behavior (withdrawn or lethargic) in children was first reported by Bradley and Bowen in 1941.[4] In some children and aggressive adults, a paradoxic calming effect was also observed. Most notably, hyperactive children tended to move more quietly, to be calmer, and less quarrelsome after treatment with amphetamine. In 1958, methylphenidate was introduced to treat hyperactivity in children.[5] These observations preceded reports on the effects of amphetamine and methylphenidate in the hyperkinetic child, which is now termed ADHD.

Amphetamine has also been prescribed in the treatment of parkinsonism, sedative abuse, alcoholism, and obesity. As the risk of abuse and dependence has been recognized, the use of amphetamine has declined. The introduction of more effective agents for these conditions has also led to fewer uses for the drug.

Structure-activity Relationships and Major Chemical Entities

Amphetamine increases energy, improves mood, prevents fatigue, increases vigilance, prevents sleep, stimulates respiration, and causes electrical and behavioral arousal from natural- or drug-induced sleep. Amphetamine has a simple chemical structure resembling endogenous catecholamines, and its backbone forms the template for a variety of pharmacologically active substances (Fig. 1). The structure of amphetamine can be divided into 3 structural components: (1) a terminal amine, (2) an aromatic nucleus, and (3) an isopropyl side chain. Minor structural modifications can result in agents having diverse effects, including nasal decongestion, anorexia, vasoconstriction, antidepressant effects, or hallucinogenic properties.

Substitution at the amine group is the most common alteration. Methamphetamine is characterized by an additional methyl group attached to the amine (a secondary substituted amine), and is more potent than amphetamine because of increased CNS penetration. In contrast, substitution on the aromatic nucleus generally produces less potent, if not entirely inactive, stimulants.[6] Substitution of 2 or more methoxy groups plus addition of ethyl, methyl, or bromine groups on the aromatic nucleus creates hallucinogens of various potencies. Ecstasy (MDMA [methylendioxymethamphetamine]) is built on a methamphetamine backbone, with a dimethoxy ring extending from the aromatic group. An intact isopropyl side chain appeared to be needed to maintain stimulant efficacy. For example, changing the propyl to an ethyl side chain creates phenylethylamine, an endogenous neuroamine. The compound is less potent with a shorter half-life than amphetamine, although it has mood- and energy-enhancing properties.

Most amphetamine derivatives have isomer-specific pharmacologic effects. These isomer-specific effects occur both at the pharmacokinetic (distribution, absorption, brain penetration, metabolism, elimination) and the pharmacodynamic (actual pharmacologic effects) level.

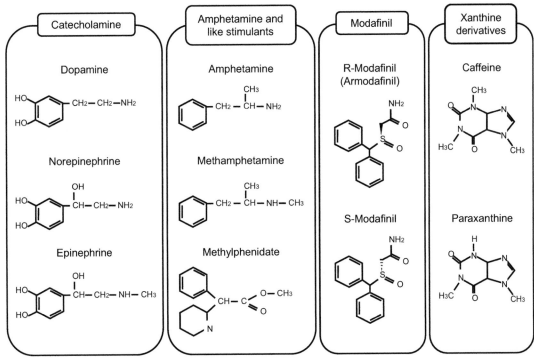

Fig. 1. Chemical structures of amphetaminelike stimulants, modafinil, and caffeine (xanthine derivatives), compared with catecholamine.

In electroencephalography (EEG) studies, D-amphetamine is 4 times more potent than L-amphetamine in inducing wakefulness.[7] However, both enantiomers are equipotent at suppressing rapid-eye movement (REM) sleep in humans and rats and at producing amphetamine psychosis, indicating that not all effects are stereospecific.

Amphetamines are highly lipophilic molecules that are well absorbed by the gastrointestinal tract. Peak levels in plasma are achieved approximately 2 hours after oral administration, with rapid tissue distribution and brain penetration. Protein binding is highly variable, with an average volume of distribution (V_d) of 5 L/kg. Amphetamines are inactivated by both hepatic catabolism and renal excretion. Amphetamine can be metabolized in the liver by either aromatic or aliphatic hydroxylation, producing biologically active metabolites parahydroxyamphetamine or norephedrine, respectively. Thirty-three percent of the oral dose is excreted unchanged in the urine. Urinary excretion of amphetamine and many amphetaminelike stimulants is greatly influenced by urinary pH. For example, at urinary pH 7.3, the elimination half-life of amphetamine is long (about 21 hours), whereas at pH 5.0 it decreases to 5 hours. Ammonium chloride shortens amphetamine action, whereas sodium bicarbonate delays excretion of amphetamine and prolongs its clinical effects (but can possibly induce toxicity).

Methylphenidate, pemoline, and fencamfamin are so-called amphetaminelike compounds; all compounds include a benzene core with an ethylamine group side chain (see **Fig. 1**). Methylphenidate is almost totally and rapidly absorbed after oral administration. Methylphenidate has low protein binding (15%) and is short acting; effects last approximately 4 hours, with a half-life of 3 hours. The primary pathway of clearance is through the urine, in which 90% is excreted. Both methylphenidate and pemoline were commonly used for the treatment of EDS in narcolepsy, but pemoline has been withdrawn from the market in several countries because of liver toxicity (**Table 1**). Although a single isomer form of D-methylphenidate is available under the trade name of Focalin, the most common form of methylphenidate commercially available is a racemic mixture of both D- and L-enantiomers. In this preparation, the D-methylphenidate mainly contributes to its clinical effects, especially after oral administration, whereas L-methylphenidate undergoes a significant first-pass effect.

Molecular Targets of Amphetamine Action

Amphetaminelike stimulants mediate complex molecular targets, which vary depending on the

Table 1
Commonly used pharmacologic compounds for EDS.

Stimulant Compound	Usual Daily Doses[a]	Half-life (h)	Side Effects and Notes
Amphetaminelike CNS Stimulants			
D-Amphetamine sulfate (II)	5–60 mg (15, 100 mg)	16–30	Irritability, mood changes, headaches, palpitations, tremors, excessive sweating, insomnia
Methamphetamine HCl[b] (II)	5–60 mg (15, 80 mg)	9–15	Same as D-amphetamine, may have a greater central over peripheral effects than D-amphetamine
Methylphenidate HCl (II)	10–60 mg (30, 100 mg)	~3	Same as amphetamines, better therapeutic index than D-amphetamine with less reduction of appetite or increase in blood pressure, short duration of action
Pemoline (IV)	20–115 mg (37.5, 150 mg)	11–13	Less sympathomimetic effect, milder stimulant, slower onset of action, occasionally produces liver toxicity, and had been withdrawn from the US market
DA/NE Uptake Inhibitor			
Mazindol (IV)	2–6 mg (na)	10–13	Weaker CNS stimulant effects, anorexia, dry mouth, irritability, headaches, gastrointestinal symptoms, mazindol is reported to have less potential for abuse
Other Agents for Treatment of EDS			
Modafinil[c] (IV)	100–400 mg (na)	9–14	No peripheral sympathomimetic action, headaches, nausea, modafinil is reported to have less potential for abuse
Armodafinil (IV)	100–300 mg (na)	10–15	Similar to those of modafinil
MAOIs with Alerting Effect			
Selegiline	5–40 mg (na)	2	Low abuse potential, partial (10%–40%) interconversion to amphetamine
Xanthine Derivative			
Caffeine[d]	100–200 mg (na)	3–7	Weak stimulant effect, 100 mg of caffeine roughly equivalent to one cup of coffee, palpitations, hypertension

All compounds except for selegiline and caffeine in the list are scheduled compounds and the class is listed in parentheses.
[a] Dosages recommended by the American Sleep Disorders Association are listed in parentheses (usual starting dose and maximal dose recommended).
[b] Methamphetamine is reported to have more central effects and may predispose more to amphetamine psychosis. The widespread misuse of methamphetamine has led to severe legal restriction on its manufacture, sale, and prescription in many countries. L-Amphetamine (dose range 20–60 mg) is not available in the United States, but probably has no advantage over D-amphetamine in the treatment of narcolepsy (slightly weaker stimulant).
[c] The half-life of s-enantiomer is short at 3 to 4 hours, and thus half-life of racemic modafinil mostly reflects the half-life of armodafinil (r-enantiomer).
[d] Caffeine can be bought without prescription in the form of tablets (No Doz, 100 mg; Vivarin 200 mg caffeine) and is used by many patients with narcolepsy before diagnosis.

specific analogue/isomer used and on the dose administered. Amphetamine per se increases catecholamine (DA and NE) release and inhibits reuptake from presynaptic terminals (**Fig. 2A**). This characteristic increases catecholamine concentrations in the synaptic cleft and enhances postsynaptic stimulation. The presynaptic modulations by amphetamines are mediated by specific catecholamine transporters.[8] Amphetamine derivatives are known to inhibit the uptake and enhance the release of DA, NE, or both, by interacting with the DAT and the NE transporter [NET]. These responsible molecules (DAT and NET) normally move DA and NE from the outside to the inside of the cell. This process is sodium-dependent; sodium and chloride binding allow the DAT/NET

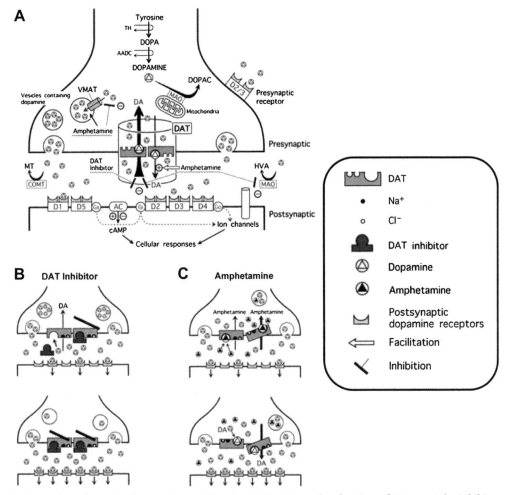

Fig. 2. Dopaminergic terminal neurotransmission in relation to mode of action of DA reuptake inhibitors and amphetamine. (*A*) DAT is one of the most important molecules located at the dopaminergic nerve terminals and regulates dopaminergic neurotransmission. Amphetamine inhibits DA uptake by virtue of the binding to the DAT. Amphetamine also facilitates DA release from the cytoplasm through the exchange diffusion mechanism (see *C*). At higher intracellular concentrations, amphetamine also disrupts vesicular storage of DA, and inhibits the MAO. (*B*) Sodium and chloride bind to the DAT to immobilize it at the extracellular surface. This process alters the conformation of the DA-binding site on the DAT to facilitate substrate binding. DAT inhibitors competitively block the DA binding, resulting in the increase of DA concentration in the synaptic cleft. (*C*) Amphetamine, in competition with extracellular DA, binds to the DAT. Substrate binding allows the movement of the DAT to the intracellular surface of the neuronal membrane, driven by the sodium and amphetamine concentration gradients. Amphetamine dissociates from the DAT, making the binding site available to cytoplasmic DA. DA binding enables the DAT to move the extracellular surface, driven by the favorable DA concentration gradient. AADC, aromatic acid decarboxylase; AC, adenylyl cyclase; cAMP, cyclic adenosine monophosphate; COMT, catechol-*O*-methyltransferase; D1-D5, DA receptors 1 to 5; DOPA, 3,4-dihydroxyphenylalanine; DOPAC, dihydroxyphenylacetic acid; Gi, Go, and Gs, protein subunits; HVA, homovanillic acid; TH, tyrosine hydroxylase.

to immobilize it at the extracellular surface and to alter the conformation of the DA/NE-binding site so that it facilitates substrate binding. Substrate binding results in the movement of the carrier to the intracellular surface of the neuronal membrane, driven by sodium concentration gradients. Most DAT inhibitors increase the DA concentration in the synaptic cleft by blocking the binding of DA (see **Fig. 2**B). In the presence of some drugs such as amphetamine, the direction of DA/NE transport seems to be reversed (see **Fig. 2**C). DA and NE are moved from the inside of the cell to the outside through a mechanism called exchange diffusion, which occurs at low doses (1–5 mg/kg) of amphetamine. Recently, an inward sodium current caused by amphetamine transport has been observed in an in vitro experiment. As intracellular sodium ions become more available, a DAT-mediated reverse transport of DA occurs. This mechanism is involved in the enhancement of extracellular catecholamine release by amphetamine, and it explains why amphetamine is in particular more potent than expected based on its low binding affinity for DAT and NET.[9,10]

At higher doses, other targets are involved. Increased 5-HT release is also observed. Moderate to high doses of amphetamine (>5 mg/kg) also interact with VMAT$_2$.[8] The vesicularization of the monoamines (DA, NE 5-HT, and histamine) in the nerve terminal is dependent on VMAT$_2$; VMAT$_2$ regulates the size of the vesicular and cytosolic DA pools. Amphetamine is highly lipophilic and easily enters nerve terminals by diffusing across plasma membranes. Once inside, amphetamine depletes vesicular monoamine stores by several mechanisms. First, albeit with low affinity, it binds directly to VMAT$_2$, thereby inhibiting vesicular uptake. Second, amphetamine, a weak base, diffuses across the vesicular membrane in its uncharged (lipophilic) form and accumulates in the granules in its charged form (because of the lower pH of the synaptic vesicle interior). As vesicular amphetamine concentration increases, the buffering capacity of the catecholamine-containing vesicle is lost. As a result, the vesicular pH gradient diminishes, followed by the decrease of vesicular monoamine uptake. Both mechanisms lead to a diffusion of the native monoamines out of the vesicles into the cytoplasm along a concentration gradient. Amphetamine can therefore be considered as a physiologic VMAT$_2$ antagonist that releases the vesicular DA/NE loaded by VMAT$_2$ into the cytoplasm. The high doses of amphetamine also inhibit MAO activity. These mechanisms, as well as the reverse transport and the blocking of reuptake of DA/NE, all lead to an increase in NE and DA synaptic concentrations,[8]

and these are independent on the phasic activity of the neurons.

Methylphenidate binds to the NET and DAT and enhances catecholamine release as well. However, it has less effect on the granular storage via VMAT than native amphetamine. Similarly, D-amphetamine has proportionally more releasing effect on the DA than the NE system compared with L-amphetamine. MDMA has more effect on 5-HT release than on catecholamine release. Other antidepressant medications acting on monoaminergic systems (eg, bupropion or mazindol; see later discussion) tend to exert their actions by blocking the reuptake mechanism. Thus, various amphetamine derivatives have slightly different effects on all these systems. In addition, MDMA shows serotonergic neurotoxicity in both humans and animals. Similarly, amphetamine derivatives with strong effects on monoamine release have neurotoxic effects on DA systems at high dose in animal studies, especially in the context of repeated administration mimicking drug abuse.

Presynaptic Modulation of the Dopaminergic System Primarily Mediates the EEG Arousal Effects

Amphetamines and other stimulants increase EEG arousal. Although amphetaminelike compounds are well known to stimulate catecholaminergic transmission, the exact mechanism by which they promote EEG arousal is still uncertain. A canine model of the sleep disorder narcolepsy has been used to explore its mechanism. Canine narcolepsy is a spontaneous animal model of the human disorder. Similar to human patients, narcoleptic dogs are excessively sleepy (ie, shorter sleep latency), have fragmented sleep patterns, and display cataplexy.[10]

In vitro studies have shown that the potency and selectivity for enhancing release or inhibiting uptake of DA and NE vary between amphetamine analogues and isomers.[11] To dissect the wake-promoting effects of amphetamine, in vivo effects of various amphetamine analogues (D-amphetamine, L-amphetamine, and L-methamphetamine) on both brain extracellular DA levels and the EEG arousal were compared in narcoleptic dogs.[12] The local perfusion of D-amphetamine raised caudate DA levels 9 times more than baseline (**Fig. 3**A). L-Amphetamine also increased DA levels by up to 7 times, but maximum DA level was obtained only at the end of the 60-minute perfusion period. L-Methamphetamine did not change DA levels under these conditions. NE was also measured in the frontal cortex during perfusion of

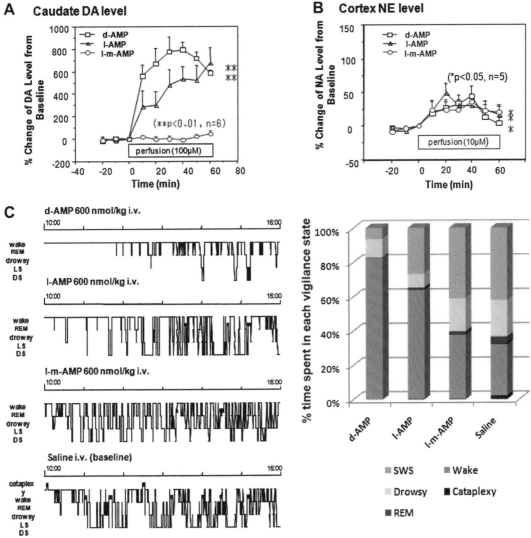

Fig. 3. Effects of amphetamine derivatives on catecholamine levels and sleep parameters in narcoleptic dogs. (A) Local perfusion of ᴅ-amphetamine (d-AMP) and ʟ-amphetamine (l-AMP) raised caudate DA levels, whereas ʟ-methamphetamine (l-m-AMP) did not change. (B) All 3 amphetamine isomers had equipotent enhancements on NE release. (C) Typical effects of amphetamine derivatives (600 nmol/kg intravenously) on sleep architecture. Representative hypnograms with and without drug treatment are shown. Recordings lasted for 6 hours, beginning at approximately 10:00 ᴀᴍ d-AMP was found to be more potent than l-AMP, and l-m-AMP was found to be the least potent, whereas all isomers equipotently reduced REM sleep.

amphetamine analogues. Although all compounds increased NE efflux, no significant difference in potency was detected among the 3 analogues (see **Fig. 3**B). In addition, EEG analysis revealed that ᴅ-amphetamine was 3 times more potent than ʟ-amphetamine, and 12 times more potent than ʟ-methamphetamine in increasing wakefulness and reducing slow-wave sleep (SWS) (see **Fig. 3**C). These results suggest that the potency of amphetamine derivatives on EEG arousal correlates with effects on DA efflux in the caudate of narcoleptic dogs. This correlation was further

confirmed by data obtained with DAT inhibitors (**Fig. 4**).

The effects of specific inhibitors for the DAT (GBR12909, bupropion, and amineptine), NET (nisoxetine and desipramine), or both the DAT and NET (mazindol and nomifensine), as well as amphetamine and a nonamphetamine stimulant modafinil, on EEG arousal were studied using narcoleptic Doberman pinschers.[9] Prototypical DAT inhibitors such as GBR12909 and bupropion dose-dependently increased EEG arousal, whereas 2 potent NET inhibitors, nisoxetine and

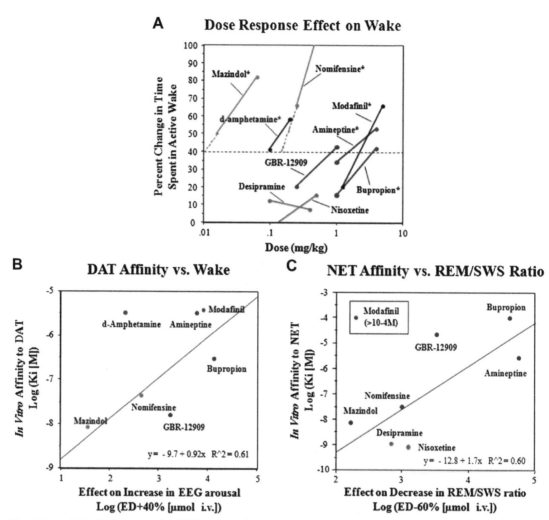

Fig. 4. Correlation between in vivo EEG arousal effects of various DAT/NET inhibitors and amphetaminelike stimulants and in vitro DAT/NET-binding affinities. (A) The effects of various compounds on daytime sleepiness were analyzed using 4-hour daytime polygraphic recordings (10:00—14:00) in 4 to 5 narcoleptic dogs. Two doses were studied for each compound. All specific inhibitors for the DAT (red), both the DAT and NET (orange), plus CNS stimulants (blue) dose-dependently increased EEG arousal and reduced SWS when compared with vehicle treatment. In contrast, 2 potent NET inhibitors (green) had no significant effect on EEG arousal at doses. (B) In vitro DAT binding was performed using [³H]WIN 35,428 onto canine caudate membranes. A significant correlation between in vivo and in vitro effects was observed for all 5 DAT inhibitors and modafinil. (C) In vitro NET binding was performed using [³H]nisoxetine. The REM/SWS ratio is considered to be a parameter of the suppression of SWS. A significant correlation between in vivo potencies on the REM/SWS and in vitro affinity to the NET suggests that presynaptic modulation of NE transmission is important for the pharmacologic control of REM sleep.

desipramine, had no effect on EEG arousal at doses that almost completely suppressed REM sleep and cataplexy (see **Fig. 4**A). Furthermore, the EEG arousal potency of various DAT inhibitors correlated tightly with in vitro DAT-binding affinities (see **Fig. 4**B), whereas a reduction in REM sleep correlated with in vitro NET-binding affinities (see **Fig. 4**C). These results suggest that DAT inhibition is critical for the EEG arousal effects of these compounds.

Considering that other amphetaminelike stimulants, such as methylphenidate and pemoline, also inhibit DA reuptake and enhance release of DA, presynaptic enhancement of DA transmission is likely to be the key pharmacologic property mediating wake promotion for all amphetamines and amphetaminelike stimulants. In contrast, there is little evidence that enhancing adrenergic transmission is wake promoting in animal studies.

Experiments using mice genetically lacking the DAT gene further assessed the role of the DA system in sleep regulation. Consistent with a role of DA in the regulation of wakefulness, these mice have reduced non-REM (NREM) sleep time and increased wakefulness consolidation (independently from locomotor effects).[13] The most striking finding was that DAT KO mice were completely unresponsive to the wake-promoting effects of methamphetamine, GBR12909, and modafinil. These results further confirm the critical role of DAT in mediating the wake-promoting effects of amphetamines and modafinil (see **Figs. 3** and **4**)[13] (see also modafinil section). DAT KO mice were also found to be more sensitive to caffeine, suggesting functional interactions between adenosinergic and DA systems in the control of sleep/wake.[13]

Anatomic Targets Mediating Dopaminergic Effects on Wakefulness

The ascending DA projections from mesencephalic DA nuclei (retrorubral [A8], SN [A9], and ventral tegmental area [VTA] [A10]) are composed of 2 major subdivisions.[14] One is the mesostriatal system, which originates in the substantia nigra (SN) and retrorubral nucleus and terminates in the dorsal striatum (principally the caudate and putamen). The other is the mesolimbocortical DA system, which consists of the mesocortical and mesolimbic DA systems. The mesocortical system originates in the VTA and the medial SN and terminates in the limbic cortex (medial prefrontal, anterior cingulated, and entorhinal cortices).

DA reuptake is physiologically important for the elimination of DA in cortical hemispheres, limbic forebrain, and striatum, but not in midbrain DA neurons.[15] Local perfusion experiments of DA compounds in rats and canine narcolepsy have suggested that the VTA, but not the SN, is critically involved in EEG arousal regulation.[16] Thus, it is possible that amphetamine, modafinil, and DA uptake inhibitors induce wakefulness by acting on DA terminals of the cortical hemispheres, limbic forebrain, and striatum. DA terminals of the mesolimbocortical DA system may be important in mediating wakefulness after DA-related CNS stimulant administration. The involvement of other, less studied dopaminergic cell groups, such as those located in the hypothalamus or in the ventral periaqueductal gray (recently suggested to be wake active[17]), is also possible and is worth further exploration.

DA agonists/antagonists typically have biphasic effects on locomotion and sleep, with DA agonists increasing locomotion and even producing stereotypes only at high doses.[18] Direct DA agonists and L-DOPA typically used in the therapy for Parkinson disease are generally not strongly wake promoting in clinical practice, but rather mildly sedative. It has been explained by the primary presynaptic effect of these compounds at low dose, an effect that may reduce DA transmission in some projection areas.[18]

Indications

Amphetamine and methylphenidate are indicated and used primarily for narcolepsy, idiopathic hypersomnia, and ADHD. Other therapeutic uses are controversial because of their abuse potential. They are classified as a schedule II substance under the Controlled Substances Act. Moreover, certain states (eg, Wisconsin) have passed even more restrictive legislation limiting the use of these substances to specific indications.[19] In the United States, the use of these compounds is highly regulated and requires triplicate prescription and monthly renewal.

Side Effects and Toxicity

Common side effects occurring during long-term treatment of narcolepsy include irritability, headache, bad temper, and profuse sweating (reported by more than one-third of subjects). Other less common side effects include anorexia, gastric discomfort, nausea, talkativeness, insomnia, orofacial dyskinesia, nervousness, palpitations, muscle jerking, chorea, and tremor. Psychiatric symptoms such as delusions or hallucinations may also occur, but are rare in narcoleptic patients who receive amphetamine. For common side effects of CNS-stimulant drugs for EDS, refer to **Table 1**.

Amphetamine releases not only DA but also NE. NE indirectly stimulates α and β-adrenergic receptors, a profile common to all indirectly acting sympathomimetic compounds. This situation results in significant cardiovascular effects. α-Adrenergic stimulation produces vasoconstriction, thereby increasing both systolic and diastolic blood pressure. Heart rate may slightly slow down in reflex at low dose, but with large doses, tachycardia and cardiac arrhythmia may occur. Cardiac output is not modulated by therapeutic doses, and cerebral blood flow is unchanged. In general, smooth muscles respond to amphetamine as they do with other sympathomimetic drugs. There is a contractile effect on the urinary bladder sphincter. Pain and difficulty in micturition may occur.

The side-effect profile of methylphenidate is similar to that of amphetamine and includes nervousness, insomnia, and anorexia, as well as dose-related systemic effects such as increased heart rate and blood pressure. Methylphenidate overdose may lead to seizures, dysrhythmias, or hyperthermia. Methamphetamine (and to a lesser extent amphetamine) can be neurotoxic to dopaminergic neurons via excess production of peroxynitrite at high doses. MDMA has a preferential effect (and toxicity) on serotonergic neurons and seems to decrease glutathione and vitamin E in the brain.

Abuse and Misuse of Amphetamine Stimulants

Tolerance is common during long-term administration of amphetamine, methamphetamine, and methylphenidate while reinforcement first occurs. These compounds are rarely problematic when used in patients with narcolepsy and hypocretin deficiency, a finding also supported by some animal data.[20] This situation may be similar to that of morphine administration in patients with pain, in whom dependence is rarely problematic after withdrawal of opiates.

Stimulants are more addictive when administered intravenously. The potential for abuse is higher when the drug is soluble and easy to inject or smoke. The mechanisms underlying abuse for amphetaminelike stimulants are complex. However, it has been shown to primarily involve stimulation of the VTA-DA systems.[21] Downstream changes in adrenergic and serotonergic systems, particularly via α-1b and 5-HT2a receptors, may be important.[22,23]

Drug-drug Interactions

A small portion of amphetamine and methylphenidate are metabolized by cytochrome P450 (CYP) 2D6. Drug-drug interactions with amphetamine and methylphenidate are generally pharmacodynamic/neurochemical in nature.[24] Theoretically, drugs that are competitively metabolized by CYP2D6 or inhibit CYP2D6 can increase plasma levels of amphetamine, but this is rarely a significant problem with therapeutic doses.

Tricyclic drugs competitively inhibit the metabolism of amphetamine and amphetaminelike stimulants and enhance behavioral effects. The combination of amphetamine with tricyclics could theoretically increase blood pressure (because of the combined effects of NE reuptake and release), but in practice amphetamine, 10 to 16 mg (and also methylphenidate, 10–60 mg, mazindol, 2–12 mg), has been safely given with imipramine and clomipramine, 10 to 100 mg, to treat narcolepsy-cataplexy. The dosage of amphetamine required to control narcolepsy may be reduced by a third by the simultaneous use of tricyclic drugs.

MAO-A inhibitors (eg, nialamide, pargyline, and tranylcypromine) inhibit the hepatic metabolism of amphetamine, and greatly potentiate the behavioral effects of amphetamine. Coadministration of MAOIs and amphetamine derivatives is generally contraindicated. In contrast to tricyclics and MAO-A inhibitors, haloperidol, reserpine, and atropine have no effect on amphetamine hydroxylation in the animal liver, although they may reduce the central effects of amphetamine.[2] Chlorpromazine, trifluoperazine, perfenazine, and thioproperazine increase the half-life of amphetamine in the brain, but inhibit central behavioral effects, such as stereotyped behavior in animals and euphoria in humans.[2] Hypnotic drugs prevent many behavioral effects of amphetamines, although chlorodiazepoxide and diazepam increase amphetamine tissue levels.[2]

MODAFINIL AND ARMODAFINIL
Structure and Pharmacokinetics

Modafinil (2-[(diphenylmethyl)sulfinyl]acetamide, see **Fig. 1**) is currently available as a racemic mixture of 2 active isomers (r- and s-modafinil) or an r-isomer only preparation (Armodafinil). Modafinil is rapidly absorbed but slowly cleared and its half-life is 9 to 14 hours. The r-enantiomer of modafinil has a considerably longer half-life of 10 to 15 hours than the s-enantiomer (3–4 hours).[25] The dual pharmacokinetic properties of the racemic mixture may explain why modafinil is often more active when taken twice per day at the beginning of therapy, during the period of drug accumulation. Modafinil has high protein binding and a Vd of 0.8 L/kg.[25] Up to 60% of modafinil is converted into inactive metabolites, modafinil acid and modafinil sulfone, primarily by CYP3A4. The compound has also been reported to inhibit CYP2C19 in vitro and induce CYP3A4 in vivo.[25]

Mechanism of Action

Modafinil/armodafinil has been shown not to bind to or inhibit receptors or enzymes for most known neurotransmitters, with the exception of the DAT.[9,26] The mechanism of action of modafinil/armodafinil is highly debated, although in our opinion it most likely involves DAT inhibition, not unlike other stimulants. In vitro, modafinil/armodafinil binds to the DAT and inhibits DA reuptake.[9,26,27] In the striatum of rats and dogs, these binding inhibitory effects have been shown to be associated with increased extracellular DA levels, suggesting functional effects. Effects of modafinil on alertness are entirely abolished in DAT KO mice,[13] and in mice lacking D1 and D2 receptors.[28] It was recently shown that modafinil was effective in noradrenaline-depleted (by DSP-4 administration)[29] and histamine-deficient (ie, histidine decarboxylase KO mice) mice,[30] also suggesting the importance of the dopaminergic system in wake promotion of modafinil. However, the data also suggest that modafinil may act on NET depending on drug dose, brain structure, and other physiologic conditions.

Recently, Madras and colleagues[31] reported in rhesus monkeys using positron emission tomography (PET) imaging that modafinil (intravenously) occupied striatal DAT sites (5 mg/kg: 35%; 8 mg/kg: 54%). In the thalamus, modafinil occupied NET sites (5 mg/kg: 16%; 8 mg/kg: 44%). The investigators also showed that modafinil inhibited [^{3}H]DA (IC_{50} [half maximal inhibitory concentration] 6.4 M) transport 5 times and 80 times more potently than [^{3}H]NE (IC_{50} 35.6 M) and [^{3}H]5-HT (IC_{50} 500 M) transport, respectively, in cell lines expressing the human DAT, NET, and 5-HT transporter. The data provide compelling evidence that modafinil occupies the DAT in the living brain of rhesus monkeys. Furthermore, a recent human PET study in 10 healthy humans with [^{11}C]cocaine (DAT radioligand) and [^{11}C]raclopride (D2/D3 radioligand sensitive to changes in endogenous DA) also showed that modafinil (200 mg and 400 mg given orally) decreased [^{11}C]cocaine-binding potential in caudate (53.8%, $P<.001$), putamen (47.2%, $P<.001$), and nucleus accumbens (39.3%, $P = .001$),[32] the results being consistent with the DAT hypothesis. In addition, modafinil also reduced [^{11}C]raclopride-binding potential in caudate (6.1%, $P = .02$), putamen (6.7%, $P = .002$), and nucleus accumbens (19.4%, $P = .02$), suggesting the increases in extracellular DA were caused by DAT blockades.[32] The investigators pointed out the potential for abuse potency of modafinil because drugs that increase DA in the nucleus accumbens have this potency.

Clinical observations also provide strong evidence that modafinil is not a primarily adrenergic compound. Amphetamine and adrenergic reuptake blockers cause dilation of the pupils by increasing NE signaling, but modafinil has no effect on pupil size. Adrenergic reuptake blockers are well known to slightly increase blood pressure and heart rate. In contrast, most clinical studies on modafinil, including a meta-analysis of 6 large clinical trials of modafinil, which is the most comprehensive study on this issue, have found no changes in heart rate or blood pressure. These clinical observations suggest that at usual clinical doses, modafinil does not increase adrenergic signaling in humans.

Indications

Since 1986, modafinil has been available in Europe. Modafinil was first approved for the treatment of narcolepsy in 1998 in the United States. More recently, it has been approved for shift-work sleep disorder and for residual sleepiness in treated patients with the obstructive sleep apnea syndrome.

Early clinical trials in France and Canada have shown that 100 to 300 mg modafinil is effective in improving EDS in narcolepsy and hypersomnia without interfering with nocturnal sleep, but has a limited efficacy on cataplexy and other symptoms of abnormal REM sleep.[33–35] A double-blind trial in 18 centers in the United States on 283 narcoleptic patients revealed that 200 mg and 400 mg of modafinil significantly reduced EDS and improved patients' overall clinical condition.[36] In canine narcolepsy, modafinil has no effects on cataplexy, whereas it significantly increases time spent in wakefulness.[37] In addition, several reports have suggested that modafinil is also effective for the treatment of ADHD, fatigue in multiple sclerosis, and EDS in myotonic dystrophy or Prader-Willi syndrome. Modafinil is also being used in the treatment of periodic hypersomnia, when treatment immediately after initiation of the episode may be critical.

Armodafinil was approved by the US Food and Drug Administration in June, 2007, for the treatment of sleepiness in association with narcolepsy, treated sleep apnea, and shift-work sleep disorder (ie, same indications as racemic modafinil).[27] Having a longer half-life, armodafinil may be useful in patients in whom modafinil once a day does not cover the entire day. Armodafinil is available at lower doses than modafinil, suggesting an improved safety profile. Although armodafinil may not be a revolutionary improvement compared with modafinil, it may have its place in the therapeutic arsenal.[27]

Side Effects

The most frequently reported side effects of modafinil are headache and nausea.[38] In patients with hepatic and renal dysfunction, modafinil should be carefully used at lower dose because of its dual hepatic and renal elimination profile and several potential drug interactions. The most substantive interactions observed in clinical studies were with ethinylestradiol and triazolam, apparently through induction of CYP3A4 by modafinil, primarily in the gastrointestinal system.[25]

For this reason, it is suggested to recommend alternative methods of contraception for women who are taking oral contraceptives in combination with modafinil.

Modafinil is an attractive alternative to amphetaminelike stimulants because of several factors. First, data obtained to date suggest that dependence is limited in humans with this compound,[33,39] although a study in rats and monkeys suggested a cocainelike discriminative stimulus and reinforcing effects of modafinil.[40] It is not liked by abusers of cocaine or stimulants, and does not have a high street value. Second, modafinil also has few effects on the neuroendocrine system. A comparison of healthy volunteers who were sleep deprived for 36 hours with those who received modafinil during sleep deprivation found no difference in cortisol, melatonin, or growth hormone levels.[41] Third, animal studies suggest that the compound does not affect blood pressure as much as amphetamines do; only high doses (800 mg) have been found to be associated with higher rates of tachycardia and hypertension. This finding suggests that modafinil might be useful for patients with a heart disease or high blood pressure.

Clinical experience suggests that the alerting effects of modafinil might be qualitatively different from those of amphetamine.[33] In general, patients feel less irritable and/or agitated with modafinil than with amphetamines and do not experience severe rebound hypersomnolence once modafinil is eliminated. This differential profile is substantiated by animal experiments.[37,42] This profile contrasts with the intense recovery sleep observed after amphetamine-induced wakefulness.[43] Considering the many advantages of modafinil over amphetamine treatment, modafinil has replaced amphetaminelike stimulants as a first-line treatment of EDS.

MAZINDOL

Mazindol is a schedule IV controlled drug and is rarely used in the United States. At 2 to 8 mg daily, mazindol produces central stimulation, a reduction in appetite, and an increase in alertness, but has little or no effect on mood or the cardiovascular system.[44] Although mazindol has a high affinity for the DAT and NET,[9] this compound has a low abuse potential. Mazindol is effective for the treatment of both EDS and cataplexy in humans[45] and in canine narcolepsy, possibly because of its blocking properties of DA and NE reuptake. However, mazindol often causes significant side effects, including anorexia, gastrointestinal discomfort, insomnia, nervousness, dry mouth, nausea,

constipation, urinary retention, and occasionally angioneurotic edema, vomiting, and tremor.

BUPROPION

Bupropion is classified as a monocyclic phenylbuthylamine of the aminoketone group, and it is a nonscheduled compound. Bupropion selectively blocks DA reuptake, and is 6 times more potent than imipramine in blocking DA reuptake. Bupropion shows a weak inhibition of NE reuptake and limited serotonergic effects. Bupropion may be useful for the treatment of EDS associated with narcolepsy at 100 mg 3 times a day.[9,46] It may be especially useful in cases associated with atypical depression.[46] Risk of convulsion increases dose-dependently (0.1% at 100–300 mg, and 0.4% at 400 mg).

SELEGILINE (L-DESPRENYL)

Selegiline is a methamphetamine derivative and a potent, irreversible, MAO-B-selective inhibitor primarily used for the treatment of Parkinson disease.[47,48] This compound is metabolized into L-amphetamine (20%–60% in urine) and L-methamphetamine (9%–30% in urine).[48] Because it is often considered as a simple MAO-B inhibitor, selegiline is indeed an amphetamine precursor. In the canine model of narcolepsy, selegiline (2 mg/kg by mouth) was shown to be an effective anticataplectic agent, but this effect was found to be mediated by its amphetamine metabolites rather than via MAO-B inhibition.[49] Several trials in human narcolepsy have shown a good therapeutic efficacy of selegiline on both sleepiness and cataplexy, with few side effects.[50,51] Although 10 mg of selegiline daily has no effect on the symptoms of narcolepsy, 20 to 30 mg improves alertness and mood, and reduces cataplexy, showing an effect comparable with D-amphetamine at the same dose. Selegiline may be an interesting alternative to the use of more classic stimulants, because its potential for abuse has been reported to be low.

ATOMOXETINE AND REBOXETINE

Atomoxetine and reboxetine (in Europe) are selective adrenergic reuptake inhibitors. Both compounds were developed as antidepressants, but atomoxetine is now mainly used in the therapy for ADHD.[52] These compounds are slightly wake promoting and reduce REM sleep, so they can be helpful in some cases of narcolepsy and idiopathic hypersomnia.[53,54] Atomoxetine needs twice-daily administration because of its short half-life. Reboxetine was shown to reduce mean sleep latency in narcoleptic patients.[54] These compounds increase heart rate and blood pressure. There is no risk of abuse, but sexual side effects are common.

CAFFEINE

Tea, cola drinks, chocolate, and cocoa all contain significant amounts of caffeine, and caffeine is probably the most popular and widely consumed CNS stimulant in the world. An average cup of coffee contains 50 to 150 mg of caffeine. Caffeine can also be bought over the counter (No Doz, 100 mg caffeine; Vivarin 200 mg caffeine). Taken orally, caffeine is rapidly absorbed. The half-life of caffeine is 3.5 to 5 hours. The physical effects of caffeine include palpitations, hypertension, increased gastric acid secretion, and increased urine output.[55] The behavioral effects of caffeine include increased mental alertness, a faster and clearer flow of thought, wakefulness, and restlessness.[55] Thus, caffeine is also commonly used by narcoleptic patients before diagnosis. However, heavy consumption (12 or more cups a day, or 1.5 g of caffeine) causes caffeine intoxication such as agitation, anxiety, tremors, rapid breathing, and insomnia.[55]

The mechanism of action of caffeine on wakefulness involves nonspecific adenosine receptor antagonism. Adenosine has been proposed to be a sleep-promoting substance, both accumulating in the brain during prolonged wakefulness[56] and possessing neuronal inhibitory effects. In animals, sleep can be induced after administration of adenosine A_1 receptor (A_1R) or A_2A receptor (A_2AR) agonist. Huang and colleagues[57] recently reported that wake-promotion effects of caffeine is abolished in A_2AR KO mice, whereas the effects were not altered in A_1R KO mice, suggesting a primary effect of caffeine through the A_2AR, at least in this species. Prostaglandin D_2, a somnogenic prostanoid highly concentrated in the brain, mediates its sleep-enhancing effects indirectly via an adenosine A_2AR-sensitive pathway.

One of the metabolites of caffeine, paraxanthine (see **Fig. 1**), significantly promoted wakefulness and proportionally reduced NREM and REM sleep in both control and narcoleptic mice.[58] The wake-promoting potency of paraxanthine (100 mg/kg by mouth) was greater than that of parent compound caffeine (92.8 mg/kg by mouth), and comparable with that of modafinil (200 mg/kg by mouth). Behavioral tests revealed that paraxanthine possessed less anxiogenic effects than caffeine. In addition, high doses of caffeine and modafinil induced hypothermia and reduced locomotor activity, whereas paraxanthine did not. These results suggest that paraxanthine may be a better wake-promoting agent for normal individuals, as well as patients suffering hypersomnia associated with neurodegenerative diseases, although further evaluation in humans is needed.

FUTURE STIMULANT TREATMENTS
Hypocretin-based Therapies

Central administration of hypocretin strongly promotes wakefulness in dogs, mice, and rats. Sleep/wake patterns and behavioral arrest episodes (equivalent to cataplexy and REM sleep onset) are normalized by central administration of hypocretin-1 in hypocretin-deficient mice.[59] Hypocretin could thus be effective to treat both sleepiness (ie, fragmented sleep/wake pattern) and cataplexy. Recently, Mishima and colleagues[60] reported that a substantial decline (by 50%−71%) in the expression level of hypocretin receptor genes was observed in hypocretin-deficient dogs and humans. The results in hypocretin-deficient mice suggested that the decline of hypocretin receptors was progressive over age. About 50% of baseline expression is still observed in old human patients. Considering these data, it is likely that an adequate ligand supplementation prevents narcolepsy in hypocretin-deficient patients even if receptors are partially nonfunctional. However, some reports suggest that stable and centrally active hypocretin analogues (possibly nonpeptidic synthetic hypocretin ligands) after peripheral administration need to be developed.[61,62]

Histaminergic H₃ Antagonists

Because H_1 antagonists are strongly sedative, histamine has long been implicated in the control of vigilance. In narcoleptic dogs, brain histamine contents are reduced.[63] Reduction of histamine contents is also observed in human narcolepsy and other hypersomnia of central origin.[64,65] The excitatory effects of hypocretins on the histaminergic system via hypocretin receptor 2 are likely to be important in mediating the wake-promoting properties of hypocretin.[66] Systemic administrations of histamine or histaminergic H_1 agonists induce various unacceptable side effects via peripheral H_1 receptor stimulation, whereas central injections of these compounds promote wakefulness. In contrast, histaminergic H_3 antagonists enhance wakefulness in normal rats and cats[67] and in narcoleptic mice models.[68] The histaminergic H_3 receptors are enriched in the CNS and are regarded as inhibitory autoreceptors. Histaminergic H_3 antagonists might be as useful as wake-promoting compounds for the treatment of EDS or as cognitive enhancers.[30]

Thyrotropin-releasing Hormone

Thyrotropin-releasing hormone (TRH) is a small peptide that penetrates the blood-brain barrier at high doses. TRH (at the high dose of several mg/kg) and its analogues have excitatory effects on motoneurons and increase alertness. It has been shown that they are wake promoting and anti-cataplectic via partially increasing DA and NE neurotransmission.[69,70] Recent electrophysiologic studies have suggested that TRH may promote wakefulness by directly interacting with the thalamocortical,[71] hypocretinergic,[72,73] and histaminergic networks.[74] TRH depolarizes thalamocortical and reticular/perigeniculate neurons in the slice preparations, and local application of TRH in the thalamus abolishes spindle-wave activity.[71] Because locomotor activation by TRH injection in the lateral hypothalamus was attenuated in hypocretin KO mice, the stimulant effects of TRH are partially mediated by stimulation of hypocretin neurons.[73] TRH also excites the histaminergic tuberomammillary nucleus.[74] Considering that TRH provokes arousal from hibernation,[75] TRH may be a potentially important wake-promoting system, although further studies are needed to disclose the roles of TRH in sleep/wake regulation.

Glutamatergic Compounds

Glutamatergic transmission is the major excitatory transmission of the mammalian brain. Compounds that are allosteric modulators of glutamatergic transmission, ampakines, are being developed as wake-promoting compounds, and may have counteracting effects on sleep deprivation.[76] Similarly, glutamine receptor subtype-specific compounds are likely to regulate sleep.[77,78] Therefore, glutamatergic transmission is increasingly believed to play a role in the generation of sleep homeostasis through changes in cortical synaptic plasticity,[79] although a more general mechanism needs to explain data across all species.

SUMMARY

Amphetaminelike stimulants have been used in the treatment of narcolepsy and various other conditions for decades, yet only recently has the mode of action of these drugs on vigilance been characterized. In almost all cases, the effects of these drugs on vigilance were found to be exerted via DAT. This finding has led to the generally widely accepted hypothesis that wake-promoting effects are impossible to differentiate from abuse-potential effects for these compounds. However, the various medications available have differential effects and potency on the DAT and on monoamine storage/release. The various stimulants available are more or less selective for DA versus other amines. Even if much work remains to be done in this area, it seems more and more likely that complex properties, for instance, the ability to release DA rather than block reuptake, plus the combined effects on other monoamines (such as 5-HT), may be important to explain abuse potential. Differential binding properties on the DAT itself may also be involved, together with drug potency and compound solubility. The lack of solubility of some low-potency compounds may result in an inability to administer the drug via snorting or intravenously. Lower abuse potential for these compounds has long been suspected in patients with narcolepsy-cataplexy, either because of the biochemical hypocretin abnormality, or because of the social aspects of treating narcolepsy as a disease.

The mode of action of the modafinil remains controversial but probably involves dopaminergic rather than nondopaminergic effects. Whatever its mode of action is, the compound is generally found to be safer and to have a lower abuse potential than amphetamine stimulants. Its favorable side-effect profile has led to increasing uses outside the narcolepsy indication, most recently in the context of shift-work sleep disorder and residual sleepiness in treated patients with sleep apnea. This recent success exemplifies the need for developing novel wake-promoting compounds with low abuse potential. A need for treating daytime sleepiness extends beyond the rare indication of narcolepsy-cataplexy.

ACKNOWLEDGMENTS

The authors thank Carl-Francis A. Deguzman for editing the manuscript.

REFERENCES

1. Snyder SH. Drugs and the brain, vol. 18. New York: Scientific American Library; 1986.
2. Parkes JD. Central nervous system stimulant drugs. In: Thorpy M, editor. Handbook of sleep disorders. New York: Marcel Dekker; 1990. p. 755.
3. Yoss RE, Daly DD. Treatment of narcolepsy with ritalin. Neurology 1959;9:171.
4. Bradley C, Bowen M. Amphetamine (benzedrine) therapy of children's behavior disorders. Am J Orthospychiatry 1941;11:92.
5. Anders TF, Ciaranello RD. Pharmacologic treatment of minimal brain dysfunction syndrome. In: Barchas JD, Berger PA, Ciaranello RD, editors. Psychopharmacology: from theory to practice. New York: Oxford University Press; 1977. p. 425.

6. Glennon RA. Psychoactive phaenylisopropylamines. In: Meltzer HY, editor. Psychopharmacology: the third generation of progress. New York: Raven; 1987. p. 1627.

7. Hartmann A, Cravens J. Sleep: effect of d- and l-amphetamine in man and rat. Psychopharmacology 1976;50:171.

8. Kuczenski R, Segal DS. Neurochemistry of amphetamine. In: Cho AK, Segel DS, editors. Psychopharmacology, toxicology and abuse. San Diego (CA): Academic Press; 1994. p. 81.

9. Nishino S, Mao J, Sampathkumaran R, et al. Increased dopaminergic transmission mediates the wake-promoting effects of CNS stimulants. Sleep Res Online 1998;1:49.

10. Nishino S, Mignot E. Pharmacological aspects of human and canine narcolepsy. Prog Neurobiol 1997;52:27.

11. Kuczenski R, Segal DS, Cho A, et al. Hippocampus norepinephrine, caudate dopamine and serotonin and behavioral responses to the stereoisomers of amphetamine and methamphetamine. J Neurosci 1995;15:1308.

12. Kanbayashi T, Nishino S, Honda K, et al. Differential effects of D-and L-amphetamine isomers on dopaminergic transmission: implication for the control of alertness in canine narcolepsy. J Sleep Res 1997; 26:383.

13. Wisor JP, Nishino S, Sora I, et al. Dopaminergic role in stimulant-induced wakefulness. J Neurosci 2001; 21:1787.

14. Björklund A, Lindvall O. Dopamine-containing systems in the CNS. In: Björklund A, Hökfelt T, editors. Handbook of chemical neuroanatomy, classical transmitter in the CNS, part I, vol. 2. Amsterdam: Elsevier; 1984. p. 55.

15. Nissbrandt N, Engberg G, Pileblad E. The effects of GBR 12909, a dopamine re-uptake inhibitor, on monoaminergic neurotransmission in rat striatum, limbic forebrain, cortical hemispheres and substantia nigra. Naunyn Schmiedebergs Arch Pharmacol 1991;344:16.

16. Honda K, Riehl J, Mignot E, et al. Dopamine D3 agonists into the substantia nigra aggravate cataplexy but do not modify sleep. Neuroreport 1999; 10:3717.

17. Lu J, Jhou TC, Saper CB. Identification of wake-active dopaminergic neurons in the ventral periaqueductal gray matter. J Neurosci 2006;26:193.

18. Monti JM, Monti D. The involvement of dopamine in the modulation of sleep and waking. Sleep Med Rev 2007;11:113.

19. Piscopo A. The impact of prescription drug diversion control systems on medical practice and patient care. In National Institute on Drug Abuse Technical Review Meeting. Bethesda, MD, May 30–June 1, 1991.

20. de Lecea L, Jones BE, Boutrel B, et al. Addiction and arousal: alternative roles of hypothalamic peptides. J Neurosci 2006;26:10372.

21. Koob GF, Nestler EJ. The neurobiology of drug addiction. J Neuropsychiatry Clin Neurosci 1997;9:482.

22. Drouin C, Darracq L, Trovero F, et al. Alpha1b-adrenergic receptors control locomotor and rewarding effects of psychostimulants and opiates. J Neurosci 2002;22:2873.

23. Salomon L, Lanteri C, Godeheu G, et al. Paradoxical constitutive behavioral sensitization to amphetamine in mice lacking 5-HT2A receptors. Psychopharmacology (Berl) 2007;194:11.

24. Markowitz JS, Patrick KS. Pharmacokinetic and pharmacodynamic drug interactions in the treatment of attention-deficit hyperactivity disorder. Clin Pharmacokinet 2001;40:753.

25. Robertson P Jr, Hellriegel ET. Clinical pharmacokinetic profile of modafinil. Clin Pharmacokinet 2003; 42:123.

26. Mignot E, Nishino S, Guilleminault C, et al. Modafinil binds to the dopamine uptake carrier site with low affinity. Sleep 1994;17:436.

27. Nishino S, Okuro M. Armodafinil for excessive daytime sleepiness. Drugs Today (Barc) 2008;44: 395.

28. Qu WM, Huang ZL, Xu XH, et al. Dopaminergic D1 and D2 receptors are essential for the arousal effect of modafinil. J Neurosci 2008;28:8462.

29. Wisor JP, Eriksson KS. Dopaminergic-adrenergic interactions in the wake promoting mechanism of modafinil. Neuroscience 2005;132:1027.

30. Parmentier R, Anaclet C, Guhennec C, et al. The brain H3-receptor as a novel therapeutic target for vigilance and sleep-wake disorders. Biochem Pharmacol 2007;73:1157.

31. Madras BK, Xie Z, Lin Z, et al. Modafinil occupies dopamine and norepinephrine transporters in vivo and modulates the transporters and trace amine activity in vitro. J Pharmacol Exp Ther 2006;319:561.

32. Volkow ND, Fowler JS, Logan J, et al. Effects of modafinil on dopamine and dopamine transporters in the male human brain: clinical implications. JAMA 2009;301:1148.

33. Bastuji H, Jouvet M. Successful treatment of idiopathic hypersomnia and narcolepsy with modafinil. Prog Neuropsychopharmacol Biol Psychiatry 1988; 12:695.

34. Besset A, Tafti M, Villemine E, et al. Effect du modafinil (300 mg) sur le sommeil, la somnolence et la vigilance du narcoleptique. Neurophysiol Clin 1993;23:47.

35. Boivin DB, Montplaisir J, Petit D, et al. Effect of modafinil on symptomatology of human narcolepsy. Clin Neuropharmacol 1993;16:46.

36. Randomized trial of modafinil for the treatment of pathological somnolence in narcolepsy. US

Modafinil in Narcolepsy Multicenter Study Group. Ann Neurol 1998;43:88.

37. Shelton J, Nishino S, Vaught J, et al. Comparative effects of modafinil and amphetamine on daytime sleepiness and cataplexy of narcoleptic dogs. Sleep 1995;18:817.

38. Fry J, Group TMs. A new alternative in the pharmacologic management of somnolence: a phase III study of modafinil in narcolepsy. Ann Neurol 1996; 40:493.

39. LaGarde D. Sustained/Continuous Operations Subgroup of the Department of Defense Human Factors Engineering Technical Group: program summary and abstracts from the 9th semiannual meeting. Pensacola, FL, July 11–12, 1989. p. 90.

40. Gold LH, Balster RL. Evaluation of the cocaine-like discriminative stimulus effects and reinforcing effects of modafinil. Psychopharmacology (Berl) 1996;126:286.

41. Brun J, Chamba G, Khalfallah Y, et al. Effect of modafinil on plasma melatonin, cortisol and growth hormone rhythms, rectal temperature and performance in healthy subjects during a 36 h sleep deprivation. J Sleep Res 1998;7:105.

42. Edgar DM, Seidel WF, Contreras P, et al. Modafinil promotes EEG wake without intensifying motor activity in the rat. Can J Physiol Pharmacol 1994; 72(S1):362.

43. Edgar DM, Seidel WF. Modafinil induces wakefulness without intensifying motor activity or subsequent rebound hypersomnolence in the rat. J Pharmacol Exp Ther 1997;283:757.

44. Parkes JD, Schachter M. Mazindol in the treatment of narcolepsy. Acta Neurol Scand 1979;60:250.

45. Iijima S, Sugita Y, Teshima Y, et al. Therapeutic effects of mazindol on narcolepsy. Sleep 1986;9: 265.

46. Rye DB, Dihenia B, Bliwise DL. Reversal of atypical depression, sleepiness, and REM-sleep propensity in narcolepsy with bupropion. Depress Anxiety 1998;7:92.

47. Golbe LI. Deprenyl as symptomatic therapy in Parkinson's disease. Clin Neuropharmacol 1988;11: 387.

48. Reynolds GP, Elsworth JD, Blau K, et al. Deprenyl is metabolized to methamphetamine and amphetamine in man. Br J Clin Pharmacol 1978;6:542.

49. Nishino S, Arrigoni J, Kanbayashi T, et al. Comparative effects of MAO-A and MAO-B selective inhibitors on canine cataplexy. J Sleep Res 1996;25: 315.

50. Hublin C, Partinen M, Heinonen EH, et al. Selegiline in the treatment of narcolepsy. Neurology 1994;44: 2095.

51. Mayer G, Meier E, Hephata K. Selegiline hydrochloride in narcolepsy: a double-blind placebo-controlled study. Clin Neuropharmacol 1995;18:306.

52. Findling RL. Evolution of the treatment of attention-deficit/hyperactivity disorder in children: a review. Clin Ther 2008;30:942.

53. Bart Sangal R, Sangal JM, Thorp K. Atomoxetine improves sleepiness and global severity of illness but not the respiratory disturbance index in mild to moderate obstructive sleep apnea with sleepiness. Sleep Med 2008;9:506.

54. Larrosa O, de la Llave Y, Bario S, et al. Stimulant and anticataplectic effects of reboxetine in patients with narcolepsy: a pilot study. Sleep 2001;24:282.

55. Rall TR. Central nervous system stimulants. In: Gilman AG, Goodman LS, Rall TW, et al, editors. The pharmacological basis of therapeutics. 7th edition. New York: Pergamon Press; 1985. p. 345.

56. Porkka-Heiskanen T, Strecker RE, Thakkar M, et al. Adenosine: a mediator of the sleep-inducing effects of prolonged wakefulness. Science 1997;276:1265.

57. Huang ZL, Qu WM, Eguchi N, et al. Adenosine A2A, but not A1, receptors mediate the arousal effect of caffeine. Nat Neurosci 2005;8:858.

58. Okuro M, Fujiki N, Kotorii N, et al. Effects of paraxanthine and caffeine on sleep, locomotor activity and body temperature in orexin/ataxin-3 transgenic narcoleptic mice. Sleep 2010;33(7):930–42.

59. Mieda M, Willie JT, Hara J, et al. Orexin peptides prevent cataplexy and improve wakefulness in an orexin neuron-ablated model of narcolepsy in mice. Proc Natl Acad Sci U S A 2004;101:4649.

60. Mishima K, Fujiki N, Yoshida Y, et al. Hypocretin receptor expression in canine and murine narcolepsy models and in hypocretin-ligand deficient human narcolepsy. Sleep 2008;31:1119.

61. Fujiki N, Ripley B, Yoshida Y, et al. Effects of IV and ICV hypocretin-1 (orexin A) in hypocretin receptor-2 gene mutated narcoleptic dogs and IV hypocretin-1 replacement therapy in a hypocretin ligand deficient narcoleptic dog. Sleep 2003;6:953.

62. Schatzberg SJ, Barrett J, Cutter KL, et al. Case study: effect of hypocretin replacement therapy in a 3-year-old Weimeraner with narcolepsy. J Vet Intern Med 2004;18:586.

63. Nishino S, Fujiki N, Ripley B, et al. Decreased brain histamine contents in hypocretin/orexin receptor-2 mutated narcoleptic dogs. Neurosci Lett 2001; 313:125.

64. Kanbayashi T, Kodama T, Kondo H, et al. CSF histamine contents in narcolepsy, idiopathic hypersomnia and obstructive sleep apnea syndrome. Sleep 2009; 32:181.

65. Nishino S, Sakurai E, Nevsimalova S, et al. Decreased CSF histamine in narcolepsy with and without low CSF hypocretin-1 in comparison to healthy controls. Sleep 2009;32:175.

66. Huang ZL, Qu WM, Li WD, et al. Arousal effect of orexin A depends on activation of the histaminergic system. Proc Natl Acad Sci U S A 2001;98:9965.

67. Lin JS, Sakai K, Vanni-Mercier G, et al. Involvement of histaminergic neurons in arousal mechanisms demonstrated with H3-receptor ligands in the cat. Brain Res 1990;523:325.

68. Shiba T, Fujiki N, Wisor J, et al. Wake promoting effects of thioperamide, a histamine H3 antagonist in orexin/ataxin-3 narcoleptic mice. Sleep 2004; 27(Suppl):A241.

69. Nishino S, Arrigoni J, Shelton J, et al. Effects of thyrotropin-releasing hormone and its analogs on daytime sleepiness and cataplexy in canine narcolepsy. J Neurosci 1997;17:6401.

70. Riehl J, Honda K, Kwan M, et al. Chronic oral administration of CG-3703, a thyrotropin releasing hormone analog, increases wake and decreases cataplexy in canine narcolepsy. Neuropsychopharmacology 2000;23:34.

71. Broberger C, McCormick DA. Excitatory effects of thyrotropin-releasing hormone in the thalamus. J Neurosci 2005;25:1664.

72. Gonzalez JA, Horjales-Araujo E, Fugger L, et al. Stimulation of orexin/hypocretin neurones by thyrotropin-releasing hormone. J Physiol 2009;587: 1179.

73. Hara J, Gerashchenko D, Wisor JP, et al. Thyrotropin-releasing hormone increases behavioral arousal through modulation of hypocretin/orexin neurons. J Neurosci 2009;29:3705.

74. Parmentier R, Kolbaev S, Klyuch BP, et al. Excitation of histaminergic tuberomammillary neurons by thyrotropin-releasing hormone. J Neurosci 2009;29: 4471.

75. Stanton TL, Winokur A, Beckman AL. Seasonal variation in thyrotropin-releasing hormone (TRH) content of different brain regions and the pineal in the mammalian hibernator, *Citellus lateralis*. Regul Pept 1982;3:135.

76. Porrino LJ, Daunais JB, Rogers GA, et al. Facilitation of task performance and removal of the effects of sleep deprivation by an ampakine (C×717) in nonhuman primates. PLoS Biol 2005;3:e299.

77. Joo DT, Xiong Z, MacDonald JF, et al. Blockade of glutamate receptors and barbiturate anesthesia: increased sensitivity to pentobarbital-induced anesthesia despite reduced inhibition of AMPA receptors in GluR2 null mutant mice. Anesthesiology 1999;91: 1329.

78. Steenland HW, Kim SS, Zhuo M. GluR3 subunit regulates sleep, breathing and seizure generation. Eur J Neurosci 2008;27:1166.

79. Tononi G, Cirelli C. Sleep function and synaptic homeostasis. Sleep Med Rev 2006;10:49.

Pharmacologic Treatment of Primary Insomnia

Janine M. Hall-Porter, PhD[a],*, D. Troy Curry, MD[a],
James K. Walsh, PhD[a,b]

KEYWORDS

- Hypnotics • Benzodiazepine receptor agonists
- Primary insomnia • Pharmacotherapy
- Pharmacologic treatment

Primary insomnia refers to persistent difficulty with initiation of sleep, maintenance of sleep, or nonrestorative sleep, in which the sleep disturbance is associated with daytime distress or impairment and cannot be attributed to a psychiatric or medical illness, another sleep disorder, or the effect of substance use (**Box 1**).[1] As is true for all insomnia disorders, difficulty with sleep is a qualitative measure, based upon a complaint or symptoms. No quantitative sleep variable (eg, sleep latency, total sleep time) is included in diagnostic criteria. Moreover, whether insomnia is "primary" is not determined by specific features, but by ruling out other conditions. Thus, primary insomnia is a symptom-based diagnosis of exclusion.

Recognizing a need for additional uniformity and precision in research to advance the understanding of insomnia and its treatments, Edinger and colleagues[2] offered standardized research diagnostic criteria (RDC) for an insomnia disorder (**Box 2**), as well as for the subtype of primary insomnia (**Box 3**). Relative to the *Diagnostic and Statistical Manual of Mental Disorders-IV (DSM-IV)* criteria, the RDC include an additional requirement of "adequate opportunity and circumstances" for sleep and provide some specificity with regard to "daytime distress or impairment" and comorbid medical and psychiatric conditions. Many researchers agree that future nosologic systems should incorporate most or all of these criteria.

PREVALENCE AND RISK FACTORS

Relatively few studies have used diagnostic criteria to establish the prevalence of insomnia. Based upon a number of studies that investigated the prevalence insomnia symptoms with some evidence of daytime impairment or distress, the *National Institutes of Health* (NIH) *State of the Science Statement*, in 2005, indicated that the best estimate was approximately 10% of the general population had an insomnia disorder.[3] Epidemiologic studies applying criteria very similar to *DSM-IV* suggest that approximately 20% have an insomnia disorder.[4,5]

Few studies have attempted to estimate the prevalence of primary insomnia. Studies by Ohayon[6,7] suggest that primary insomnia accounts for about 2% to 4% of the general population; however, these reports also estimate the prevalence for *DSM-IV*–defined insomnia to be much lower than most studies, ranging from 4.4% to 6.4%.[7] Somewhat restrictive criteria were used to define *DSM-IV* insomnia in these studies, undoubtedly influencing the estimates of prevalence. Thus, an accurate estimate of the population prevalence of primary insomnia is not currently available.

Risk factors specific to primary insomnia have not been studied systematically. However, sex and age are two demographics that influence risk, with females and older adults having an

[a] Sleep Medicine and Research Center, St Luke's Hospital, 232 South Woods Mill Road, Chesterfield, MO 63017, USA
[b] Department of Psychology, Saint Louis University, 3511 Laclede Avenue, St Louis, MO 63103, USA
* Corresponding author.
E-mail address: Janine.Hall@stlukes-stl.com

Sleep Med Clin 5 (2010) 609–625
doi:10.1016/j.jsmc.2010.08.006
1556-407X/10/$ — see front matter © 2010 Elsevier Inc. All rights reserved.

Box 1
Diagnostic and Statistical Manual of Mental Disorders-IV-Text Revision criteria for primary insomnia

- The predominant complaint is difficulty initiating or maintaining sleep, or nonrestorative sleep, for at least 1 month.
- The sleep disturbance (or associated daytime fatigue) causes clinically significant distress or impairment in social, occupational, or other important areas of functioning.
- The sleep disturbance does not occur exclusively during the course of narcolepsy, breathing-related sleep disorder, circadian rhythm sleep disorder, or a parasomnia.
- The disturbance does not occur exclusively during the course of another mental disorder (eg, major depressive disorder, generalized anxiety disorder, a delirium).
- The disturbance is not due to the direct physiologic effects of a substance (eg, a drug of abuse, a medication) or a general medical condition.

Box 2
Research diagnostic criteria for insomnia disorder

The individual reports one or more of the following sleep related complaints:

1. Difficulty initiating sleep
2. Difficulty maintaining sleep
3. Waking up too early
4. Sleep that is chronically nonrestorative or poor in quality.

The above sleep difficulty occurs despite adequate opportunity and circumstances for sleep.

At least one of the following forms of daytime impairment related to the nighttime sleep difficulty is reported by the individual:

1. Fatigue or malaise
2. Attention, concentration, or memory impairment
3. Social or vocational dysfunction or poor school performance
4. Mood disturbance or irritability
5. Daytime sleepiness
6. Motivation or energy or initiative reduction
7. Proneness for errors or accidents at work or while driving
8. Tension headaches or gastrointestinal symptoms in response to sleep loss
9. Concerns or worries about sleep

Box 3
Research diagnostic criteria for primary insomnia

- The individual meets the criteria for insomnia disorder.
- The insomnia has been present for at least 1 month.
- One of the following conditions applies:

    1. There is no current or past mental or psychiatric disorder.
    2. There is a current or past mental or psychiatric disorder, but the temporal course of the insomnia shows some independence from the temporal course of the mental or psychiatric condition.

- One of the following conditions applies:

    1. There is no current or past sleep-disruptive medical condition.
    2. There is a current or past sleep-disruptive medical condition, but the temporal course of the insomnia shows some independence from the temporal course of the medical condition.

- The insomnia cannot be attributed exclusively to another primary sleep disorder (eg, sleep apnea, narcolepsy, or parasomnia) or to an unusual sleep-wake schedule or circadian rhythm disorder.
- The insomnia cannot be attributed to a pattern of substance abuse or to use or withdrawal of psychoactive medications.

increased risk of insomnia.[3] Women nearly always have significantly higher odds of insomnia than men, with odds ratios from 1.2 to 1.7 for both insomnia symptoms and insomnia diagnoses.[5,7–9] The insomnia and age association is more complex. Several studies document a higher prevalence of insomnia symptoms in the elderly,[7,9,10] although others find no association with age.[11,12] In fact, a recent report found that nocturnal insomnia symptoms increase in people who are over the age of 65, without a corresponding rise in daytime impairment; thus, the number of individuals meeting diagnostic criteria for insomnia was not increased in that age group.[5]

ETIOLOGIC BASIS AND PATHOPHYSIOLOGY

Because insomnia was viewed for many years as a symptom of other medical, psychiatric, and behavioral conditions, research probing the cause or pathophysiology of insomnia was essentially nonexistent. More recently, researchers are conceptually and experimentally focusing upon mechanisms that may contribute to insomnia.

Ideally, this will lead to an understanding of the biology of insomnia and, eventually, a sign-based diagnostic approach, as well as the development of novel therapies. Most of the current conceptual models apply to both primary insomnia and co-morbid insomnia and include a common theme of physiologic hyperarousal.

The etiologic basis for hyperarousal is unknown, with some investigators focused on origins that are biologic,[13–15] while others emphasize cognitive and emotional factors.[16–18] Some believe that both neurobiologic and cognitive-behavioral factors contribute to the hyperarousal and that, regardless of the cause, biologic processes are involved.[19]

A number of years ago, psychological assessments of insomnia patients linked personality characteristics to arousal. Kales and colleagues[20,21] found that the personality patterns of insomniacs consistently showed more depression, rumination, anxiety, inhibition of emotions, and inability to discharge anger outwardly. The researchers concluded that this internalization of emotions and difficulty handling stress produce emotional arousal and physiologic activation that may be the underlying mechanism of insomnia.[20,21]

More recently, Espie and colleagues[17] have provided a model that emphasizes the cognitive mechanisms that accompany or underlie the assumed hyperarousal in insomnia patients. The model explains the development and maintenance of chronic insomnia via an attention-intention-effort pathway. The investigators propose that normal sleep is largely an automatic and involuntary process that can be inhibited or compromised by (1) selectively directing attention to sleep, (2) an explicit intention to sleep, and (3) increased effort to fall asleep and the subsequent development of maladaptive sleep-preventing behaviors in response to the frustration from poor sleep.[17]

Several lines of evidence indicate that insomniacs have elevated sympathetic nervous system activity. Increased heart rate before and during sleep,[22,23] as well as decreased heart rate variability during sleep,[24] have been reported for insomniacs as compared with normal sleepers. In addition, body temperature and whole body metabolic rate of insomniacs are elevated throughout the 24-hour day.[25,26] Compared to normals (individuals without any sleep problems or complaints), insomniacs have increased norepinephrine levels,[27] increased cortisol secretion,[28,29] and increased adrenocorticotropic hormone secretion,[29] suggesting hypothalamic-pituitary-adrenal (HPA) axis overactivity.

Measures of insomniacs' central nervous system (CNS) activity also indicate relative hyperarousal compared with sound sleepers.

Physiologic sleepiness during the daytime can be viewed as a measure of brain activation. Despite poor sleep at night, a number of studies have demonstrated that adult patients with insomnia have a similar[30–32] or lower[25,33,34] sleep tendency during the day relative to normals, although this may not be true for elderly primary insomniacs.[35] In addition, spectral analysis of the electroencephalogram (EEG) of insomnia patients during nocturnal sleep has demonstrated increased beta activity compared with normals in several investigations.[36–41] Increased gamma[36,39] and decreased delta[37,38] power have also been described. Since cortical electrophysiological signals in the beta and gamma band have been hypothesized to be a main feature of coherent cortical processing of sensory information, these EEG power increases may indicate cortical hyper-activity or hyperarousal.[41]

Functional neuroimaging demonstrates elevated whole-brain cerebral metabolism in insomnia patients, compared with normals, during sleep and while awake.[42] Furthermore, a smaller decline is seen in relative metabolism from waking to sleeping states in the reticular activating system, hypothalamus, thalamus, insular cortex, anterior cingulate cortex, medial prefrontal cortex, amygdala, and hippocampus for insomniacs, suggesting that brain areas involved in arousal and in emotional control are not "turned off" when insomniacs sleep. A subsequent study indicated that wake time during sleep was positively correlated with brain metabolic rate in emotional areas of the brain during sleep.[43]

INSOMNIA AND RISK OF IMPAIRMENT OR POOR HEALTH

At a symptomatic level, chronic insomnia has also been associated with fatigue and perceived impairment in mood, cognition, energy, and motivation. However, research with primary insomniacs has generally been unable to consistently demonstrate deficits in neuropsychological performance,[44–47] psychomotor function,[48] or executive functioning.[48] Studies evaluating measures of attention yield inconsistent results, as some have found slower reaction times[44] and impaired vigilance[31,49,50] with insomniacs, whereas others found no impairments.[46,47,51] However, a small number of investigations have consistently found impairments in insomniacs on more complex attention tasks.[50,52] Inconsistencies have also been found among working memory studies, with some reporting impairments[25,49] and others a lack of impairment[46] in insomniacs. Interestingly, two studies investigating overnight sleep-dependent memory consolidation found impairments in both procedural[53] and declarative[54] memory consolidation for primary insomniacs compared with good sleepers.   .

Substantial evidence demonstrates an association between insomnia and depression. Multiple studies show that insomnia is a precursor and often an independent risk factor for depression.[55–57] Furthermore, residual insomnia is associated with a higher rate of relapse or recurrence of depression,[58] and insomnia has been linked to suicide and suicidal behavior.[59,60] Depression is not the only psychiatric condition with a link to insomnia. Patients with primary insomnia have reported subclinical anxiety symptoms, and a correlation between anxiety level and sleep disruption has been found.[61] Some evidence suggests that insomnia is associated with an increased risk for developing an anxiety disorder.[57,62] Insomniacs are also more likely to develop alcohol (1.72 odds ratio) and drug (7.18 odds ratio) abuse or dependence disorders.[55] Relapse rates of alcoholics also are higher when significantly disrupted sleep is perceived.[63]

Chronic insomniacs consistently report reduced quality of life in multiple domains. For example, Zammit and colleagues[64] found statistically significant decrements in all eight domains of Short Form-36 (SF-36) for insomniacs relative to controls. Katz and McHorney[65] have reported that severe insomnia decreases quality of life in some domains of the SF-36 to a degree comparable to conditions such as chronic heart failure or depression.

Survey and epidemiology studies have demonstrated increased health care use and cost burden,[66–68] higher rate of absenteeism,[66,69] reduced work productivity,[69] and increased risk of accidents[66,68] associated with chronic insomnia or poor sleep.

As mentioned above, hyperarousal in insomnia has been associated with increased sympathetic nervous system activity and HPA activation,[24,29] and such increased activation may elevate cardiovascular risk.[70] In recent years, insomnia symptoms and polysomnographic measures have been associated with an increased risk for the development of hypertension.[71,72] Other studies suggest that insomniacs have an increased risk for negative cardiac events such as first myocardial infarct or cardiac mortality.[73,74]

PHARMACOLOGIC TREATMENT OF PRIMARY INSOMNIA

Pharmacologic treatment is one area of insomnia research that has specifically focused upon primary insomnia, rather than insomnia symptoms or nonspecific insomnia disorder. For example, a large percentage of the investigations of benzodiazepine receptor agonists (BzRAs) for insomnia during the past 25 years or more enrolled only primary insomniacs. Thus, the knowledge level of the efficacy and safety of drug treatments for primary insomnia greatly exceeds that of comorbid insomnia.

Drugs currently used for insomnia include those with an US Food and Drug Administration (FDA) indication for treatment of insomnia (nine BzRAs, the melatonin-receptor agonist ramelteon, and the histamine-1 antagonist doxepin; **Table 1**), sedating antidepressants, and antipsychotics. Below is a review of the mechanism of action, efficacy, and safety of these drugs with an emphasis on BzRAs, as relatively little is known about treatment of primary insomnia with antidepressant and antipsychotic drugs.

BzRA Hypnotics

The BzRA hypnotics are generally recommended as first-line therapeutic agents for several reasons. All the BzRA hypnotics have been shown to be efficacious, although there are some differences between drugs, associated with pharmacokinetic properties and marketed dose. Compared with other CNS drug classes, the margin of safety or therapeutic index (ie, the effective dose relative to lethal dose) is wide.[75] For example, barbiturates have margins of safety of two to four times the effective dose, whereas the margin of safety can be as great as 100 for BzRAs. Abuse or dependence is infrequent with BzRAs in the therapeutic context. However, some risk factors for benzodiazepine dependence have been identified and include higher doses, longer duration of use, younger age, and a history of drug or alcohol abuse.[76]

BzRAs are a group of drugs with a well-described common mechanism of action (see elsewhere in this issue for a detailed discussion of the pharmacology of drugs used as hypnotics). Briefly, BzRAs act as allosteric modulators of γ-aminobutyric acid (GABA) activity by binding to benzodiazepine sites on the $GABA_A$ receptor complex, further opening chloride ion channels and facilitating GABA inhibitory activity.[77–79] Some BzRAs have a benzodiazepine chemical structure (ie, estazolam, flurazepam, quazepam, temazepam, triazolam) and others do not (ie, eszopiclone, zaleplon, zolpidem). BzRAs with a benzodiazepine chemical structure appear to be non-selective, having comparable affinity for $GABA_A$ receptor complexes that contain one of four alpha subunits ($alpha_1$, $alpha_2$, $alpha_3$, and $alpha_5$).[77] BzRAs that are nonbenzodiazepines

Table 1
Drugs with an FDA indication for insomnia

Generic Name	Trade Name	Mechanism of Action	Dose(s) (mg)	Metabolic Enzymes	Elimination Half-life (hours)	T_{max} (hours)
Estazolam	ProSom	BzRA	1, 2	CYP3A4[195]	10–24	0.5–6
Flurazepam	Dalmane	BzRA	15, 30	CYP3A4 (probable)[196]	47–100[a]	0.5–1
Temazepam	Restoril	BzRA	7.5, 15, 22.5, 30	Conjugation with glucuronic acid	3.5–18.4	1.2–1.6
Triazolam	Halcion	BzRA	0.125, 0.25	CYP3A4[197]	1.5–5.5	2
Quazepam	Doral	BzRA	7.5, 15	CYP3A4 (minor: CYP2C9, CYP2C19)[198]	39–73[a]	2
Zolpidem	Ambien	BzRA	5, 10	CYP3A4, CYP2C9[199]	1.4–4.5	1.6
Zolpidem CR	Ambien CR	BzRA	6.25, 12.5	CYP3A4, CYP2C9[199]	2.8	1.5
Zaleplon	Sonata	BzRA	5, 10, 20	aldehyde oxidase (minor: CYP3A4)	1	1
Eszopiclone	Lunesta	BzRA	1, 2, 3	CYP3A4, CYP2E1	6	1
Ramelteon	Rozerem	MtRA	8	CYP1A2 (minor: CYP2C, CYP3A4)	1–2.6	0.75
Doxepin	Silenor	H_1Ant	3, 6	CYP2C19, CYP2D6 (minor: CYP1A2, CYP2C9)	15.3–31[b]	3.5

Table data were obtained from the prescribing information for each drug, unless otherwise indicated.
Abbreviations: H1Ant, Histamine-1Antagonist; MtRA, melatonin receptor agonist.
[a] Half-life of active metabolite(s).
[b] Half-life of parent drug and active metabolite.

are typically more selective. For example, zolpidem and zaleplon are highly selective for the alpha$_1$ subunit, which is thought to mediate sedation. While eszopiclone appears less selective, with comparable affinity for alpha$_1$, alpha$_2$, alpha$_3$, and alpha$_5$ subunits, there is evidence to suggest that it binds differently than benzodiazepines.[80] It is important to recognize that the functional significance of the binding differences among BzRAs for effect on sleep in humans remains unclear, although the nonselective binding of benzodiazepines is thought to lead to increased side effects.[77]

The most clinically relevant differences among BzRAs are associated with pharmacokinetic properties of the drugs, particularly duration of drug action. Elimination half-life, drug dose, and formulation (eg, extended release, sublingual absorption) are the most significant factors in determining duration of action. Individual variability in the metabolism and elimination of BzRAs produces individual differences in efficacy and safety among patients.[77]

It should be noted that it is not uncommon for benzodiazepines without an indication for insomnia to be used as hypnotics (eg, lorazepam, clonazepam, and alprazolam). The pharmacologic properties of these drugs are similar to the benzodiazepine hypnotics; thus, although efficacy in insomnia has not been as extensively studied with these drugs, they appear to have similar effects on sleep. However, their half-lives are relatively long, ranging from about 11 to 40 hours.[77]

Efficacy and effectiveness in primary insomnia
Most insomnia clinical trials have documented the hypnotic efficacy using patient reports or polysomnography (PSG) in patients with primary insomnia. A meta-analysis of clinical trials with benzodiazepines and zolpidem found that these drugs in aggregate produce reliable improvements in the sleep of persons with chronic insomnia,[81] although it should be noted that the median duration of the studies included in the analysis was only 1 week. Other meta-analyses largely concur regarding short-term efficacy of BzRAs.[82–84] However, meta-analyses have significant limitations, often combining data from multiple drugs with widely different pharmacokinetics or multiple doses of the same drug (which impacts the outcome variables examined in the meta-analysis). Although meta-analyses allow generalizations to be made about a group of drugs,

studies examining individual drugs are more informative and may be particularly useful when determining which drug is best for a given patient. Below, although similarities among BzRAs are discussed, important differences among drugs will be emphasized.

All BzRA hypnotics reduce sleep latency and most increase total sleep time, when used at appropriate doses. One exception is zaleplon, which does not significantly increase total sleep time in most trials.[85] The reduction of sleep latency produced by BzRAs is attributable to a rapid onset of hypnotic effect. Specific sleep maintenance variables, other than total sleep time, have begun to receive attention in recent years. Investigations assessing number of awakenings or wake-after-sleep onset (WASO) typically find that the longer the drug's duration of action (ie, the longer the half-life or higher the dose), the more likely the drug will show efficacy on these measures. At doses within the therapeutic range, a dose response effect is observed on efficacy measures, and generally there is little additional effect apparent at supratherapeutic doses.

Tolerance is defined as a reduction of a drug effect with repeated administration of a constant dose, or the need to increase dose to sustain a specific level of effect. Despite frequent speculations in the medical literature, tolerance to the hypnotic effects of BzRAs does not develop in the vast majority of studies, at least for therapeutic doses and for the periods of time that have been studied. Nearly 30 years ago, Oswald and colleagues[86] reported that lormetazepam and nitrazepam, two benzodiazepines available in some European countries, retained their effect according to some patient estimates of hypnotic efficacy during 24 weeks of nightly use. More recently, in rigorous PSG studies, zolpidem 10 mg and zaleplon 10 mg were shown to retain efficacy for 5 weeks of nightly use.[85,87] A study of several hundred patients with primary insomnia showed continued hypnotic efficacy of eszopiclone for 6 months of nightly use.[88] Patient reports of sleep latency, WASO, total sleep time, number of awakenings, and sleep quality were significantly reduced with eszopiclone 3 mg as compared with placebo at each monthly time point. These 6-month findings have been replicated,[89] and examination of open-label extension data has indicated sustained efficacy of eszopiclone for a total of 12 months.[90] Other evidence for sustained efficacy of nightly BzRA use includes a 3-month trial with indiplon, a nonmarketed hypnotic.[91]

A non-nightly treatment schedule has been evaluated for zolpidem 10 mg for up to 12 weeks.[92,93] Ratings of sleep latency, total sleep time, number of awakenings, and sleep quality were all improved on nights when zolpidem was taken, as compared with placebo (average self-administration of 3–4 nights per week for both). Additionally, investigator global ratings, which considered both medication nights and no-medication nights, indicated reduced insomnia severity with zolpidem.[92] More recently, a 6-month study examining an extended-release formulation of zolpidem, administered 3 to 7 nights per week for 6 months, generated similar results over the study duration.[94]

In addition to efficacy studies, some reports provide information on hypnotic use in the general population that may approximate reports of clinical investigations of effectiveness. Using epidemiologic methodology, Ohayon and colleagues[95] reported that 67% of chronic insomniacs with long-term use of hypnotic medications rated their sleep quality as improved "a lot" and only 14.4% reported little or no improvement with medication. Balter and Uhlenhuth[96] interviewed individuals who, in the prior year, had significant trouble with insomnia or had taken a medication to help them sleep. High satisfaction rates among hypnotic users were found. Specifically, 84% taking triazolam, 82% taking flurazepam, and 74% taking temazepam reported they would take the medication again for the same purpose.

Long-term, open-label studies conducted in both adult and elderly subjects in outpatient settings also provide some information about the effectiveness of BzRAs.[90,97–100] In general, patients and physicians report sustained benefit of BzRAs over periods of 6 to 12 months, without adverse reactions unique to long-term use. Again, the ability to generalize results and the confidence level regarding any conclusions drawn must be tempered by the self-selection of those remaining in these open-label studies.

Elimination or reduction of the daytime symptoms of insomnia could be viewed as evidence of treatment benefit. The few studies that have systematically assessed patient-reported daytime measures in primary insomniacs generally show improvement. For example, in two 6-month studies of patients with primary insomnia, patient reports of daytime alertness, ability to function during the daytime, and physical sense of well-being were all significantly better in the eszopiclone group than in the placebo group.[88,89]

Safety in primary insomnia

Adverse reactions to BzRAs in clinical trials or in clinical practice are seen in a minority of patients and severity ratings are typically mild. The median rate of adverse events among hospital inpatients using any hypnotic was found to be about 1 in every 10,000 doses.[101] Many of the side effects associated with BzRAs are mediated by their desired pharmacologic activity of sedation.[102] Residual sedation, which is a prolongation of the hypnotic effect of the drug into the wake period, results in adverse reactions such as drowsy feelings, sleepiness, and impairment in psychomotor performance and driving. The likelihood of residual sedation is determined by the duration of drug activity, which in turn is determined by the elimination half life and the dose of the drug. When used at recommended doses in healthy adults, the most rapidly eliminated hypnotics have durations of action in the range of 1 to 6 hours (eg, triazolam, zaleplon, zolpidem, eszopiclone, ramelteon), whereas the slowly eliminated drugs (and their active metabolites) have durations of action of 24 hours or more (eg, flurazepam, quazepam). Such long half-lives may cause residual sedation and drug accumulation (toxicity) may occur with chronic use. Drugs that have intermediate durations of action from 8 to 24 hours (eg, estazolam and temazepam) may also produce residual daytime sedation.[77]

Anterograde amnesia, or memory for information presented after drug administration, is potentially observed with any sedative, including the BzRAs, alcohol, and barbiturates. The severity of amnesia is related to the plasma concentration of the drug, such that the proximity of information input to peak plasma concentration determines the degree of amnesia.[103,104] Higher doses, which increase plasma concentration, are associated with a greater degree of amnesia and a higher prevalence of amnesiac events.[103,104]

The most frequently described discontinuation effect of BzRAs is rebound insomnia, which is defined as a worsening of sleep relative to the patient's status before treatment initiation. Unlike other discontinuation effects, rebound insomnia is brief and typically lasts only 1 to 2 nights after the hypnotic is discontinued.[105] This differs from a withdrawal syndrome, which is the appearance of a new cluster of symptoms (not present before treatment) that are unpleasant and generally last a few days to a few weeks rather than 1 or 2 days. Rebound insomnia has been reported when a hypnotic is abruptly discontinued after just 1 or 2 nights of use[106]; however, there is no evidence that it increases in severity with the number of repeated nights of use.[105,106] Rebound insomnia is more likely to occur after high doses of short- and intermediate-acting benzodiazepines, but it can be minimized by gradually tapering the dose over a few nights and reducing the frequency of administration.[106,107] It appears that rebound insomnia does not occur with long-acting hypnotics because of the gradual decline in plasma concentration that is inherent to the pharmacology of such drugs.[108] Rebound insomnia is typically not observed with the newer nonbenzodiazepine hypnotics, even though these are short- and intermediate-acting drugs. One study demonstrated that rebound insomnia occurred after the abrupt discontinuation of triazolam but not zolpidem, indicating that short-acting nonbenzodiazepines at appropriate doses may not produce rebound insomnia.[109] Another study found no evidence of rebound insomnia when zolpidem 10 mg was self-administered "as needed" for 8 weeks, as total sleep time was not decreased on no-pill nights that immediately followed a pill night.[92] In a 6-month study comparing zolpidem-CR to placebo, rebound insomnia was not observed on the 3 nights following discontinuation.[110,111] Abrupt discontinuation of zaleplon also does not appear to produce rebound insomnia in adult[85,112–114] or elderly[115] patients after periods of up to 5 weeks of nightly use. Results of one study indicated that eszopiclone (2 mg) produced rebound insomnia only on the first night after treatment discontinuation,[116] whereas another study found no rebound insomnia.[117]

Dependence on BzRAs continues to be a concern despite only anecdotal supporting evidence. Epidemiologic data from representative population samples indicate that the majority of insomnia patients do not continue taking hypnotics for long periods of time, as about 70% use them for 2 weeks or less.[118,119] Approximately 36% of individuals taking prescription hypnotics report regular use (ie, longer than one month),[120] but it is unlikely that this pattern of persistent use reflects drug dependence (physical or psychological dependence). Studies investigating hypnotic self-administration among insomniacs indicate that dose escalation does not occur,[121] daytime use is infrequent (ie, it does not occur outside the therapeutic context),[122] and the rate of self-administration varies as a function of the severity of the sleep problem.[123] Additional studies show that BzRAs have a low-to-moderate behavioral dependence liability, suggesting that hypnotic self-administration in insomniac patients is best explained as therapy-seeking behavior, rather than drug dependence.[119,121,124]

Virtually all investigations assessing the risk of falls with BzRA use have involved elderly individuals, the majority of whom do not have primary insomnia because they are either institutionalized or have one or more physical or psychiatric conditions associated with age. Therefore, it is difficult to attribute any increased fall risk to the drugs alone. Interestingly, recent studies appear to indicate that insomnia, but not hypnotic use, increases fall risk in the elderly,[125,126] although these studies cannot be considered definitive.

Idiosyncratic side effects associated with BzRA hypnotics, such as somnambulism and sleep-related eating, have been described in the media, based upon anecdotal reports. A few published case reports provide more detail and presumably more accurate information, including assessment of other contributing factors; however, until placebo-controlled investigations are conducted, the actual risk of complex behaviors in sleep will remain unknown. Somnambulism[127,128] and sleep-related eating disorder[129,130] have been reported with BzRAs at two to three times the clinical doses of the drug, in individuals who have a prior history of somnambulism or brain injury, or when taken in combination with antidepressant medications and alcohol.

Melatonin Receptor Agonist

Ramelteon, a melatonin receptor agonist, was the first non-BzRA and non-scheduled substance approved by the FDA for insomnia. Indicated for insomnia characterized by sleep-onset difficulty, ramelteon is rapidly absorbed and eliminated.[131,132] It has agonist properties at both melatonin type 1 and melatonin type 2 receptors,[133,134] which are located in various tissues including the suprachiasmatic nucleus (SCN), an area of the brain involved in sleep regulation and circadian rhythms. Evidence suggests that agonists of melatonin type 1 receptors inhibit SCN wake-promoting activity, thus promoting sleep.[135] Melatonin type 2 receptors appear to be involved in sleep-wake timing.[135–138]

Both polysomnographic and subjective data indicate that ramelteon (from 4–32 mg) decreases sleep latency in adult[139] and elderly[140,141] primary insomniacs. Long-term efficacy studies demonstrate that sleep latency improvements are maintained with ramelteon after 5 weeks (8 and 16 mg),[142] 6 months (8 mg),[143] and 1 year (8 and 16 mg).[144] Improvements in total sleep time and sleep efficiency are small and appear to be accounted for by the reduction in sleep latency, with no observable impact on sleep maintenance variables such as wake after sleep onset.[141] Ramelteon also appears to have chronobiotic properties at doses from 1 to 4 mg, facilitating a phase shift of the circadian rhythm, measured as melatonin offset after morning awakening, when subjects underwent a 5-hour phase advance in their sleep-wake cycles.[145] Ramelteon has not been directly compared with other sleep-promoting drugs, nor has it been evaluated in broad clinical populations.

The most common adverse events with ramelteon are headache, somnolence, dizziness, fatigue, and nausea.[146] Clinical trials at various doses have indicated no residual sedation or cognitive impairment,[139,147,148] as well as no evidence of rebound insomnia or withdrawal symptoms after discontinuation of ramelteon.[140,149] Because of low abuse potential,[148,150] ramelteon may have a role in the treatment of insomnia in individuals with a history of chemical dependence; however, there are no published reports with that population.

Histamine-1 Antagonist

Recently, the FDA approved low-dose (3 mg and 6 mg) doxepin for the treatment of insomnia characterized by sleep maintenance difficulty. For many years, doxepin has been available as an antidepressant (generally at doses from 25–600 mg) and has been used off-label to promote sleep. At very low doses, the majority of doxepin's pharmacologic activity appears to be antagonism of histamine-1 receptors. The safety issues associated with higher doses of doxepin are apparently not an issue at these very low doses, predominantly because the anticholinergic activity is negligible.

Only a few studies of the approved compound have been published to date.[151–153] These acute administration PSG studies demonstrate, in both adult and elderly primary insomniacs, that 3 and 6 mg doses reduce WASO throughout the sleep period and increase total sleep time (TST). The 6 mg dose also has a significant but modest effect in reducing sleep latency. Despite the reduction of WASO, even in the last hour of the night, residual sedation was not observed. It has been hypothesized that this relates to the circadian pattern of endogenous histamine release, with the rising histamine levels around the time of awakening overcoming the antagonism of the drug.[151] Subjective data largely mirror the PSG findings. The type and frequency of adverse events were largely similar to those with placebo in these trials.[151–153] Studies as long as three months of nightly use show the same reduction in WASO and increase in TST, with no evidence of tolerance or significant safety concerns.[153] Doxepin is not a scheduled drug and is not known to have abuse potential; therefore it may be a therapeutic option for individuals with history of substance abuse. However, to the authors' knowledge, no studies have been conducted in this population.

Sedating Antidepressants Used as Hypnotics

Sedating antidepressants are commonly used "off-label" to treat insomnia, despite limited efficacy data and potentially significant safety concerns. In fact, treatment with benzodiazepines decreased by 54% from 1987 to 1996, while use of sedating antidepressants increased by 146%.[154] In 2002, trazodone was the second most prescribed drug for insomnia, with amitriptyline and mirtazapine ranked as third and fourth, respectively.[155] Only 4 of the 16 most commonly used drugs for insomnia had an FDA indication for insomnia.[155] Data supplied by Verispan, Inc, for 2005 through 2007 suggest that prescribing patterns may be changing slightly. Use of trazodone and amitriptyline has begun to decline while use of BzRAs and ramelteon has increased.[156] Although sedating antidepressants may be used for insomnia coexistent with a mood disorder, their use is not limited to that situation. The majority of antidepressants used for insomnia in 2002 were prescribed at doses that are subtherapeutic for depression, suggesting that antidepressants are being used to treat insomnia alone, and not depression with comorbid insomnia.[155]

The neural mechanism mediating the sedating activity of these antidepressants is not identified, but it is unlikely that one common mechanism is involved. Trazodone is a weak inhibitor of serotonin reuptake and an antagonist of 5-HT2, 5-HT1A, 5-HT1C, and alpha-adrenergic receptors.[157–160] Amitriptyline inhibits the reuptake of serotonin and norepinephrine and blocks acetylcholine and histamine binding[157,161,162] Mirtazapine antagonizes 5-HT2A, 5-HT2C, 5-HT3, histamine1, and alpha1-adrenergic receptors.[163,164] The sedating effect of antidepressant is likely associated with multiple mechanisms, including the antagonism of histamine type 1 receptor, serotonin type 2 receptor, and alpha-adrenergic receptor. The adrenergic, histaminergic, and cholinergic systems in the brainstem, midbrain, and basal forebrain all are implicated strongly in the promotion and maintenance of wakefulness, and antagonizing these systems is likely to result in sedation. The serotonergic system plays a more controversial, less established, and perhaps more complicated role in wakefulness.

Efficacy in primary insomnia

The hypnotic efficacy of trazodone in primary insomnia has been investigated in two studies. The first examined the effect of trazodone (50 mg) on subjective sleep measures as compared with zolpidem (10 mg) and placebo in a 2-week, parallel-group design. Trazodone and zolpidem shortened latency to sleep onset and increased total sleep time, but improvements with zolpidem were greater than trazodone.[165] In an earlier study of nine individuals taking trazodone (150 mg a night for 3 weeks), there was no improvement in sleep latency or total sleep time, but there was a reduction in stage 1 sleep and wakefulness, along with an increase in stage 3-4 sleep.[166] Subjectively, there was an improvement in sleep quality. These findings suggest that trazodone may have some sleep-promoting effect in primary insomnia, at least short-term, but efficacy is not well established and the optimal dose remains undetermined.

Amitriptyline and mirtazapine are also used frequently as hypnotics for insomniacs who are not depressed,[164,167–169] despite the lack of published studies demonstrating their efficacy in this group of patients.

Safety in primary insomnia

Although the majority of safety data for the sedating antidepressants have been acquired from their use in mood or anxiety disorders at doses higher than those used for insomnia, antidepressants have more frequent and significant side effects than BzRAs.[166,170] In fact, these side effects are the primary reason why selective serotonin reuptake inhibitors are frequently preferred over tricyclics and other sedating antidepressants when treating depression.[171] Furthermore, the margin of safety (lethal dose to effective dose) is much smaller for sedating antidepressants compared with BzRAs.[172] Just as evidence for efficacy is lacking, the safety of antidepressants at doses typically used to treat insomnia has not been adequately evaluated in insomniac populations. Of the studies that have been conducted using primary insomnia patients, there are reports of leucopenia, thrombocytopenia, increased liver enzymes with doxepin[173]; dizziness, dry mouth, and nausea with trimipramine[174,175]; and daytime somnolence, dizziness, and weight gain with mirtazapine.[175] The safety of trazodone has not been extensively evaluated in patients with insomnia,[176] but one study has observed carry-over sedation among primary insomniacs taking 50 mg of trazodone.[165] In studies of depressed patients, side effects of trazodone include orthostatic hypotension, priapism, and cardiac arrhythmias and conduction abnormalities.[176–178]

Currently, there is insufficient data demonstrating the efficacy or safety of sedating antidepressants for primary insomnia, thus these medications have not been recommended as preferred treatment options.[176,179] Their frequent use for insomnia may have more to do with regulatory issues and misperceptions regarding the risks of BzRAs, despite available data that show risks are minimal.

Other Medications Used for Insomnia

Other drugs used off-label for the treatment of insomnia include antihistamines (ie, diphenhydramine, hydroxyzine), antipsychotics (ie, quetiapine, olanzepine), and muscle relaxants (eg, cyclobenzaprine). Little is known regarding their hypnotic efficacy for primary insomnia and safety concerns exist. In a few studies, diphenhydramine (at doses from 25 to 50 mg) was found to improve subjective measures such as global ratings,[180] number of awakenings,[181] as well as sleep latency and sleep quality.[182] However, tolerance to the sedative effect of diphenhydramine (25 to 50 mg, two or three times per day) has been shown to develop within 3 to 4 days,[183,184] and cognitive and psychomotor impairments have also been demonstrated.[185]

The atypical antipsychotics, quetiapine and olanzepine, have multiple mechanisms of action, including antagonism of serotonin, histaminergic, dopaminergic, and adrenergic receptors. Efficacy data for use in treating insomnia is quite limited. Small open-label studies lacking a placebo-control have shown that various dosages of quetiapine and olanzapine improved subjective measures of sleep in patients with primary[186] and comorbid insomnia.[187,188] Although the sedative property of these medications makes them potentially useful, their broad activity across the CNS results in several undesirable side effects, making them less tolerable.[77] Moreover, concerns regarding increased risk of metabolic syndrome exist.[189] Both of these antipsychotics reach peak plasma levels relatively slowly and have half-lives that make residual sedation likely.

CONSIDERATIONS FOR PHARMACOTHERAPY

The following information regarding pharmacotherapy for insomnia was extracted from previously published guidelines.[179,190] Hypnotic therapy should be considered for insomnia when the patient is significantly distressed by the presence or possibility of disturbed sleep, or when the physician judges the sleep disturbance to be deleterious to the patients' overall safety or health. The 2005 NIH *State of the Science* report on the management of chronic insomnia concluded that BzRAs are the only medications with an established scientific basis (ie, clearly defined risk benefit by dose) for treating insomnia.[3] At the time of this NIH report, ramelteon had not yet been FDA-approved for insomnia, but recent guidelines include this drug with the short- and intermediate-acting BzRAs, recommending these medications as preferable treatments for chronic insomnia.[179] There is also widespread agreement that a BzRA or ramelteon is an appropriate therapy for short-term insomnia. The recently approved doxepin can now be considered as an appropriate treatment option as well.

When selecting the specific hypnotic for treatment, the pharmacokinetics of the drug and the patient characteristics (eg, age, nature of the sleep problem, concurrent illness) should be considered. Other factors to consider are symptom pattern, treatment goals, past treatment responses, and cost. The dose and treatment regimen should be individualized and closely monitored by the physician, particularly in the first few days or weeks. The hypnotic should be taken only at the time and frequency prescribed. The initial dose should be the lowest clinically indicated dose, and the physician should determine effectiveness of that dose soon after initiation of treatment (eg, after 3–5 nights). The dose can then be adjusted as appropriate based on both efficacy and safety reports from the patient.

Hypnotics can be prescribed to be taken nightly, on a predetermined intermittent schedule (eg, every third night), or as needed.[92,93,191] With the exception of zaleplon, all medications should be taken only when the patient has the opportunity to stay in bed 7 to 8 hours. Zaleplon has been evaluated in middle-of-the-night dosing protocols (ie, medication is administered with 5 hours or less of bedtime remaining) and been found to improve sleep in the remaining bedtime without residual effects the next morning, although middle-of-the-night administration is not part of zaleplon's FDA indication.[192,193] If nightly hypnotic use is not desirable for a patient, they can be instructed to attempt sleep without medication and, if unsuccessful, to take the drug later, provided there are 4 to 5 hours remaining before they must arise. Thus, in cases of sleep maintenance insomnia characterized only by a middle-of-the-night awakening, or in cases of intermittent sleep-onset insomnia, middle-of-the-night administration could be considered.

The physician should specifically inquire about the aspects of sleep and daytime function that were most problematic for the patient before treatment, rather than relying solely on global statements. A sleep diary can be helpful for comparing pretreatment and posttreatment symptoms. Patient behavior and lifestyle factors should always be addressed with hypnotic therapy. Treatment should be accompanied by patient education of appropriate behavioral interventions (eg, inadequate sleep hygiene and excessive stimulation near bedtime magnifies nocturnal arousal). For primary insomniacs, who are otherwise reasonably healthy, monthly visits should be sufficient to identify most potential adverse effects. After longer-term use, gradual discontinuation, via dose tapering at a rate of one clinical dose per week, is a reasonable practice.

The primary contraindications to BzRA and ramelteon therapy are concomitant illnesses, such as obstructive sleep apnea, substance abuse disorder, or advanced hepatic disease. All sedative medications have the potential to worsen sleep apnea by blunting arousal from sleep, although central apnea has been reduced by a BzRA in some investigations.[194] The dependence liability of BzRAs and other sedative drugs, although not high, leads to the conclusion that most patients with a history of alcoholism or drug abuse should not receive BzRAs in outpatient settings without close supervision. Caution is advised for moderate users of alcohol because of additive sedative effects with hypnotics, which narrows the wide margin of safety described earlier. Because most BzRAs undergo hepatic metabolism, advanced liver disease requires the use of a lower dose or avoidance of these medications. Ramelteon might be considered when there are concerns regarding substance abuse, particularly if the complaint is sleep initiation difficulty; however, this drug has not been specifically evaluated in the substance abuse population.

Pharmacotherapy for insomnia during pregnancy is also contraindicated; the teratogenic effects of all psychoactive drugs are a matter of concern. People who may be required to awaken and perform duties in the middle of the night should avoid CNS-depressant drugs when "on call." All hypnotics have the potential to disrupt alertness and cognitive function for the duration of the sedative activity of the drug, and they may impact motor function.

SUMMARY

The BzRAs remain the most effective, safe, and well-understood therapeutic agents for the treatment of primary insomnia, as well as comorbid and transient insomnia. Pharmacokinetic characteristics are the most clinically relevant differences among the BzRAs. The melatonin receptor antagonist, ramelteon, is an alternative for some patients with only sleep onset difficulty. Use of other drugs for the treatment of primary insomnia is not supported by empirical evidence.

REFERENCES

1. American Psychiatric Association. Diagnostic and Statistical Manual of Mental Disorders. 4th edition. Text revision: Washington, DC: American Psychiatric Publishing, Inc; 2000.
2. Edinger JD, Bonnet MH, Bootzin RR, et al. Derivation of research diagnostic criteria for insomnia: report of an American Academy of Sleep Medicine work group. Sleep 2004;27(8):1567–96.
3. National Institutes of Health. National Institutes of Health State of the Science Conference Statement: manifestations and management of chronic insomnia in adults. Sleep 2005;28:1049–57.
4. Leger D, Guilleminault C, Dreyfus JP, et al. Prevalence of insomnia in a survey of 12,778 adults in France. J Sleep Res 2000;9(1):35–42.
5. Roth T, Coulouvrat C, Hajak G, et al. Differences in the prevalence and perceived health associated with insomnia based on DSM-IV-TR, ICD-10, and RDC/ICSD-2 criteria: results from the America Insomnia Survey (AIS). Biological Psychiatry, in press.
6. Ohayon MM. Prevalence of DSM-IV diagnostic criteria of insomnia: distinguishing insomnia related to mental disorders from sleep disorders. J Psychiatr Res 1997;31(3):333–46.
7. Ohayon MM. Epidemiology of insomnia: what we know and what we still need to learn. Sleep Med Rev 2002;6(2):97–111.
8. Ram S, Seirawan H, Kumar SKS, et al. Prevalence and impact of sleep disorders and sleep habits in the United States. Sleep Breath 2010; 14(1):63–70.
9. Ohayon MM, Roth T. What are the contributing factors for insomnia in the general population? J Psychosom Res 2001;51:745–55.
10. Weyerer S, Dilling H. Prevalence and treatment of insomnia in the community: results from the Upper Bavarian Field Study. Sleep 1991;14(5):392–8.
11. Sutton DA, Moldofsky H, Badley EM. Insomnia and health problems in Canadians. Sleep 2001;24(6): 665–70.
12. Chevalier H, Los F, Boichut D, et al. Evaluation of severe insomnia in the general population: results of a European multinational survey. J Psychopharmacol 1999;13(4 Suppl 1):S21–4.
13. Bonnet MH, Arand DL. Hyperarousal and insomnia. Sleep Med Rev 1997;1(2):97–108.
14. Benoit O, Aguirre A. Homeostatic and circadian aspects of sleep regulation in young poor sleepers. Clin Neurophysiol 1996;26:40–50.
15. Vgontzas AN, Zoumakis M, Papanicolaou DA, et al. Chronic insomnia is associated with a shift of interleukin-6 and tumour necrosis factor secretion from nighttime to daytime. Metabolism 2002;51: 887–92.

16. Perlis ML, Giles DE, Mendelson WB, et al. Psycho-physiological insomnia: the behavioural model and a neurocognitive perspective. J Sleep Res 1997;6: 179–88.

17. Espie CA, Broomfield NM, MacMahon K, et al. The attention-intention-effort pathway in the development of psychophysiologic insomnia: a theoretical review. Sleep Med Rev 2006;10:215–45.

18. Harvey AG. A cognitive model of insomnia. Behav Res Ther 2002;40:869–93.

19. Riemann D, Spiegelhalder K, Feige B, et al. The hyperarousal model of insomnia: a review of the concept and its evidence. Sleep Med Rev 2010; 14(1):19–31.

20. Kales A, Caldwell AB, Soldatos CR, et al. Biopsychobehavioral correlates of insomnia. II. Pattern specificity and consistency with the Minnesota Multiphasic Personality Inventory. Psychosom Med 1983;45(4):341–56.

21. Kales A, Caldwell AB, Preston TA, et al. Personality patterns in insomnia. Arch Gen Psychiatry 1976;33: 1128–34.

22. Monroe LJ. Psychological and physiological differences between good and poor sleepers. J Abnorm Psychol 1967;72:255–64.

23. Stepanski E, Glinn M, Zorick FJ, et al. Heart rate changes in chronic insomnia. Stress Med 1994; 10:261–6.

24. Bonnet MH, Arand DL. Heart rate variability in insomniacs and matched normal sleepers. Psychosom Med 1998;60(5):610–5.

25. Bonnet MH, Arand DL. 24-Hour metabolic rate in insomniacs and matched normal sleepers. Sleep 1995;18(7):581–8.

26. Bonnet MH, Arand DL. Physiological activation in patients with sleep state misperception. Psychosom Med 1997;59:533–40.

27. Irwin M, Clark C, Kennedy B, et al. Nocturnal catecholamines and immune function in insomniacs, depressed patients, and control subjects. Brain Behav Immun 2003;17:365–72.

28. Rodenbeck A, Hajak G. Neuroendocrine dysregulation in primary insomnia. Rev Neurol 2001;157: S57–61.

29. Vgontzas AN, Bixler EO, Lin H, et al. Chronic insomnia is associated with nyctohemeral activation of the hypothalamic-pituitary axis: clinical implications. J Clin Endocrinol Metab 2001;86: 3787–94.

30. Lichstein KL, Wilson NM, Noe SL, et al. Daytime sleepiness in insomnia: behavioral, biological and subjective indices. Sleep 1994;17(8):693–702.

31. Sugerman JL, Stern JA, Walsh JK. Daytime alertness in subjective and objective insomnia: some preliminary findings. Biol Psychiatry 1985;20(7):741–50.

32. Seidel WF, Ball S, Cohen S, et al. Daytime alertness in relation to mood, performance, and nocturnal sleep in chronic insomniacs and noncomplaining sleepers. Sleep 1984;7(3):230–8.

33. Stepanski E, Zorick F, Roehrs T, et al. Daytime alertness in patients with chronic insomnia compared with asymptomatic control subjects. Sleep 1988; 11(1):54–60.

34. Rosa R, Bonnet M. Reported chronic insomnia is independent of poor sleep as measured by electroencephalography. Psychosom Med 2000; 62:474–82.

35. Ancoli-Israel S, Martin JL. Insomnia and daytime napping in older adults. J Clin Sleep Med 2006; 2(3):333–42.

36. Perlis ML, Smith MT, Andrews PJ, et al. Beta/gamma EEG activity in patients with primary and secondary insomnia and good sleeper controls. Sleep 2001;24(1):110–7.

37. Merica H, Blois R, Gaillard J-M. Spectral characteristics of sleep EEG in chronic insomnia. Eur J Neurosci 1998;10:1826–34.

38. Krystal AD, Edinger JD, Wohlgemuth WK, et al. Non-REM sleep EEG frequency spectral correlates of sleep complaints in primary insomnia subtypes. Sleep 2002;25:630–40.

39. Buysse DJ, Germain A, Hall ML, et al. EEG spectral analysis in primary insomnia: NREM period effects and sex differences. Sleep 2008;31:1673–82.

40. Freedman RR. EEG power spectra in sleep-onset insomnia. Electroencephalogr Clin Neurophysiol 1986;63:408–13.

41. Perlis ML, Merica H, Smith MT, et al. Beta EEG activity and insomnia. Sleep Med Rev 2001;5(5): 363–74.

42. Nofzinger EA, Buysse DJ, Germain A, et al. Functional neuroimaging evidence for hyperarousal in insomnia. Am J Psychiatry 2004;161(11):2126–8.

43. Nofzinger EA, Nissen C, Germain A, et al. Regional cerebral metabolic correlates of WASO during NREM sleep in insomnia. J Clin Sleep Med 2006; 2(3):316–22.

44. Hauri PJ. Cognitive deficits in insomnia patients. Acta Neurol Belg 1997;97:113–7.

45. Mendelson WB, Garnett D, Linnoila M. Do insomniacs have impaired daytime functioning? Biol Psychiatry 1984;19:1261–4.

46. Varkevisser M, Van Dongen HP, Van Amsterdam JG, et al. Chronic insomnia and daytime functioning: an ambulatory assessment. Behav Sleep Med 2007; 5(4):279–96.

47. Orff HJ, Drummond SP, Nowakowski S, et al. Discrepancy between subjective symptomatology and objective neuropsychological performance in insomnia. Sleep 2007;30(9):1205–11.

48. Vignola A, Lamoureux C, Bastien CH, et al. Effects of chronic insomnia and use of benzodiazepines on daytime performance in older adults. J Gerontol B Psychol Sci Soc Sci 2000;55(1):P54–62.

49. Varkevisser M, Kerkhof GA. Chronic insomnia and performance in a 24-h constant routine study. J Sleep Res 2005;14(1):49–59.

50. Altena E, Van Der Werf YD, Strijers RL, et al. Sleep loss affects vigilance: effects of chronic insomnia and sleep therapy. J Sleep Res 2008;17(3):335–43.

51. Broman J-E, Lundh L-G, Aleman K, et al. Subjective and objective performance in patients with persistent insomnia. Cogn Behav Ther 1992;21(3):115–26.

52. Edinger JD, Means MK, Carney CE, et al. Psychomotor performance deficits and their relation to prior nights' sleep among individuals with primary insomnia. Sleep 2008;31(5):599–607.

53. Nissen C, Kloepfer C, Nofzinger EA, et al. Impaired sleep-related memory consolidation in primary insomnia. Sleep 2006;29:1068–73.

54. Backhaus J, Junghanns K, Born J, et al. Impaired declarative memory consolidation during sleep in patients with primary insomnia: influence of sleep architecture and nocturnal cortisol release. Biol Psychiatry 2006;60:1324–30.

55. Breslau N, Roth T, Rosenthal L, et al. Sleep disturbance and psychiatric disorders: a longitudinal epidemiological study of young adults. Biol Psychiatry 1996;39:411–8.

56. Ford DE, Kamerow DB. Epidemiologic study of sleep disturbances and psychiatric disorders: an opportunity for prevention? J Am Med Assoc 1989;262:1479–84.

57. Weissman MM, Greenwald S, Nino-Murcia G, et al. The morbidity of insomnia uncomplicated by psychiatric disorders. Gen Hosp Psychiatry 1997;19:245–50.

58. Cho HJ, Lavretsky H, Olmstead R, et al. Sleep disturbance and depression recurrence in community-dwelling older adults: a prospective study. Am J Psychiatry 2008;165(12):1543–50.

59. Agargun MY, Kara H, Solmaz M. Sleep disturbances and suicidal behavior in patients with major depression. J Clin Psychiatry 1997;58(6):249–51.

60. Fawcett J, Scheftner WA, Fogg L, et al. Time-related predictors of suicide in major affective disorder. Am J Psychiatry 1990;147(9):1189–94.

61. Spira AP, Friedman L, Aulakh JS, et al. Subclinical anxiety symptoms, sleep, and daytime dysfunction in older adults with primary insomnia. J Geriatr Psychiatry Neurol 2008;21:149–53.

62. Neckelmann D, Mykletun A, Dahl AA. Chronic insomnia as a risk factor for developing anxiety and depression. Sleep 2007;30:873–80.

63. Conroy DA, Arnedt TJ, Brower KJ, et al. Perception of sleep in recovering alcohol-dependent patients with insomnia: relationship with future drinking. Alcohol Clin Exp Res 2006;30(12):1992–9.

64. Zammit GK, Weiner J, Damato N, et al. Quality of life in people with insomnia. Sleep 1999;22(Suppl 2):S379–85.

65. Katz DA, McHorney CA. The relationship between insomnia and health-related quality of life in patients with chronic illness. J Fam Pract 2002;51(3):229–35.

66. Chilcott LA, Shapiro CM. The socioeconomic impact of insomnia: an overview. Pharmacoeconomics 1996;10(Suppl 1):1–14.

67. Ozminkowski RJ, Wang S, Walsh JK. The direct and indirect costs of untreated insomnia in adults in the United States. Sleep 2007;30(3):263–73.

68. Balter MB, Uhlenhuth EH. New epidemiologic findings about insomnia and its treatment. J Clin Psychiatry 1992;53(Suppl 12):34–9.

69. Kuppermann M, Lubeck DP, Mazonson PD, et al. Sleep problems and their correlates in a working population. J Gen Intern Med 1995;10(1):25–32.

70. Bonnet MH, Arand DL. Hyperarousal and insomnia: state of the science. Sleep Med Rev 2010;14:9–15.

71. Suka M, Yoshida K, Sugimori H. Persistent insomnia is a predictor of hypertension in Japanese male workers. J Occup Health 2003;45:344–50.

72. Vgontzas AN, Liao D, Bixler EO, et al. Insomnia with objective short sleep duration is associated with a high risk for hypertension. Sleep 2009;32:491–7.

73. Bonnet MH, Arand DL. Cardiovascular implications of poor sleep. Sleep Med Clin 2007;2:529–38.

74. Schwartz S, Anderson WM, Cole SR, et al. Insomnia and heart disease: a review of epidemiologic studies. J Psychosom Res 1999;47:313–33.

75. Greenblatt DJ, Shader RI. Benzodiazepines in clinical practice. New York: Raven Press; 1974.

76. Kan CC, Hilberink SR, Breteler MH. Determination of the main risk factors for benzodiazepine dependence using a multivariate and multidimensional approach. Compr Psychiatry 2004;45:88–94.

77. Stahl S. Stahl's essential psychopharmacology: neuroscientific basis and practical applications. 3rd edition. New York: Cambridge University Press; 2008.

78. Sieghart W. Structure and pharmacology of gamma-aminobutyric acid A receptor subtypes. Pharmacol Rev 1995;47:181–234.

79. Nutt D. GABA-A receptors: subtypes, regional distribution, and function. J Clin Sleep Med 2006;2:S7–11.

80. Doble A, Canton T, Malgouris C, et al. The mechanism of action of zopiclone. Eur Psychiatry 1995;10(Suppl 3):117S–28S.

81. Nowell PD, Mazumdar S, Buysse DJ, et al. Benzodiazepines and zolpidem for chronic insomnia: a meta-analysis of treatment efficacy. JAMA 1997;278:2170–7.

82. Holbrook AM, Crowther R, Lotter A, et al. Meta-analysis of benzodiazepine use in the treatment of insomnia. Can Med Assoc J 2000;162(2): 225–33.

83. Dündar Y, Dodd S, Strobl J, et al. Comparative efficacy of newer hypnotic drugs for the short-term management of insomnia: a systematic review and meta-analysis. Hum Psychopharmacol 2004; 19(5):305–22.

84. Smith MT, Perlis ML, Park A, et al. Comparative meta-analysis of pharmacotherapy and behavior therapy for persistent insomnia. Am J Psychiatry 2002;159(1):5–11.

85. Walsh JK, Vogel GW, Scharf M, et al. A five week, polysomnographic assessment of zaleplon 10 mg for the treatment of primary insomnia. Sleep Med 2000;1:41–9.

86. Oswald I, French C, Adam K, et al. Benzodiazepine hypnotics remain effective for 24 weeks. Br Med J (Clin Res Ed) 1982;284:860–3.

87. Scharf MB, Roth T, Vogel GW, et al. A multicenter, placebo-controlled study evaluating zolpidem in the treatment of chronic insomnia. J Clin Psychiatry 1994;55:192–9.

88. Krystal AD, Walsh JK, Laska E, et al. Sustained efficacy of eszopiclone over 6 months of nightly treatment: results of a randomized, double-blind, placebo-controlled study in adults with chronic insomnia. Sleep 2003;26:793–9.

89. Walsh JK, Krystal AD, Amato DA, et al. Nightly treatment of primary insomnia with eszopiclone for six months: effect on sleep, quality of life and work limitations. Sleep 2007;30:959–68.

90. Roth T, Walsh J, Krystal A, et al. An evaluation of the efficacy and safety of eszopiclone over 12 months in patients with chronic primary insomnia. Sleep Med 2005;6:487–95.

91. Scharf MB, Black J, Hull S, et al. Long-term nightly treatment with indiplon in adults with primary insomnia: results of a double-blind, placebo-controlled, 3-month study. Sleep 2007;30:743–52.

92. Walsh JK, Roth T, Randazzo AC, et al. Eight weeks of non-nightly use of zolpidem for primary insomnia. Sleep 2000;23:1087–96.

93. Perlis M, McCall WV, Krystal A, et al. Long-term, non-nightly administration of zolpidem in the treatment of patients with primary insomnia. J Clin Psychiatry 2004;65:1128–37.

94. Krystal AD, Erman M, Zammit GK, et al. ZOLONG Study Group. Long-term efficacy and safety of zolpidem extended-release 12.5 mg, administered 3 to 7 nights per week for 24 weeks, in patients with chronic primary insomnia: a 6-month, randomized, double-blind, placebo-controlled, parallel-group, multicenter study. Sleep 2008;31:79–90.

95. Ohayon MM, Caulet M, Arbus L, et al. Are prescribed medications effective in the treatment of insomnia complaints? J Psychosom Res 1999; 47:359–68.

96. Balter MB, Uhlenhuth EH. The beneficial and adverse effects of hypnotics. J Clin Psychiatry 1991;52(Suppl):16–23.

97. Kummer J, Linden J, Eich FX, et al. Long-term polysomnographic efficacy and safety of zolpidem in elderly psychiatric in-patients with insomnia. J Int Med Res 1993;21:171–84.

98. Maarek L, Cramer P, Coquelin JP, et al. The safety and efficacy of zolpidem in insomnia patients: a long-term open study in general practice. J Int Med Res 1991;20:162–70.

99. Schlich D, L'Heritier C, Coquelin JP, et al. Long-term treatment of insomnia with zolpidem: a multicentre general practitioner study of 107 patients. J Int Med Res 1991;19:271–9.

100. Ancoli-Israel S, Richardson GS, Mangano RM, et al. Long-term use of sedative hypnotics in older patients with insomnia. Sleep Med 2005;6: 107–13.

101. Mendelson WB, Thompson C, Franko T. Adverse reactions to sedative/hypnotics: three years' experience. Sleep 1996;19:702–6.

102. Roth T, Roehrs T. Issues in the use of benzodiazepine therapy. J Clin Psychiatry 1992;53:S14–8.

103. Roth T, Roehrs TA, Stepanski EJ, et al. Hypnotics and behavior. Am J Med 1990;8:43S–6S.

104. Greenblatt D, Harmatz JS, Shapiro L, et al. Sensitivity to triazolam in elderly. N Engl J Med 1991; 324:1691–8.

105. Merlotti L, Roehrs T, Zorick F, et al. Rebound insomnia: duration of use and individual differences. J Clin Psychopharmacol 1991;11:368–73.

106. Roehrs T, Vogel G, Roth T. Rebound insomnia: its determinants and significance. Am J Med 1990; 88:39S–42S.

107. Roehrs T, Merlotti L, Zorick F, et al. Rebound insomnia in normals and patients with insomnia after abrupt and tapered discontinuation. Psychopharmacology 1992;108:67–71.

108. Woods JH, Katz JL, Winger G. Benzodiazepines: use, abuse, and consequences. Pharmacol Rev 1992;44(2):151–347.

109. Silvestri R, Ferrillo F, Murri L, et al. Rebound insomnia after abrupt discontinuation of hypnotic treatment: double-blind randomized comparison of zolpidem versus triazolam. Hum Psychopharmacol 1996;11(3):225–33.

110. Erman M, Krystal A, Zammit G, et al. Long-term efficacy of zolpidem extended-release in the treatment of sleep maintenance and sleep onset insomnia with improvements in next-day functioning. Sleep 2007;30(Suppl):A241.

111. Erman M, Krystal A, Zammit G, et al. No evidence of rebound insomnia in patients with chronic insomnia treated with zolpidem extended-release

12.5 mg administered as needed 3–7 nights/week for 6 months. Sleep 2007;30(Suppl):A241–2.

112. Elie R, Ruther E, Farr I, et al. Sleep latency is shortened during 4 weeks of treatment with zaleplon, a novel non-benzodiazepine hypnotic. Zaleplon Clinical Study Group. J Clin Psychiatry 1999;60(8):536–44.

113. Fry J, Scharf M, Mangano R, et al. Zaleplon improves sleep without producing rebound effects in outpatients with insomnia. Zaleplon Clinical Study Group. Int Clin Psychopharmacol 2000; 15(3):141–52.

114. Walsh JK, Fry J, Erwin CW, et al. Efficacy and tolerability of 14-day administration of zaleplon 5 mg and 10 mg for the treatment of primary insomnia. Clin Drug Investig 1998;16(5):347–54.

115. Ancoli-Israel S, Walsh JK, Mangano RM, et al. Zaleplon: a novel nonbenzodiazepine hypnotic, effectively treats insomnia in elderly patients without causing rebound effects. Prim care companion. J Clin Psychiatry 1999;1(4):114–20.

116. Zammit GK, McNabb LJ, Caron J, et al. Efficacy and safety of eszopiclone across 6-weeks of treatment for primary insomnia. Curr Med Res Opin 2004;20(12):1979–91.

117. Krystal A, Walsh JK, Rubens R, et al. Efficacy and safety of six-months of nightly eszopiclone in patients with primary insomnia: a second long term placebo-controlled study. Sleep 2006; 29(Suppl):A249.

118. Mellinger GD, Balter MB, Uhlenhuth EH. Insomnia and its treatment. Arch Gen Psychiatry 1985;42: 225–32.

119. Roehrs T, Hollebeek E, Drake C, et al. Substance use for insomnia in Metropolitan Detroit. J Psychosom Res 2002;53:571–6.

120. Johnson EO, Roehrs T, Roth T, et al. Epidemiology of alcohol and medication as aids to sleep in early adulthood. Sleep 1998;21(2):178–86.

121. Roehrs T, Pedrosi B, Rosenthal L, et al. Hypnotic self administration and dose escalation. Psychopharmacology 1996;127:150–4.

122. Roehrs T, Bonahoom A, Pedrosi B, et al. Nighttime versus daytime hypnotic self-administration. Psychopharmacology 2002;161:137–42.

123. Roehrs T, Bonahoom A, Pedrosi B, et al. Disturbed sleep predicts hypnotic self administration. Sleep Med 2002;3:61–6.

124. Roehrs T, Merlotti L, Zorick F, et al. Rebound insomnia and hypnotic self administration. Psychopharmacology 1992;107:480–4.

125. Brassington GS, King AC, Bliwise DL. Sleep problems as a risk factor for falls in a sample of community-dwelling adults aged 64–99 years. J Am Geriatr Soc 2000;48(10):1234–40.

126. Avidan AY, Fries BE, James ML, et al. Insomnia and hypnotic use, recorded in the minimum data set, as predictors of falls and hip fractures in Michigan nursing homes. J Am Geriatr Soc 2005;53(6): 955–62.

127. Yang W, Dollear M, Muthukrishnan SR. One rare side effect of zolpidem—sleepwalking: a case report. Arch Phys Med Rehabil 2005;86:1265–6.

128. Liskow B, Pikalov A. Zaleplon overdose associated with sleepwalking and complex behavior. J Am Acad Child Adolesc Psychiatry 2004;43:927–8.

129. Morgenthaler TI, Silber MH. Amnestic sleep-related eating disorder associated with zolpidem. Sleep Med 2002;3:323–7.

130. Vetrugno R, Manconi M, Ferini-Strembi LF, et al. Nocturnal eating: sleep-related eating disorder or nocturnal eating syndrome? A videopolysomnographic study. Sleep 2006;29:949–54.

131. Karim A, Tolbert D, Cao C. Disposition kinetics and tolerance of escalating single doses of ramelteon, a high-affinity MT1 and MT2 melatonin receptor agonist indicated for treatment of insomnia. J Clin Pharmacol 2006;46:140–8.

132. Hibberd M, Stevenson SJ. A phase-I open-label study of the absorption, metabolism, and excretion of (14C)-ramelteon (TAK-375) following a single oral dose in healthy male subjects. Sleep 2004; 27:A54.

133. Kato K, Hirai K, Nishiyama K, et al. Neurochemical properties of ramelteon (TAK-375), a selective MT1/MT2 receptor agonist. Neuropharmacology 2005;48(2):301–10.

134. Uchikawa O, Fukatsu K, Tokunoh R, et al. Synthesis of a novel series of tricyclic Indian derivatives as melatonin receptor agonists. J Med Chem 2002; 45:4222–39.

135. Liu C, Weaver DR, Jin X, et al. Molecular dissection of two distinct actions of melatonin on the suprachiasmatic circadian clock. Neuron 1997;19:91–102.

136. Dubocovich ML. Selective MT2 melatonin receptor antagonists block melatonin-mediated phase advances of circadian rhythms. FASEB J 1998;12: 1211–20.

137. Dubocovich ML. Molecular pharmacology, regulation and function of mammalian melatonin receptors. Front Biosci 2003;8:d1093–108.

138. Von Gall C, Stehle JH, Weaver DR. Mammalian melatonin receptors: molecular biology and signal transduction. Cell Tissue Res 2002;309: 151–62.

139. Erman M, Seiden D, Zammit G, et al. An efficacy, safety, and dose-response study of ramelteon in patients with chronic primary insomnia. Sleep Med 2006;7:17–24.

140. Roth T, Seiden D, Sainati S, et al. Effects of ramelteon on patient-reported sleep latency in older adults with chronic insomnia. Sleep Med 2006;7: 312–8.

141. Roth T, Seiden D, Wang-Weigand S, et al. A 2-night, 3-period crossover study of ramelteon's

efficacy and safety in older adults with chronic insomnia. Curr Med Res Opin 2007;23:1005–14.

142. Zammit G, Erman M, Wang-Weigand S, et al. Evaluation of the efficacy and safety of ramelteon in subjects with chronic insomnia. J Clin Sleep Med 2007;3:495–504.

143. Mayer G, Wang-Weigand S, Roth-Schechter B, et al. Efficacy and safety of 6-month nightly ramelteon administration in adults with chronic primary insomnia. Sleep 2009;32(3):351–60.

144. DeMicco M, Wang-Weigand S, Zhang J. Long-term therapeutic effects of ramelteon treatment in adults with chronic insomnia: a 1 year study. Sleep 2006; 29(Suppl):A234.

145. Richardson GS, Zee PC, Wang-Weigand S, et al. Circadian phase-shifting effects of repeated ramelteon administration in healthy adults. J Clin Sleep Med 2008;4(5):456–61.

146. Borja NL, Daniel KL. Ramelteon for the treatment of insomnia. Clin Ther 2006;28:1540–55.

147. Roth T, Stubbs C, Walsh J. Ramelteon (TAK-375), a selective MT1/MT2 receptor agonist, reduces latency to persistent sleep in a model of transient insomnia related to a novel sleep environment. Sleep 2005;28(3):303–7 [erratum in: Sleep 2006; 29(4):417].

148. Griffiths R, Suess P, Johnson M. Ramelteon and triazolam in humans: behavioral effects and abuse potential. Sleep 2005;28:A44.

149. Zammit G, Roth T, Erman M, et al. Double-blind, placebo-controlled polysomnography and outpatient trial to evaluate the efficacy and safety of ramelteon in adult patients with chronic insomnia. Sleep 2005;28(Suppl):A228–9.

150. Johnson MW, Suess PE, Griffiths RR. Ramelteon: a novel hypnotic lacking abuse liability and sedative adverse effects. Arch Gen Psychiatry 2006; 63:1149–57.

151. Roth T, Rogowski R, Hull S, et al. Efficacy and safety of doxepin 1 mg, 3 mg, and 6 mg in adults with primary insomnia. Sleep 2007;30(11):1555–61.

152. Scharf M, Rogowski R, Hull S, et al. Efficacy and safety of doxepin 1 mg, 3 mg, and 6 mg in elderly patients with primary insomnia: a randomized, double-blind, placebo-controlled crossover study. J Clin Psychiatry 2008;69(10):1557–64.

153. Owen RT. Selective histamine H(1) antagonism: a novel approach to insomnia using low-dose doxepin. Drugs Today (Barc) 2009;45(4):261–7.

154. Walsh JK, Schweitzer PK. Ten year trends in the pharmacologic treatment of insomnia. Sleep 1999; 22:371–5.

155. Walsh JK. Drugs used to treat insomnia in 2002: regulatory-based rather than evidence-based medicine. Sleep 2004;27(8):1441–2.

156. Schweitzer PK, Curry DT, Eisenstein RD, et al. Pharmacological treatment of insomnia. In: Attarian HP,

Schuman C, editors. Clinical handbook of insomnia. 2nd edition. New York (NY): Humana Press, c/o Springer Science + Business Media LLC; 2010. p. 297–316.

157. Frazer A. Pharmacology of antidepressants. J Clin Psychopharmacol 1997;17(Suppl 1):2S–18S.

158. Marek GJ, McDougle CJ, Price LH, et al. A comparison of trazodone and fluoxetine: implications for a serotonergic mechanism of antidepressant action. Psychopharmacology 1992;109(1–2):2–11.

159. Cusak B, Nelson A, Richelson E. Binding of antidepressants to human brain receptors: focus on newer generation compounds. Psychopharmacology 1994;114(4):559–65.

160. Brogden RN, Heel RC, Speight TM, et al. Trazodone: a review of its pharmacologic properties and therapeutic use in depression and anxiety. Drugs 1981;21:401–29.

161. Preskorn SH. Pharmacokinetics of antidepressants: why and how they are relevant to treatment. J Clin Psychiatry 1993;54(Suppl):14–34.

162. Richelson E. The pharmacology of antidepressants at the synapse: focus on newer compounds. J Clin Psychiatry 1994;55(Suppl A):34–9.

163. De Boer T. The pharmacological profile of mirtazapine. J Clin Psychiatry 1996;57(Suppl 4):19–25.

164. Radhakishun FS, van den Bos J, van der Heijden BC, et al. Mirtazapine effects on alertness and sleep in patients as recorded by interactive telecommunication during treatment with different dosing regimens. J Clin Psychopharmacol 2000;20(5):531–7.

165. Walsh JK, Erman M, Erwin CW, et al. Subjective hypnotic efficacy of trazodone and zolpidem in DSM-III-R primary insomnia. Hum Psychopharmacol 1998;13:191–8.

166. Montgomery I, Oswald I, Morgan K, et al. Trazodone enhances sleep in subjective quality but not in objective duration. Br J Clin Pharmacol 1983; 16:139–44.

167. Gillin JC, Wyatt RJ, Fram D, et al. The relationship between changes in REM sleep and clinical improvement in depressed patients treated with amitriptyline. Psychopharmacology (Berl) 1978;59:267–72.

168. Hartmann E, Cravens J. The effects of long-term administration of psychotropic drugs on human sleep: III. The effects of amitriptyline. Psychopharmacologia 1973;33:185–202.

169. Schmid DA, Wichniak A, Uhr M, et al. Changes of sleep architecture, spectral composition of sleep EEG, the nocturnal secretion of cortisol, ACTH, GH, prolactin, melatonin, ghrelin, and leptin, and the DEX-CRH test in depressed patients during treatment with mirtazapine. Neuropsychopharmacology 2006;31:832–44.

170. Sharpley AL, Cowen PJ. Effects of pharmacologic treatments on the sleep of depressed patients. Biol Psychiatry 1995;37:85–98.

171. Peretti S, Judge R, Hindmarch I. Safety and tolerability considerations: tricyclic antidepressants vs serotonin reuptake inhibitors. Acta Psychiatr Scand 2000;101(Suppl 403):17−25.

172. Bliwise DL. Treating insomnia: pharmacological and nonpharmacological approaches. J Psychoactive Drugs 1991;23(4):335−41.

173. Hajak G, Rodenbeck A, Voderholzer U, et al. Doxepin in the treatment of primary insomnia: a placebo-controlled, double-blind, polysomnographic study. J Clin Psychiatry 2001;62:453−63.

174. Riemann D, Voderholzer U, Cohrs S, et al. Trimipramine in primary insomnia: results of a polysomnographic double-blind controlled study. Pharmacopsychiatry 2002;35:165−74.

175. Mir S, Taylor D. The adverse effects of antidepressants [mood disorders]. Curr Opin Psychiatry 1997;10:88−94.

176. Mendelson WB. A review of the evidence for the efficacy and safety of trazodone in insomnia. J Clin Psychiatry 2005;66(4):469−76.

177. Haria M, Fitton A, McTavish D. Trazodone: a review of its pharmacology, therapeutic use in depression Drugs Aging 1994;4:331−55.

178. Golden RN, Dawkins K, Nicholas L. Trazodone and nefazodone. In: Schatzberg A, Nemeroff CB, editors. The American Psychiatric Publishing Textbook of Psychopharmacology. 4th edition. Washington, DC: American Psychiatric Publishing; 2009. p. 403−14.

179. Schutte-Rodin S, Broch L, Buysse D, et al. Clinical guideline for the evaluation and management of chronic insomnia in adults. J Clin Sleep Med 2008;4(5):487−504.

180. Kudo Y, Kurihara M. Clinical evaluation of diphenhydramine hydrochloride for the treatment of insomnia in psychiatric patients: a double-blind study. J Clin Pharmacol 1990;30:1041−8.

181. Glass JR, Sproule BA, Herrmann N, et al. Effects of 2-week treatment with temazepam and diphenhydramine in elderly insomniacs: a randomized, placebo-controlled trial. J Clin Psychopharmacol 2008;28(2):182−8.

182. Rickels K, Morris RJ, Newman H, et al. Diphenhydramine in insomniac family practice patients: a double- blind study. J Clin Pharmacol 1983; 23(5−6):234−42.

183. Schweitzer PK, Muehlbach MJ, Walsh JK. Sleepiness and performance during three-day administration of cetirizine or diphenhydramine. J Allergy Clin Immunol 1994;94:716−24.

184. Richardson GS, Roehrs TA, Rosenthal L, et al. Tolerance to daytime sedative effects of H1 antihistamines. J Clin Psychopharmacol 2002;22:511−5.

185. Basu R, Dodge H, Stoehr GP, et al. Sedative-hypnotic use of diphenhydramine in a rural, older adult, community-based cohort: effects on cognition. Am J Geriatr Psychiatry 2003;11:205−13.

186. Wiegand M, Landry T, Bruckner T, et al. Quetiapine in primary insomnia: a pilot study. Psychopharmacology 2008;196:337−8.

187. Juri C, Chana P, Tapia J, et al. Quetiapine for insomnia in Parkinson disease: results from an open-label trial. Clin Neuropharmacol 2005;28(4):185−7.

188. Estivill E, de la Fuente V, Segarra F, et al. The use of olanzapine in sleep disorders. An open trial with nine patients. Rev Neurol 2004;38(9):829−31.

189. Cates ME, Jackson CW, Feldman JM, et al. Metabolic consequences of using low-dose quetiapine for insomnia in psychiatric patients. Community Ment Health J 2009;45(4):251−4.

190. Curry DT, Eisenstein RD, Walsh JK. Pharmacologic management of insomnia: past, present, and future. Psychiatr Clin North Am 2006;29:871−93.

191. Hajak G, Cluydts R, Declerck A, et al. Continuous versus non-nightly use of zolpidem in chronic insomnia: results of a large-scale, double-blind, randomized, outpatient study. Int Clin Psychopharmacol 2002;17:9−17.

192. Walsh JK, Pollak CP, Scharf MB, et al. Lack of residual sedation following middle-of-the-night zaleplon administration in sleep maintenance insomnia. Clin Neuropharmacol 2000;23:17−21.

193. Danjou P, Paty I, Fruncillo R, et al. A comparison of the residual effects of zaleplon and zolpidem following administration 5 to 2 hrs before awakening. Br J Clin Pharmacol 1999;48:367−74.

194. Bonnet MH, Dexter JR, Arand DL. The effect of triazolam on arousal and respiration in central sleep apnea patients. Sleep 1990;13(1):31−41.

195. Miura M, Otani K, Ohkubo T. Identification of human cytochrome P450 enzymes involved in the formation of 4-hydroxyestazolam from estazolam. Xenobiotica 2005;35(5):455−65.

196. D'Empaire I, Preskorn SH. CYP enzyme system and its relevance to the pharmacology of sleep. In: Pandi-Perumal SR, Verster JC, Monti JM, et al, editors. Sleep disorders: diagnosis and therapeutics. London: Informa Healthcare; 2008. p. 133−9.

197. Lilja JJ, Kivisto KT, Backman JT, et al. Effect of grapefruit juice dose on grapefruit juice-triazolam interaction: repeated consumption prolongs triazolam half-life. Eur J Clin Pharmacol 2000;56:411−5.

198. Miura M, Ohkubo T. In vitro metabolism of quazepam in human liver and intestine and assessment of drug interactions. Xenobiotica 2004;34(11−12): 1001−11.

199. von Moltke LL, Greenblatt DJ, Granda BW, et al. Zolpidem metabolism in vitro: responsible cytochromes, chemical inhibitors, and in vivo correlations. Br J Clin Pharmacol 1999;48:89−97.

Comorbid Insomnia: Reciprocal Relationships and Medication Management

Robert N. Glidewell, PsyD[a],*, William H. Moorcroft, PhD[b],
Teofilo Lee-Chiong Jr, MD[c]

KEYWORDS

- Comorbid • Insomnia • Depression • Pain
- Obstructive sleep apnea • Combination therapy

Historically, this [comorbid insomnia] has been termed "secondary insomnia." However, the limited understanding of mechanistic pathways in chronic insomnia precludes drawing firm conclusions about the nature of these associations or direction of causality. Furthermore, there is concern that the term secondary insomnia may promote under treatment. Therefore, we propose that the term "comorbid insomnia" may be more appropriate.[1]

As reported in the previous chapter, insomnia is the most prevalent sleep disorder in the general population. Most cases of insomnia are comorbid insomnia.[1,2] Up to 86% of patients with insomnia have a comorbid medical condition; 27% to 45% have a comorbid psychiatric condition.[3–6] Accordingly, comorbid insomnia is the rule rather than the exception, and sleep clinicians should become well versed in its clinical implications and management.

A variety of reciprocal relationships between insomnia and comorbidities have been proposed and researched. Insomnia is documented to increase risk for, or even cause, a variety of medical and psychiatric conditions.[6,7] Insomnia also exacerbates certain comorbidities and is associated with reduced efficacy of treatment of comorbid disorders such as depression.[8,9] Clinical trials of comorbid insomnia have shown that targeted treatment of insomnia results in improvements in insomnia as well as improved treatment outcomes in the comorbid disorder.[10–13] Several studies have documented the persistence of chronic insomnia despite effective management or remission of comorbid conditions.[14–17]

Given the current evidence base, it is no longer acceptable to consider insomnia only as a symptom of a comorbid disorder. This article reviews the literature on the reciprocal interactions between insomnia and medical and psychiatric illness and on pharmacotherapy approaches for comorbid insomnia. The focus is on several of the comorbidities that are most common or relevant for the sleep clinician, including major depressive disorder (MDD), chronic pain, obstructive sleep apnea (OSA), chronic obstructive pulmonary

No financial support was received for preparation of this article.
The authors have nothing to disclose.
[a] Sleep Medicine and Research Program, Lynn Institute For Healthcare Research, 1625 Medical Center Point, Suite 260, Colorado Springs, CO 80907, USA
[b] Northern Colorado Sleep Consultants, 4443 Vista Drive, Fort Collins, CO 80526, USA
[c] Division of Sleep Medicine, National Jewish Health, University of Colorado Denver School of Medicine, 1400 Jackson Street, Room J221 Denver, CO 60206, USA
* Corresponding author.
E-mail address: rglidewell@lhsi.net

disease (COPD), end-stage renal failure, dementia, alcohol use disorders (AUD), and comorbid insomnia during terminal illness.

ASSESSMENT AND DIAGNOSIS

Given the extremely high rates of comorbidity, all patients presenting with insomnia should be thoroughly evaluated for comorbid medical (including other sleep disorders) and psychological conditions.[18,19] A full medical and psychiatric history and review of medical records is the standard for assessment of comorbid medical and psychiatric illnesses. Possible medication effects should also be a prominent feature of the assessment (see elsewhere in this issue for the effect of medications on sleep-wake processes). Alternately, the existing evidence on the rate of insomnia in patients with medical and psychiatric illness suggests that insomnia should be thoroughly evaluated in this population as well.[6] A variety of assessment methods and instruments have been recommended to standardize the assessment of insomnia.[20]

Diagnosis of comorbid insomnia is similar to diagnosis of primary insomnia, with the added requirement of determining and making a judgment regarding the relationship between insomnia and the comorbid conditions and its implication for treatment.[21] In most cases, insomnia is a clinical diagnosis based on subjective complaints of problems falling asleep, staying asleep, waking too early, or of generally unrefreshing sleep.[22,23] These symptoms must be accompanied by daytime symptoms or impairment (ie, problems with attention, memory, fatigue, mood and so forth) that is attributed to the patient's sleep disturbance. A minimum duration criteria of 30 days to 6 months is also required. Usually there is little, if anything, that can be added by overnight polysomnography (PSG).[24] However, PSG is indicated in some cases of chronic refractory insomnia if occult sleep-related breathing or movement disorders are suspected.

INTERACTIONS: INSOMNIA AND COMORBID MEDICAL AND PSYCHIATRIC DISORDERS

Sleep disturbance is broadly associated with deregulation of mood, cognition, and behavior as well as a variety of biologic systems.[25] From this perspective, it is easy to suspect insomnia as playing a causal or exacerbating role in comorbid medical and psychiatric illness. Control of sleep and wakefulness is broadly distributed throughout the brain.[26] With this knowledge, the probability for insomnia (or hypersomnia) is high in the context of medical and psychiatric illness that affects the central nervous system either directly or indirectly. For example, it is common for a man in his 50s or 60s to present at the sleep clinic for evaluation of insomnia complaining of sleep fragmentation related to frequent nocturnal urination. He is diagnosed with a prostate abnormality or overactive bladder and is prescribed medication for these conditions. Regardless, he continues to complain of insomnia. On clinical evaluation, he may attribute his insomnia directly to the need to urinate, or he may state that he gets up to urinate because he is awake.

Bliwise and colleagues[27] found that 53% of their sample of older adults listed nocturia as a perceived cause of sleep disturbance every night or almost every night. Multivariate logistic analysis of their data revealed nocturia as an independent predictor of self-reported insomnia and reduced sleep quality with 75% and 71% increased risk for these symptoms respectively. These findings clearly identify a relationship between insomnia and nocturia. However, in the case described earlier, the nature of the relationship for this patient is still unknown. Is the urinary disorder ineffectively treated? Is there a functionally independent (ie, conditioned) insomnia that results in increased perception of normal bladder sensation? Is there another condition, such as OSA, that is the promoting the symptoms of insomnia and nocturia? Is there an ongoing urological condition causing abnormal bladder sensation or perception? These relationships and interactions between insomnia and various comorbid medical and psychiatric illnesses are discussed later.

Prevalence and Risk of Psychiatric Disorders in Individuals with Insomnia

Of all patients diagnosed with insomnia caused by a mental disorder, approximately half had a comorbid diagnosis of a depressive disorder and half had a comorbid diagnosis of an anxiety disorder.[3,28–31] Conversely, of individuals diagnosed with primary insomnia (as defined in 1988 before the 2005 NIH Consensus Conference endorsing the term comorbid insomnia), 45% reported depressive symptoms, 6% reported anxiety symptoms, 40% reported anxiety and depression symptoms, and only 9% reported no psychiatric symptoms.[3]

Of patients presenting with a predominant complaint of insomnia who failed to meet criteria for insomnia, 6% were diagnosed with a depressive disorder and 14% were diagnosed with an anxiety disorder.[3] This reminds us that (1) a complaint of insomnia does not equal a diagnosis of insomnia, and (2) sometimes, the primary treatment target may be the psychiatric disorder.

Breslau and colleagues[30] examined the relationships between insomnia and psychiatric comorbidities in a 1200-person sample of 21- to 30-year-old adults using the Diagnostic Interview Schedule-Revised. Compared with those with no history of insomnia, individuals with a history of insomnia are more likely to have major depression (odds ratio [OR] = 16.6), generalized anxiety disorder (OR = 7.0), panic disorder (OR = 5.3), and AUD (OR = 2.0). In recognition of the problems related to sleep disturbance being a part of the diagnostic criteria for major depression, the investigators calculated ORs, "... using a definition of major depression that excludes sleep from the list of criteria." This calculation resulted in an OR of 10.4 for having MDD.

In this same study, the investigators also presented results of their examination of the incidence of new psychiatric disorders in individuals with a history of insomnia compared with individuals without a history of insomnia.[30] This prospective examination allows the investigators to make judgments regarding risk of psychiatric morbidity associated with sleep disturbance and the predictive validity of sleep disturbances for the development of other psychiatric disorders. Regarding the risk of psychiatric morbidity, the investigators found that (1) the risk of MDD was fourfold (OR = 3.95) for individuals with a history of insomnia, (2) history of insomnia significantly increased the risk for any anxiety disorder (OR = 1.97) or AUD (OR = 1.72). Regarding the predictive value of insomnia for MDD, the investigators stated, "... the value of insomnia (but not hypersomnia) for predicting subsequent major depression was higher than any other single depressive symptom...."

Based on this information, it can be concluded that many, if not most, patients with insomnia will present with psychiatric symptoms. The work for the clinician is to determine their relationship to insomnia and role in the treatment of insomnia. Regardless of the nature of the relationship and its effects, clinicians should be diligent in the investigation of psychiatric comorbidities in all patients presenting with a prominent complaint of insomnia. In addition, openness to the possibility that the sleep complaint may not represent a sleep disorder may lead to improved treatment of psychiatric disorders.

INSOMNIA COMORBID WITH MDD
Temporal Relationships Between Insomnia and Psychiatric Symptoms

One study examined the temporal relationship between onset of insomnia and onset of depressive and anxiety disorders in a sample of 14,915 subjects from the general population aged 15 to 100 years.[4] Data from this study are represented in **Fig. 1**. Insomnia symptoms preceded a first episode of MDD in 40% of cases. Based on these findings as well as the data regarding the risk for development of depression, it has been proposed that insomnia may be a prodromal feature of MDD and possibly play a causal role in the development of new first episodes of MDD. In patients with anxiety disorders, insomnia symptoms were much more likely to begin at the same time as (38%) or follow (42%) the onset of anxiety symptoms. This pattern of temporal relationships may suggest a causal role for anxiety in insomnia symptoms, with insomnia being a symptom of anxiety or a consequence of prolonged anxiety.

Insomnia and Relapse in MDD

Several studies have examined the relationship between insomnia symptoms and relapse in MDD.[4,32–34] One study reported a survival analysis of 47 elderly patients with remitted depression who participated in maintenance treatment of psychotherapy or monthly medication clinic for 1 year.[35] Overall, patients in the psychotherapy group were more likely to experience sustained remission. Of patients in the psychotherapy maintenance treatment, 90% of patients with good

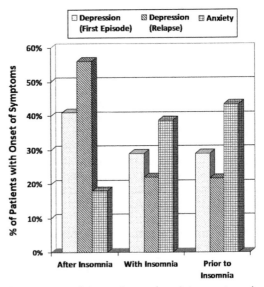

Fig. 1. Onset of depression and anxiety symptoms in relation to the onset of insomnia symptoms. (*Data from* Ohayon MM, Roth T. Place of chronic insomnia in the course of depressive and anxiety disorders. J Psychiatr Res 2003;37:13.)

sleep quality remained remitted, whereas only 33% of patients with poor sleep quality remained remitted. Of patients in the medication clinic group, 31% of patients with good sleep quality remained remitted, whereas only 17% of patients with poor sleep quality remained remitted.

Two studies examined the temporal relationship between insomnia symptoms and relapse in MDD. In 56% of cases, insomnia preceded relapse into an additional major depressive episode (see **Fig. 1**).[4] In explanation of this finding, the investigators propose that chronic insomnia as a residual symptom of MDD represents a risk for relapse. Perlis and colleagues[36] found that disturbed sleep precedes the recurrence of MDD symptoms by several weeks. The investigators propose that these findings suggest a role for sleep disturbance in the pathogenesis of MDD and that routine self-monitoring of sleep in patients with history of depression may be an effective way to initiate early intervention and possibly prevent relapse.

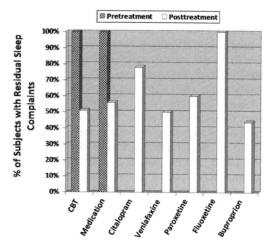

Fig. 2. Residual sleep complaints in patients with MDD following remission. (*Data from* Carney CE, Segal ZV, Edinger JD, et al. Comparison of rats of residual insomnia symptoms following pharmacotherapy or cognitive therapy for major depressive disorder. J Clin Psychiatry 2007;68:258.)

Persistence of Insomnia Following Remission in MDD

Carney and colleagues[17] reported on the rates of residual insomnia symptoms following remission of depression in response to 6 months of either pharmacotherapy or cognitive-behavioral therapy (CBT) for depression. Remission in this study was defined as having a posttreatment Hamilton Rating Scale for Depression (HAM-D), 17-item version, score of 7 or less. All subjects had MDD with comorbid insomnia at the beginning of the study. Overall, 53% of subjects had residual insomnia following remission of depression. Rates of residual insomnia for CBT versus pharmacotherapy and for various specific pharmacotherapies are presented in **Fig. 2**. Another study examined the residual symptoms of patients with MDD treated with 8 weeks of fluoxetine 20 mg.[37] Of the 215 subjects, 108 were considered full responders, defined as a posttreatment HAM-D score of 7 or less. More than 80% of full responders experienced residual symptoms, and their findings regarding residual sleep symptoms were similar to those in the Carney and colleagues[17] study described earlier.

Sleep Disturbance, Depression Severity, and Treatment Response in MDD

Several studies suggest that the presence of sleep disturbance is associated with, and may contribute to, depression severity.[38,39] Walker[25] has proposed a possible mechanism for this relationship. He proposes that increased rapid eye movement (REM) sleep percentage found in

depression may increase consolidation of negative memories, which predominate because of the negative bias in many individuals with depression. In possible support of this hypothesis, another study found that increased REM sleep was associated with increased intensity of daytime emotion.[40]

"Subjective and objective (electroencephalographic) sleep disturbances are associated with slower and lower rates of remission from depression."[41] This statement is supported by evidence from several studies. Dew and colleagues[9] examined the patterns and predictors of recovery from major depression in 95 older adults. In addition to other psychosocial, demographic, and disease-specific variables, poorer subjective and PSG documented sleep parameters were associated with delayed and poorer response to depression treatments. Another study found that addition of lorazepam to concurrent pharmacotherapy and psychotherapy for depression was associated with a higher likelihood of response to treatment.[8]

INSOMNIA COMORBID WITH AUD

Insomnia is prevalent in alcoholism, with 36% to 72% of alcoholic patients having a clinically significant insomnia complaint.[16] Compared with the general population, individuals with an insomnia complaint have a greater incidence of AUD (7% vs 3.8%).[42] Insomnia symptoms persist for months to years after discontinuing alcohol consumption, and the presence of persistent insomnia is an independent risk factor for relapse in alcoholic patients.[43,44] Fifty percent of alcoholics report presence of sleep problems before onset of alcohol dependence.[44] Individuals with insomnia are more likely to use alcohol as a sleep aid than individuals without insomnia. Evidence on these relationships between insomnia and alcohol use and dependence is reviewed later.

Use of Alcohol as a Hypnotic and the Effect of Alcohol on Sleep in Nonalcoholic Individuals

Before the development of dependence, alcohol can be experienced as, and is often used as, a hypnotic.[45] Thirteen percent of the general population use alcohol to get to sleep, and 15% of these individuals (2% of the general population) report regular use of alcohol for sleep lasting more than 1 month.[46] Compared with normal sleepers, individuals with an insomnia complaint are more likely to use alcohol as a sleep aid and may prefer alcohol to nonalcoholic beverages when they have a choice.[45]

In support of this popular preference for alcohol as a sleep aid, multiple studies have examined the effect of alcohol on polysomnographic sleep variables in nonalcoholic individuals and suggest that these effects resemble those of a short-acting hypnotic drug.[45,47] In their study the effects of alcohol on PSG documented sleep in normal sleepers, Feige and colleagues[47] found that alcohol consumption resulting in a blood alcohol level (BAL) of 0.03% had no meaningful effect on polysomnographic sleep. However, with alcohol consumption sufficient to achieve a BAL of 0.1%, a clear dual effect was documented. In the first half of the night alcohol consumption was associated with shortened sleep latency, increased slow wave sleep (SWS), reduced REM density, reduced number of awakenings, and reduced stage 1 sleep. In the second half of the night, a clear increase in stage 1 sleep was documented.[47] Roehrs and colleagues[45] evaluated the effects of alcohol on the PSG documented sleep of normal sleepers and subjects with insomnia. In this study, 0.5 g/kg alcohol reduced REM sleep percentage in both groups, whereas only the insomnia group experienced increased SWS and reduced stage 1 sleep during the first half of the night.[45]

Multiple epidemiologic studies have found that chronic insomnia is a risk factor for development of an AUD. In these studies, adults with insomnia were 1.7 to 2.4 times more likely to develop an alcohol use disorder compared with adults without insomnia.[48–50]

Sleep in Alcoholic Individuals During Active Drinking and Acute and Protracted Withdrawal

Sixty-one percent of alcoholics complain of symptomatic insomnia during the active drinking phase of the disease.[43] Compared with nonalcoholic patients, consumption of alcohol is associated with prolonged sleep onset latency, decreased total sleep time, increased SWS%, decreased REM sleep, and increased REM sleep latency. Accordingly, although the sleep onset latency is now prolonged compared with prior alcohol use, the benefit of increased SWS is maintained throughout the active drinking period.[16]

Between 58% and 72% of alcoholic patients have insomnia complaints during the acute withdrawal phase ($\leq$14 days of abstinence).[51–53] Compared with the active drinking phase, the sleep of alcoholics during acute withdrawal is characterized by persistently prolonged sleep onset latency and reduced total sleep time, reduced SWS%, and REM sleep rebound in the form of reduced REM sleep latency and increased REM sleep percentage.[16]

For most individuals with alcoholism, insomnia persists into the period of protracted abstinence (2 weeks to several years after the cessation of alcohol). The findings of Drummond and colleagues[54] indicate that although the sleep of abstinent alcoholics improves slowly during the first year of abstinence, persistent sleep structure abnormalities were documented after 27 months of abstinence.

To summarize, alcohol is frequently used as a hypnotic self-medication. Compared with normal sleepers, individuals with insomnia are more likely to use alcohol to induce sleep and experience greater sleep structure changes in response to alcohol consumption. Although alcohol use is associate with reduced sleep onset latency and increased SWS, once dependence on alcohol is achieved, much of the hypnotic effect is lost. Once the decision to discontinue use of alcohol is made, it is likely that subjectively and objectively disturbed sleep will persist for months to years of abstinence.

Insomnia and Relapse in Alcoholism

A growing body of evidence has identified insomnia as an independent predictor of relapse in alcoholic patients. Complaint of prolonged sleep latency during acute withdrawal is a significant predictor of relapse at 12 weeks after cessation of alcohol, and complaints of prolonged sleep onset latency and poor sleep quality at the 12-week follow-up were also associated with relapse.[15] In another study, alcoholics with insomnia relapsed at twice the rate (60%) compared with alcoholics without insomnia (30%) within 5 months of cessation of alcohol (χ^2 = 6.16, df = 1, P = .02).[43] In this study, insomnia remained a statistically significant independent predictor of relapse even after controlling for severity of alcohol dependence, depression severity, wake after sleep onset durations, and rates of using alcohol for self-medication. Another study found that greater sleep onset latency and reduced sleep efficiency at 19 weeks of abstinence differentiated alcoholics who relapse from those who did not relapse by 14 months of abstinence.[54] In this study, baseline values of age, years of alcohol dependence, frequency or quantity of alcohol consumption, and depression scores were not statistically significantly different between relapse and nonrelapse groups.

Insomnia and Alcoholism: A Reciprocal Relationship

The research reviewed earlier suggests multiple relationships between insomnia and alcoholism. Chronic insomnia may lead to the development of an alcohol use disorder. Insomnia during the active drinking phase of alcoholism may compel individuals to increased amount and frequency of evening and nocturnal alcohol consumption. Persistence of insomnia throughout acute and protracted abstinence is a predictor of relapse to drinking. A model of these relationships is depicted and described in **Fig. 3**.

INSOMNIA COMORBID WITH OSA

Based on a literature review published by Luyster and colleagues[55] in 2010, 39% of patients with OSA meet criteria for insomnia and 42% to 55% report at least 1 insomnia symptom. Conversely, 29% of patients with insomnia have an apnea-hypopnea index of 15 or greater, and 43% to 67% have an apnea-hypopnea index (AHI) of 5 or greater. Despite this high level of comorbidity, there has been little research on the relationships between insomnia and OSA.[55] The relationships between insomnia and OSA, insomnia and positive airway pressure (PAP) therapy, and the effect of OSA on treatments for insomnia are discussed later.

Insomnia and OSA

Sleep maintenance insomnia is the most common insomnia complaint in patients with OSA, whereas a minority of patients with OSA without insomnia complain of difficulty initiating sleep.[56–58] Krakow

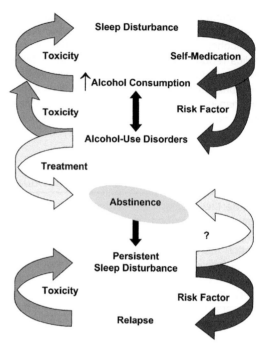

Fig. 3. A model of the reciprocal relationships between heavy alcohol consumption and sleep disturbances. Sleep disturbance may lead to increased alcohol consumption for self-medication. At the same time, alcohol consumption, through its effects on brain chemicals (ie, neurotoxicity), may lead to sleep disturbance. Sleep disturbance is also a risk factor for developing alcohol use disorders (ie, alcohol abuse and alcohol dependence). Treatment of these disorders can lead to abstinence, but sleep disturbances may persist even during recent and sustained abstinence. Sleep disturbances at the time of treatment are risk factors for relapse to drinking. In turn, relapse contributes to alcohol neurotoxicity and persistent sleep disturbances. The question mark represents the untested hypothesis that treatment of sleep disturbances as an adjunct to alcoholism treatment can facilitate abstinence and decrease the risk of relapse. Purple arrows indicate processes that favor unhealthy patterns of drinking, blue arrows indicate processes that favor sleep disturbance, and yellow arrows represent treatment processes that may favor abstinence. (*From* Brower KJ. Alcohol's effects on sleep in alcoholics. Alcohol Res Health 2001;25:116.)

and colleagues[58] examined the prevalence of insomnia in patients with OSA with and without insomnia. In this study, insomnia was determined by a locally developed questionnaire and OSA was defined as an AHI of 5 or greater and daytime sleepiness, or 2 or more additional symptoms. Statistically significant differences were found between insomnia and no-insomnia groups on polysomnographic measures of sleep latency

(64.94 vs 16.99 minutes, F = 51.84, $P<.0001$), total sleep time (5.56 vs 7.22 hours, F = 51.75, $P<.0001$), and sleep efficiency (75.06% vs 92%, F = 50.04, $P<.001$). There were no significant differences in PSG or questionnaire-based indices of sleep-related breathing including body mass index (BMI), snoring, minimum arterial oxygen concentration (Sao_2), or AHI. Smith and colleagues[59] reported similar findings. Another study failed to reproduce these findings.[57] However, the definitions of insomnia in this failed study were not as rigorous as those in the Krakow and colleagues[58] study and these discrepant findings likely reflect heterogeneity within the 2 groups as opposed to the absence of differences in patients with OSA with and without insomnia.

Insomnia and PAP Therapy

Difficulty initiating or maintaining sleep with use of PAP therapy is a frequent complaint. However, There is little evidence to support a causal role for insomnia in the nonadherence or nonacceptance of PAP therapy. One study found that pretreatment insomnia complaints were negatively correlated with mean continuous positive airway pressure (CPAP) use duration (r = −0.35; $P<.01$).[60] In a study by Aloia and colleagues,[61] 15% of inconsistent users endorsed "sleeps poorly with it" as a CPAP side effect, compared with only 2% of consistent users (χ^2 = 7.61, P = .01). In another study, patients who were nonadherent to PAP therapy (average nightly use, all nights, <4 hours) had higher rates of moderate to severe persistent insomnia (defined as an Insomnia Severity Index score of ≥15) than adherent patients at 30 to 60 days after initiation of PAP therapy.[14] This study also found that 40% of patients reported persistent insomnia despite adherence to PAP therapy (average nightly use, all nights, ≥4 hours).

These studies clearly show a relationship between insomnia and PAP use. However, does insomnia lead to nonadherence or does adherence lead to reduced insomnia? Research is needed to better understand this relationship and develop guidelines regarding the course of treatment of insomnia comorbid with OSA. In combination, these data and those in the previous section suggest that, although sleep apnea may be the cause of insomnia in some cases (as indicated by the resolution of insomnia with adherence to PAP therapy), there is clearly a significant minority of patients with OSA for whom insomnia is an independent clinical entity, which persists despite the effective treatment of OSA. Based on PSG data, patients with OSA with insomnia seem to be a distinct group compared with patients with OSA without insomnia and may require unique approaches to assessment and treatment.

Does OSA Interfere with Treatment of Insomnia?

To our knowledge, there is no research on the effect of sleep apnea on the effectiveness of insomnia treatment ,whether it is cognitive-behavioral, pharmacologic, or other types of treatment. Occult OSA may be common in patients with insomnia, and standard clinical practice demands laboratory assessment to rule out sleep-related breathing and movement disorders in cases of chronic refractory insomnia.[19,24,62] Logically and by implication of the practice discussed earlier, it is reasonable to speculate that there is a subpopulation of patients with insomnia who fail to respond or who experience only partial benefit from insomnia treatments because of the neurologic and physiologic effects of occult respiratory disturbance. Although there is an absence of clinical research on this subject, a recently published case report and general clinical experience strongly supports the likelihood that OSA impairs the effectiveness of treatments for insomnia in some patients.[10]

INSOMNIA COMORBID WITH CHRONIC PAIN

Pain is frequently mentioned in lists of what contributes to insomnia. It seems logical that people with chronic pain would have problems with their sleep; survey results support this.[63–65] Between 10% and 30% of the general population complain of chronic pain. Of these, more than half also complain of poor sleep. Conversely, approximately 50% of people who complain of poor sleep also complain of chronic pain.[6]

Reciprocal Relationships Between Chronic Pain and Sleep Disturbance

It has long been held that pain and insomnia have a reciprocal relationship. A night of poor sleep results in more pain during subsequent waking periods, and poor sleep increases as the intensity of pain increases.[65] Smith and colleagues[66] reviewed extant literature on the relationship between sleep and pain in patients with osteoarthritis and presented a conceptual model of putative mechanisms underlying the relationship. In this model, they propose that sleep directly interacts with central nervous system (CNS) pain processing and inflammatory processes. They also propose that sleep has an indirect effect on mood and physical function, which can exacerbate pain. However, this model cannot be generalized to all chronic pain conditions, because some evidence suggests that the relationships and mechanisms of the pain-sleep relationship vary according to the type of pain and nature of the sleep disturbance.[64] Although people with chronic pain sleep less than healthy sleepers, sleep fragmentation has been proposed as the more salient influence on increased pain sensitivity.[67]

Evidence for the Effect of Pain on Sleep Behavior and Architecture

Some investigators have proposed a behavioral mechanism for the pain-sleep relationship. Specifically, sleep and sleep-related behaviors used to self-manage pain may alter circadian and homeostatic drives and may promote negative associations with the bed/bedroom, resulting in development of psychophysiologic insomnia.[68] Clinical experience and observation suggest that overactivity caused by obligations, psychological factors associated with rest/inactivity, or other psychosocial factors may also play a role.

Pain has been shown to negatively affect sleep architecture in several ways.[63] Compared with people with insomnia and no pain, people with periodic leg movement syndrome (PLMS), or healthy sleepers, individuals with insomnia and pain tend to have lower average sleep efficiency, typically ranging from 75% to 85%. They sometimes have more stage 1 but less stage 3 to 4 sleep and their sleep is more fragmented.

Several studies have documented that sleep disturbance can alter pain processing. Sleep fragmentation seems to compromise the normal pain inhibitory functions, thereby increasing the perception of pain.[67] Roehrs and colleagues[69] found that sleep deprivation in general, and REM sleep deprivation in particular, results in hyperalgesia during the subsequent awake period. The effect of insomnia on waking pain sensitivity may contribute to idiopathic pain disorders.[70]

Pain-sleep Relationships in Fibromyalgia, Musculoskeletal, and Other Pain Disorders

Sleep problems, especially nonrestorative sleep, occur in 73% to 76% of patients with fibromyalgia (FM) and sleep symptoms seem to play an important role in the other symptoms of this syndrome.[71] One study documented that, compared with healthy sleepers, patients with FM had higher scores on a standardized measure of dysfunctional sleep beliefs.[72] Additionally, the scores recorded by patients with FM indicated dysfunctional beliefs equal to or exceeding those of patients with primary insomnia. Another study

examined the differences in PSG recorded sleep between women with FM versus a control group of healthy women.[73] In this study, patients with FM had significantly more sleep stage transitions than controls (126 ± 27 vs 107 ± 22, $P = .042$) and lower stage 2 durations ($P = .006$). The investigators also reported a correlation between reduced stage 2 durations and pain diary scores (Spearman $\rho = -.56$, $P = .0014$) and current pain intensity ($\rho = -.71$, $P<.0001$). Similar sleep structure differences and sleep-pain correlations were also documented by Landis and colleagues.[74]

As stated earlier, sleep is proposed to have direct and indirect effects on osteoarthritis.[66] Hawker and colleagues[75] examined relationships between sleep quality, fatigue, and osteoarthritis in 613 older adults. Independent correlates of poor sleep quality in this sample included higher pain severity (OR = 1.3, $P<.0001$), having 3 or more comorbid medical conditions (OR = 1.98, $P<.02$), depressed mood (OR = 1.09, $P<.0001$), and restless legs syndrome (RLS; OR = 1.92, $P<.01$). Another study found that the presence of osteoarthritis pain increased the odds of having insomnia (OR = 1.29) and sleep deprivation (OR = 1.35).[76]

Insomnia and sleep complaints have also been documented in most other pain conditions. Tension-type headaches in young adults increase sleep problems, and sleep problems are a trigger for headaches.[68] Temporomandibular joint disorder is frequently associated with insomnia.[70] Other pain conditions that interact with sleep disturbance include neuropathic pain such as oral, facial, or dental pain.[77,78]

INSOMNIA COMORBID WITH COPD

COPD is characterized by progressive and not fully reversible air flow limitation that develops because of injury to the small airways and alveoli from noxious particles or gases. Patients with COPD commonly present with dyspnea and/or chronic cough. Sleep-related complaints, such as repetitive awakenings, insomnia, early awakenings, and nonrestorative sleep, are common within this population. In one study that used postal questionnaire surveys of Icelandic men, subjects with chronic bronchitis had a higher prevalence of awakening by breathlessness compared with healthy controls [35.2% vs 6%].[79] Another study, the Tucson Epidemiologic Study of Chronic Lung Disease, reported that more than 50% of subjects with COPD had insomnia. The prevalence of insomnia differed with the number of symptoms: 28% in asymptomatic subjects, 39%

in those with 1 symptom (cough or wheezing) 39%, and 53% in subjects who had 2 symptoms.[80] Several possible mechanisms might explain the development of sleep disturbance in persons with COPD, and the cause of insomnia is often multifactorial. These factors include nocturnal coughing, wheezing, or dyspnea; orthopnea; increased work of breathing; and medication use. Medications that have been implicated in insomnia in patients with COPD include, methylxanthines, β-adrenergic agonists, theophylline, corticosteroids, bronchodilators, and anticholinergic agents.[81–87]

Sleep disturbance in persons with COPD can also result from concurrent OSA, RLS, or PLMS. In one study of 87 subjects with COPD versus 110 controls, the prevalence of RLS was 36% and 11% for COPD and controls, respectively ($P<.001$).[88] In addition, both the severity of RLS (based on the International Restless Legs Syndrome Study Group criteria) and daytime sleepiness (based on the Epworth Sleepiness Scale) were worse in subjects with COPD and RLS compared with subjects with RLS alone. Another study reported that periodic limb movements during sleep associated with arousals are common in persons with COPD.[89]

INSOMNIA COMORBID WITH END-STAGE RENAL DISEASE

Sleep complaints, including insomnia and excessive sleepiness, can complicate the clinical course of patients with end-stage renal disease (ESRD). One study estimated an insomnia prevalence of 66% in this patient population.[90] Polysomnographic features may include diminished sleep efficiency, reduced total sleep time, sleep maintenance insomnia, and early morning awakenings. Insomnia can arise from metabolic derangements (eg, increased levels of phosphate and urea levels), hyperparathyroidism, pruritus, pain, or concurrent primary sleep disorders.[91–93] Abnormalities in melatonin production can also potentially contribute to sleep disturbance, and administration of exogenous melatonin has been reported to improve sleep onset latency, total sleep time, and sleep efficiency.[94,95]

INSOMNIA COMORBID WITH DEMENTIA

Dementia can give rise to several sleep-related disturbances including repetitive arousals and awakenings, sleep fragmentation, and reversal of sleep-wake rhythms. These disturbances may be caused by the disorder itself, or by the development of sleep disorders (eg, sleep apnea or periodic limb movement disorder) or depression, the prevalence of which is greater in this patient group.

INSOMNIA COMORBID WITH TERMINAL ILLNESS

Persons with terminal illness often complain of sleep disturbance, and insomnia has been described in patients with advanced heart failure, terminal cancer, and amyotrophic lateral sclerosis, as well as those admitted for hospice care.[96–99] Aside from the underlying medical illness, other causes of poor sleep quality in this palliative care population include psychological distress and posttraumatic experience.[99,100]

PHARMACOTHERAPY APPROACHES TO COMORBID INSOMNIA
Pharmacotherapy for Insomnia Comorbid with MDD

Insomnia and MDD are commonly comorbid and there is a reciprocal relationship between these conditions. The presence and persistence of insomnia is a risk factor for onset and relapse in MDD. Insomnia requires independent, targeted assessment, monitoring, and treatment when comorbid with MDD. Mounting evidence exists to guide clinical practice regarding the pharmacologic managements of this particular comorbidity.

In his review of literature on the comorbidity of insomnia and depression, Staner[32] provides a cogent discussion of various treatment approaches and combinations and their rationale. He states that our knowledge of the reciprocal relationships should actively drive our treatment decisions. For example, when insomnia precedes depression, targeted treatment of insomnia may have a preventative role in depression. In cases in which insomnia and depression manifest concurrently, consideration of a common cause and common treatment may be most effective. When a common cause is not apparent, targeted treatment of each comorbidity may be the optimal approach.

Antidepressant Monotherapy for Insomnia Comorbid with Depression

Jindal[101] produced a detailed review of current evidence on the effects of specific antidepressant monotherapies and pharmacologic combination therapies for treatment of sleep in depression.

In terms of antidepressant monotherapy, the important points of this review are as follows:

- Tricyclic antidepressants (TCA) have a generally sedating and REM suppressant effect, and controlled studies have found these medications to improve mood and sleep in patients with insomnia who are depressed.
- The sleep effect of selective serotonin reuptake inhibitors (SSRI) varies greatly from drug to drug, and some SSRI drugs are known to cause onset or worsening of insomnia.
- Although mirtazipine has proven positive effects on sleep and mood symptoms, it is frequently not tolerated because of a high likelihood of weight gain associated with its use.
- Other popular antidepressants are also variable in their effectiveness for treatment of sleep symptoms as well as their side effect profiles.

In summary, antidepressant monotherapy for comorbid insomnia and depression can be effective. However, an intimate knowledge of the neurotransmitter profiles and documented efficacy for sleep and mood symptoms is necessary when choosing this treatment approach.

Combination Therapies for Insomnia Comorbid with Depression

Several forms of combination therapy have also proved effective in the treatment of insomnia and comorbid depression.[32,101] These combination therapies include coprescription of multiple antidepressants, coprescription of antidepressants and benzodiazepines or nonbenzodiazepine hypnotics, and coprescription of antidepressants with over-the-counter medications.

Several studies have found that combination therapy in the form of hypnotic medication or CBT for insomnia with pharmacotherapy for depression improves insomnia and enhances depression outcomes. Fava and colleagues[11] examined the effect of eszopiclone coadministered with fluoxetine in patients with insomnia and MDD. Compared with placebo plus fluoxetine, subjects in the eszopiclone plus fluoxetine group experienced significantly greater improvements in sleep latency, wake after sleep onset durations, total sleep time, subjective sleep quality, and depth of sleep ($P<.05$ for all variables). Additionally the eszopiclone plus fluoxetine group experienced significantly greater improvements in depression symptoms as measured by the HAM-D-17. There

were also more depression responders (59% vs 48%, $P = .009$) and remitters (42% vs 33%, $P = .03$) in the eszopiclone plus fluoxetine group.

Another group performed a similar study evaluating the efficacy of cognitive-behavioral treatment of insomnia (CBT-I) plus escitalopram compared with placebo plus escitalopram.[41] Compared with placebo, subjects in the CBT-I plus escitalopram group experienced greater rates of remission of depression (61.5% vs 33.3%) and remission of insomnia (50% vs 8%). CBT-I subjects also experienced larger improvements in sleep diary and actigraphy measures.

As a follow-up to the Fava and colleagues[11] study discussed earlier, Krystal and colleagues[102] evaluated the effect of eszopiclone discontinuation on adverse events and maintenance of treatment gains following 8 weeks of fluoxetine and concurrent treatment with either eszopiclone or placebo. They documented no difference in the rate of CNS, or potential CNS, adverse events (8.8% vs 9.8%) between placebo and eszopiclone groups. The advantage for the eszopiclone group in regard to greater improvements in depression symptoms, as well as higher rates of response and remission, were maintained at 10 weeks (2 weeks after discontinuation of eszopiclone). Improvements in sleep latency, wake after sleep onset, and total sleep time durations were also maintained 2 weeks after discontinuing eszopiclone.

Another study examined the combination of SSRI plus zolpidem 10 mg HS versus SSRI plus placebo for 4 weeks in 190 patients with persistent insomnia despite effectively treated depression.[103] This was a randomized, double-blind, placebo-controlled study. Compared with placebo, subjects receiving zolpidem experienced improvements in total sleep time (TST), subjective sleep quality, and number of awakenings ($P<.05$ for all variables). Rebound insomnia was documented only on the first night after placebo substitution for zolpidem. Although treatment gains in terms of the number of awakenings were maintained, all other sleep variables returned to pretreatment levels. There was no difference in adverse events between the zolpidem and placebo groups (74% vs 83%).

PHARMACOTHERAPY FOR INSOMNIA COMORBID WITH ALCOHOL DEPENDENCE

"Data from this review that either pharmacological or cognitive behavioural treatment of insomnia could reduce the risk of relapse in substance dependence were substantially lacking"[104]

This statement by Roth[104] is the product of a workshop and subsequent literature review performed in

2008 to evaluate whether treatment of sleep disorders could reduce rates of substance use disorders or risk of relapse. Accordingly, given the current evidence, treatment of comorbid insomnia is intended primarily to relieve insomnia symptoms. However, given the well-documented relationship between insomnia and relapse, treatment of comorbid insomnia should be seriously considered.

Controversy exists regarding the use of pharmacotherapy for the treatment of alcoholism and psychiatric comorbidities.[42,105,106] The pharmacologic treatment of comorbid insomnia is often at the core of this controversy because first-line treatments for insomnia (benzodiazepine and nonbenzodiazepine hypnotics) are commonly associated with tolerance, dependence, and abuse in AUDs. Although some clinicians state that pharmacotherapy in alcoholic patients is contraindicated in patients with disorders of abuse and dependence, others believe that leaving a comorbid condition untreated represents the greater concern, especially for relapse, as discussed earlier. There has been little research to validate or invalidate concerns on either side.

Although tolerance, dependence, and abuse are certainly issues with the traditional benzodiazepines, extended clinical trials of nonbenzodiazepine hypnotics, such as zolpidem and eszopiclone, have failed to show these characteristics in individuals with pure primary insomnia (see the article by Roth elsewhere in this issue for further exploration of this issue). However, patterns of tolerance, dependence, and abuse for these drugs have not been investigated in alcoholic patients.[42] A PubMed search of the terms zolpidem, eszopiclone, alcoholic, alcoholism, alcohol recovery, and alcohol dependence produced only 1 study of the risks of tolerance, dependence, and abuse associated with these drugs in alcoholic patients.[107] This study of dependence on legal psychotropic drugs among alcoholics found that, compared with the general population, alcoholism is associated with a increased rate of dependence on psychotropic drugs. Although benzodiazepines were the most common psychotropic drug, only 17% of benzodiazepine-dependent alcoholics developed high-dose benzodiazepine-dependence.

Three-hundred and eleven physicians (35% psychiatry, 21% family medicine, 18% internal medicine, and 27% other specialties) who were members of the American Society for Addiction Medicine were surveyed regarding their prescribing practices for treatment of sleep complaints in recovering alcoholics.[106] In this study, 64% of physicians had offered pharmacotherapy for treatment of insomnia to alcoholic patients with an insomnia complaint. However, this was not a standard practice: only 22% of these physicians offered pharmacotherapy to more than half these patients. When pharmacotherapy was offered, 38% of physicians chose trazodone (mean starting dose 61.1 mg, SD 28.1 mg) as the first-line treatment, whereas 12% chose other sedating antidepressants (amitriptyline, doxepin, mirtazipine, nefazodone, and imipramine), and another 12% chose antihistamines (diphenhydramine, doxylamine, hydroxyzine, and promethazine). Only 3.5% of respondents indicated selection of nonbenzodiazepine hypnotics (zolpidem or zaleplon) as a first-line treatment, and only 2.6% offered benzodiazepines, with temazepam, flurazepam, and clonazepam being the only benzodiazepines offered.

At least 2 studies have examined the effectiveness of the anticonvulsant gabapentin for the treatment of comorbid insomnia in alcoholic patients. Karam-Hage and Brower[108] completed an open-label study comparing the effects of gabapentin (N = 34) and trazodone (N = 16) for treatment of insomnia in outpatients with alcoholism. Sleep was evaluated using the Sleep Problems Questionnaire (SPQ).[109] Compared with pretreatment SPQ scores, significant improvements in sleep were documented for trazodone ($t = 7.1$, $df = 15$, $P<.001$) and gabapentin ($t = 12.7$, $df = 33$, $P<.001$). However, the improvements in the gabapentin group were significantly greater that those of the trazodone group (8.8 ± 4.0 vs 6.1 ± 3.4, $t = -2.35$, $df = 48$, $P = .023$).

Brower and colleagues[12] completed a randomized, double-blind, placebo-controlled trial of gabapentin for treatment of comorbid alcohol dependence and insomnia. Their sample was composed of alcoholic patients in early abstinence (2–8 weeks after cessation of drinking) and who were randomized to either placebo (N = 11) or gabapentin (N = 10) treatment for 6 weeks. Sleep variables were measured using the SPG, PSG, and sleep diary. Patients in the gabapentin group relapsed at a significantly lower rate than those in the placebo group (30% vs 82%, Fisher's exact test, $P = .03$) and relative risk (RR) for relapse was lower for the gabapentin group (Cox regression, $RR = 0.25$, $P = .047$). However, there were no statistically significant between-group or group/time differences for SPQ, PSG, or sleep diary measured sleep variables. For some variables, trends toward improved sleep favored the placebo group.

Cognitive-Behavioral Treatment of Insomnia Comorbid with Alcohol Dependence

Given the apprehension regarding the prescription of hypnotics and the lack of evidence for use of sedating antidepressants and antihistamines for the treatment of insomnia, cognitive-behavioral treatment of insomnia (CBT-I) may be a viable alternative. Three published studies have evaluated the efficacy of CBT-I in alcoholic patients.

In a 2005 review of studies of CBT-I for comorbid insomnia, Smith and colleagues[110] identified a single study evaluating the effectiveness of a 10-session progressive relaxation treatment. At the end of treatment, diary ratings of sleep quality were significantly improved (effect size = 2.2) compared with the wait-list controls (effect size = 0.22).

Arnedt and colleagues[111] delivered an 8-week multicomponent CBT-I intervention to 7 alcoholics with comorbid insomnia. After treatment, sleep diary and standardized questionnaire ratings of sleep onset latency (SOL) ($F_{(2,10)}$ = 14.4, $P<.001$), wake after sleep onset (WASO) ($F_{(2,10)}$ = 7.7, $P<.009$), sleep efficiency (SE) ($[F_{(2,10)}$ = 28.3, $P<.001$), insomnia severity index (ISI) scores, and dysfunctional beliefs and attitudes about sleep were significantly improved.

Currie and colleagues[112] investigated the efficacy of a 7-week CBT-I treatment or a self-help insomnia treatment compared with a wait-list control in 60 recovering alcoholics. Subjects receiving either treatment were more improved than controls and reported statistically significant improvements in sleep quality, SE, SOL, and number of awakenings (NWAK).

PHARMACOTHERAPY FOR INSOMNIA COMORBID WITH OSA

No research exists to provide guidance regarding the course of treatment of insomnia that is comorbid with OSA. Should insomnia be treated first because it may cause intolerance or nonadherence to OSA treatments? Should the OSA be treated first because it may be the cause of the insomnia? Should treatments be provided concurrently? Although several groups are actively researching this issue, currently these decisions must be made on a case-by-case basis. Two aspects of pharmacotherapy for insomnia comorbid with OSA are here: (1) the effect of hypnotic medications on respiratory function in patients with OSA on CPAP, and (2) the usefulness of hypnotic medications as a treatment of CPAP nonadherence.

Oral Hypnotics in the Treatment of Insomnia in Patients with OSA

There have been anecdotal reports that use of benzodiazepine and nonbenzodiazepine hypnotics may negatively affect respiration during sleep and are, therefore, contraindicated in patients with OSA. However, several studies have shown that hypnotic medications can be effective and do not worsen OSA in patients treated with CPAP. A polysomnographic examination of the effect of an oral hypnotic on CPAP efficacy found that use of zolpidem 10 mg caused no significant change in AHI, non-REM AHI, TST, or REM sleep while patients used CPAP at prescribed levels.[113] These findings must be interpreted with caution because this initial report included data from only 4 subjects.

Rosenberg and colleagues[114] performed a similar, but more robust, examination of the effects of eszopiclone on OSA in 22 subjects using a double-blind, randomized, crossover design. They found no significant differences in mean total AHI, total arousals, respiratory arousals, duration of apnea or hypopnea episodes, or oxygen saturation in subjects treated with eszopiclone versus controls. In addition, several PSG documented sleep variables were improved. Compared with placebo, patients receiving eszopiclone had fewer spontaneous arousals (13.6 vs 11.4, 90% confidence interval = −3.7 to −0.7), greater sleep efficiency (85.1% vs 88.4%, P = .0075), and lower wake after sleep onset durations (61.8 vs 48.1 minutes, P = .0125). The investigators of both studies concluded that oral hypnotic medication can be used safely in patients with OSA.

Series and colleagues[115] reviewed studies of the use of clonazepam and temazepam in patients with comorbid insomnia and OSA, both of which failed to document any exacerbation of nocturnal respiratory function with use of these drugs. Studies of flurazepam, triazolam, and nitrazepam were also reviewed and none of these studies documented worsening of OSA associated with medication use.

Oral Hypnotics may be Useful for Treatment of PAP Nonadherence

Two studies have examined the ability of oral hypnotic medications to improve CPAP adherence. In a prospective, randomized, placebo-controlled study, Bradshaw and colleagues[116] investigated the use of the oral hypnotic medication zolpidem to improve CPAP compliance during the first 14 days of treatment in 72 male patients with moderate to severe OSA. In this study, patients in the zolpidem group did not show greater CPAP use frequency or average nightly use duration than placebo or standard care groups. More recently, Lettieri and colleagues[13] used a prospective, randomized, placebo-controlled study design to investigate the use of eszopiclone administered during the initial 14 days of treatment to improve CPAP compliance in 154 patients with OSA. In this study, patients in the eszopiclone group used CPAP on more nights and for more hours per night than controls. Compared with control subjects, fewer patients in the eszopiclone group discontinued CPAP.

These findings are contradictory and should be interpreted with caution for several reasons. First, CPAP adherence is influenced by many diverse variables including side effects, equipment features such as humidification, and psychological factors.[117,118] Hypnotic medication would not be expected to influence all of these factors. Second, multiple studies have clearly shown 2 distinct naturally occurring groups of CPAP users.[61,119] In the study by Aloia and colleagues,[61] a group of consistent users used PAP an average of 6 days or more per week for the first 6 months, whereas intermittent users used PAP an average of less than 6 days per week for 6 months. Compared with intermittent users, consistent users also had greater average duration of use per night during the first 6 months of treatment (5.98 ± 1.4 hours vs 2.13 ± 1.7 hours, $P<.000$). These data indicate the presence of a group of PAP users who will achieve a therapeutic level of PAP use independently. Hypnotic use in these patients is unwarranted. Neither study differentiated patients with OSA with insomnia from those without insomnia. Hypnotic medication could reasonably be expected to improve sleep and CPAP adherence in patients with OSA with (1) a prominent insomnia complaint, and (2) who use CPAP at subtherapeutic levels. However, in our view, there is no justification for the general use of hypnotics in all patients with OSA on PAP.

PHARMACOTHERAPY FOR INSOMNIA COMORBID WITH CHRONIC PAIN

Because pain and insomnia are so entwined, combined treatment may be necessary.[120] However, there is no agreement about how to adequately manage comorbid pain and sleep.[64] Accordingly, this article discusses the evidence regarding pharmacologic monotherapies and combined therapies for treatment of insomnia comorbid with pain.

Pharmacologic Monotherapy for Insomnia Comorbid with Chronic Pain

Numerous studies have examined or documented the efficacy of single nonhypnotic medications for management of comorbid insomnia and pain. Based on a review of 10 studies examining the effect of long-acting opioid analgesics in patients with osteoarthritis, the investigators state, "In each of the 10 placebo-controlled studies identified, concurrent improvements in pain intensity and sleep disturbances were observed…"[121] However, this statement must be applied with caution, because the findings of Dimsdale and colleagues[122] may indicate clinically significant effects of long-acting opioids on sleep architecture and daytime fatigue. Although a meta-analysis of studies of opioids for pain identified no statistically significant sleep improvements, several studies have documented a positive effect of opioids on insomnia related to pain.[123–125]

Gilron[126] recently reviewed studies on the use of the α-2 calcium channel binding medications gabapentin and pregabalin for the treatment of neuropathic and postsurgical pain. He concluded that these drugs positively affected pain and sleep and that these improvements resulted in improved quality of life. One randomized, placebo-controlled, double-blind, multicenter study examined the efficacy of gabapentin for treatment of traumatic nerve injury pain in 120 patients.[127] Compared with controls, patients receiving gabapentin reported reductions in pain and less pain interference of sleep ($P = .0016$). Straub and colleagues[128] completed a responder analysis for patients with FM treated with pregabalin. They also found improved pain and reduced pain interference of sleep.

Combination Therapy: Use of Sedative-Hypnotics for Insomnia Comorbid with Chronic Pain

There is some evidence to suggest that hypnotics do not have direct analgesic effects or indirect effects on subjective pain ratings, although some studies have examined this question in patients with fibromyalgia and in animal models.[129,130] However, studies have found that benzodiazepine and nonbenzodiazepine hypnotics improve sleep despite the presence of multiple types of pain. Moldofsky and colleagues[130] reported improvements in SOL, TST, NWAK, and overall sleep improvement with use of zolpidem 5 to 15 mg. A comparison of the response rates to zolpidem versus temazepam in patients with pain found that 52% of patients treated with temazepam experienced complete response, whereas only 22% of patients in the zolpidem group achieved complete response.[131] Roth and colleagues[132] investigated the effect of eszopiclone for treatment of insomnia comorbid with rheumatoid arthritis and found that eszopiclone improved all subjectively reported sleep variables ($P<.05$ vs placebo).

PHARMACOTHERAPY FOR INSOMNIA COMORBID WITH COPD

Therapy for insomnia generally consists of sleep hygiene education, nonpharmacologic therapy, and the use of pharmacologic agents. Selection of hypnotic agents should be individualized and both drug efficacy and safety monitored closely.[133–135] The use of the melatonin receptor agonist, ramelteon, has been studied in patients with COPD. In a double-blind, crossover study involving 25 subjects with moderate (forced expiratory volume in 1 second [FEV_1] 50%–80% and FEV_1/forced vital capacity [FVC]<70%) to severe (FEV_1<50% and FEV_1/FVC <70%) COPD and no history of insomnia, ramelteon at a dose of 8 mg improved sleep compared with placebo (TST 389 vs 348 min, $P = .019$; sleep efficiency 81 vs 72%, $P = .019$; and sleep onset latency 23 vs 57 min, $P = .051$). However, there were no significant changes in self-reported measures of sleep onset latency, TST, awakenings, or sleep quality with the agent.[136]

PHARMACOTHERAPY FOR INSOMNIA COMORBID WITH END-STAGE RENAL DISEASE

Zaleplon, a nonbenzodiazepine benzodiazepine receptor agonist, has been shown in a randomized, double-blind, placebo-controlled crossover study to significantly improve sleep quality (change in score based on the Pittsburg questionnaire; $P<.03$), reduce sleep onset latency ($P<.01$), and increase sleep efficiency ($P<.05$) in 10 patients on HD for ESRD who have insomnia.[137]

PHARMACOTHERAPY FOR INSOMNIA COMORBID WITH DEMENTIA

Medications that have been used to improve sleep in patients with dementia include risperidone and melatonin. In a study involving 338 patients, risperidone treatment improved total nighttime sleep hours (5.5 vs 7.1 hours) and wake time in bed at night (2.3 vs 1.2 hours) compared with baseline. Reports of insomnia decreased from 40.1% to 8.4%.[138] There are conflicting data on the efficacy of melatonin in this population group. Although one study reported significantly improved sleep quality and decreased nighttime agitated behavior (sundowning) and frequency of awakenings following melatonin administered at bedtime in patients with dementia, another study noted no statistically significant differences in objective sleep measures between baseline and treatment in patients with Alzheimer disease suffering from insomnia.[139,140]

PHARMACOTHERAPY FOR INSOMNIA COMORBID WITH TERMINAL ILLNESS

There is a paucity of reports on the indications for hypnotic agents among the terminally ill with complaints of insomnia. Matsuo and Morita[141] described the use of intravenous midazolam and flunitrazepam for insomnia on patients in palliative care units when oral administration was not possible. In a national survey of Japanese physicians in palliative care units, 112 respondents reported that midazolam or flunitrazepam was used in 79% and 53% of units, respectively, but administration protocols varied widely. Twelve percent of palliative care units used both agents. Eight percent did not use either agent.[141] In another report, the same investigators compared the efficacy and safety of these 2 agents in the treatment of insomnia in patients with terminal cancer, and noted no differences between the agents in efficacy, delirium, withdrawal symptoms or treatment-related death; respiratory depression was more common with flunitrazepam.[142]

SUMMARY

The relationships between insomnia comorbid with medical and psychiatric illness are complex and remain poorly understood. The relationship varies according to the specific comorbidity, as do the relevant treatment options and their effects. Identification and management of comorbid insomnia would be improved simply through the recognition of the pervasive role it has in the course of general medical and psychiatric illness. Key points that may help to guide future practice include:

- Insomnia that persists despite effective control of comorbid illness warrants thorough targeted assessment and treatment
- Treatment resistant insomnia should be accompanied by a thorough evaluation of comorbid conditions and consideration of modification of current therapeutic regimens for those conditions
- In many cases, combination treatment of comorbid insomnia and comorbidities can improve insomnia and result in enhanced treatment gains in the comorbid condition
- In some cases, effective management of insomnia and its comorbid condition may be achieved with the use of monotherapies such as antidepressants for mood and anxiety disorders and anticonvulsants for chronic pain.

Similar relationships with comorbid insomnia have been documented in neurologic disorders, gastrointestinal disorders, menopause and perimenopause, cancer, and anxiety disorders including generalized anxiety, panic, and posttraumatic stress disorders. Because of space constraints, we are unable to give full attention to each of these conditions. However, the references provide a solid introduction for the interested reader.[143–151]

REFERENCES

1. NIH State of the Science Conference statement on Manifestations and Management of Chronic Insomnia in Adults statement. J Clin Sleep Med 2005;1(4):412–21.

2. Roth T, Roehrs T. Insomnia: epidemiology, characteristics, and consequences. Clin Cornerstone 2003;5(3):5–15.

3. Ohayon MM, Caulet M, Lemoine P. Comorbidity of mental and insomnia disorders in the general population. Compr Psychiatry 1998;39(4):185–97.

4. Ohayon MM, Roth T. Place of chronic insomnia in the course of depressive and anxiety disorders. J Psychiatr Res 2003;37(1):9–15.

5. Sarsour K, Morin CM, Foley K, et al. Association of insomnia severity and comorbid medical and psychiatric disorders in a health plan-based sample: Insomnia severity and comorbidities. Sleep Med 2010;11(1):69–74.

6. Taylor DJ, Mallory LJ, Lichstein KL, et al. Comorbidity of chronic insomnia with medical problems. Sleep 2007;30(2):213–8.

7. Staner L, Boeijinga P, Danel T, et al. Effects of acamprosate on sleep during alcohol withdrawal: a double-blind placebo-controlled polysomnographic study in alcohol-dependent subjects. Alcohol Clin Exp Res 2006;30(9):1492–9.

8. Buysse DJ, Reynolds CF, Houck PR, et al. Does lorazepam impair the antidepressant response to nortriptyline and psychotherapy? J Clin Psychiatry 1997;58(10):426–32.

9. Dew MA, Reynolds CF, Houck PR, et al. Temporal profiles of the course of depression during treatment. Predictors of pathways toward recovery in the elderly. Arch Gen Psychiatry 1997;54(11):1016–24.

10. An H, Chung S. A case of obstructive sleep apnea syndrome presenting as paradoxical insomnia. Psychiatry Investig 2010;7(1):75–8.

11. Fava M, McCall WV, Krystal A, et al. Eszopiclone co-administered with fluoxetine in patients with insomnia coexisting with major depressive disorder. Biol Psychiatry 2006;59(11):1052–60.

12. Brower KJ, Myra Kim H, Strobbe S, et al. A randomized double-blind pilot trial of gabapentin versus placebo to treat alcohol dependence and comorbid insomnia. Alcohol Clin Exp Res 2008;32(8):1429–38.

13. Lettieri CJ, Shah AA, Holley AB, et al. Effects of a short course of eszopiclone on continuous positive airway pressure adherence: a randomized trial. Ann Intern Med 2009;151(10):696–702.

14. Glidewell R, Roby E, Orr W. The course of insomnia prior to and following treatment of obstructive sleep apnea. Sleep 2010;33(Abstract Supplement):A171.

15. Foster JH, Peters TJ. Impaired sleep in alcohol misusers and dependent alcoholics and the impact upon outcome. Alcohol Clin Exp Res 1999;23(6):1044–51.

16. Brower KJ. Alcohol's effects on sleep in alcoholics. Alcohol Res Health 2001;25(2):110–25.

17. Carney CE, Segal ZV, Edinger JD, et al. A comparison of rates of residual insomnia symptoms following pharmacotherapy or cognitive-behavioral therapy for major depressive disorder. J Clin Psychiatry 2007;68(2):254–60.

18. Doghramji K. Common comorbidies of insomnia. 2009. Available at: http://cme.medscape.com/viewarticle/585753. Accessed November 11, 2010.

19. Chesson A, Hartse K, Anderson WM, et al. Practice parameters for the evaluation of chronic insomnia. An American Academy of Sleep Medicine report. Standards of Practice Committee of the American Academy of Sleep Medicine. Sleep 2000;23(2):237–41.

20. Buysse DJ, Ancoli-Israel S, Edinger JD, et al. Recommendations for a standard research assessment of insomnia. Sleep 2006;29(9):1155–73.

21. Roth T. Comorbid insomnia: current directions and future challenges. Am J Manag Care 2009;15(Suppl):S6–13.

22. American Psychiatric Association, Association AP, American Psychiatric Association Task Force on DSM-IV, editors. Diagnostic and statistical manual of mental disorders. Washington, DC: American Psychiatric Publishing; 2000. p. 943.

23. American Academy of sleep Medicine, editor. The international classification of sleep disorders. Westchester (IL): American Academy of Sleep Medicine; 2005. p. 297.

24. Littner M, Hirshkowitz M, Kramer M, et al. Standards of Practice Committee of the American Academy of Sleep Medicine. Practice parameters for using polysomnography to evaluate insomnia: an update for 2002. Sleep 2003;26(6):754–60.

25. Walker MP. The role of sleep in cognition and emotion. Ann N Y Acad Sci 2009;1156:168–97.

26. Saper CB, Chou TC, Scammell TE. The sleep switch: hypothalamic control of sleep and wakefulness. Trends Neurosci 2001;24(12):726–31.

27. Bliwise DL, Foley DJ, Vitiello MV, et al. Nocturia and disturbed sleep in the elderly. Sleep Med 2009;10(5):540–8.

28. Tan TL, Kales JD, Kales A, et al. Biopsychobehavioral correlates of insomnia. IV: Diagnosis based on DSM-III. Am J Psychiatry 1984;141(3):357–62.

29. Buysse DJ, Reynolds CF, Kupfer DJ, et al. Clinical diagnoses in 216 insomnia patients using the

International Classification of Sleep Disorders (ICSD), DSM-IV and ICD-10 categories: a report from the APA/NIMH DSM-IV Field Trial. Sleep 1994;17(7):630–7.

30. Breslau N, Roth T, Rosenthal L, et al. Sleep disturbance and psychiatric disorders: a longitudinal epidemiological study of young adults. Biol Psychiatry 1996;39(6):411–8.

31. Soldatos CR. Insomnia in relation to depression and anxiety: epidemiologic considerations. J Psychosom Res 1994;38(Suppl 1):3–8.

32. Staner L. Comorbidity of insomnia and depression. Sleep Med Rev 2010;14(1):35–46.

33. Judd LL, Akiskal HS, Maser JD, et al. Major depressive disorder: a prospective study of residual subthreshold depressive symptoms as predictor of rapid relapse. J Affect Disord 1998; 50(2–3):97–108.

34. Paykel ES, Ramana R, Cooper Z, et al. Residual symptoms after partial remission: an important outcome in depression. Psychol Med 1995;25(6): 1171–80.

35. Reynolds CF, Frank E, Houck PR, et al. Which elderly patients with remitted depression remain well with continued interpersonal psychotherapy after discontinuation of antidepressant medication? Am J Psychiatry 1997;154(7):958–62.

36. Perlis ML, Giles DE, Buysse DJ, et al. Self-reported sleep disturbance as a prodromal symptom in recurrent depression. J Affect Disord 1997; 42(2–3):209–12.

37. Nierenberg AA, Keefe BR, Leslie VC, et al. Residual symptoms in depressed patients who respond acutely to fluoxetine. J Clin Psychiatry 1999;60(4):221–5.

38. Manber R, Chambers AS. Insomnia and depression: a multifaceted interplay. Curr Psychiatry Rep 2009;11(6):437–42.

39. McCall WV, Reboussin BA, Cohen W. Subjective measurement of insomnia and quality of life in depressed inpatients. J Sleep Res 2000;9(1):43–8.

40. Nofzinger EA, Schwartz RM, Reynolds CF, et al. Affect intensity and phasic REM sleep in depressed men before and after treatment with cognitive-behavioral therapy. J Consult Clin Psychol 1994;62(1):83–91.

41. Manber R, Edinger JD, Gress JL, et al. Cognitive behavioral therapy for insomnia enhances depression outcome in patients with comorbid major depressive disorder and insomnia. Sleep 2008; 31(4):489–95.

42. Arnedt JT, Conroy DA, Brower KJ. Treatment options for sleep disturbances during alcohol recovery. J Addict Dis 2007;26(4):41–54.

43. Brower KJ, Aldrich MS, Robinson EA, et al. Insomnia, self-medication, and relapse to alcoholism. Am J Psychiatry 2001;158(3):399–404.

44. Currie SR, Clark S, Rimac S, et al. Comprehensive assessment of insomnia in recovering alcoholics using daily sleep diaries and ambulatory monitoring. Alcohol Clin Exp Res 2003;27(8):1262–9.

45. Roehrs T, Papineau K, Rosenthal L, et al. Ethanol as a hypnotic in insomniacs: self administration and effects on sleep and mood. Neuropsychopharmacology 1999;20(3):279–86.

46. Johnson EO, Roehrs T, Roth T, et al. Epidemiology of alcohol and medication as aids to sleep in early adulthood. Sleep 1998;21(2):178–86.

47. Feige B, Gann H, Brueck R, et al. Effects of alcohol on polysomnographically recorded sleep in healthy subjects. Alcohol Clin Exp Res 2006;30(9): 1527–37.

48. Ford DE, Kamerow DB. Epidemiologic study of sleep disturbances and psychiatric disorders. An opportunity for prevention? JAMA 1989;262(11): 1479–84.

49. Weissman MM, Greenwald S, Niño-Murcia G, et al. The morbidity of insomnia uncomplicated by psychiatric disorders. Gen Hosp Psychiatry 1997; 19(4):245–50.

50. Gillin JC. Are sleep disturbances risk factors for anxiety, depressive and addictive disorders? Acta Psychiatr Scand Suppl 1998;393:39–43.

51. Mello NK, Mendelson JH. Behavioral studies of sleep patterns in alcoholics during intoxication and withdrawal. J Pharmacol Exp Ther 1970; 175(1):94–112.

52. Caetano R, Clark CL, Greenfield TK. Prevalence, trends, and incidence of alcohol withdrawal symptoms: analysis of general population and clinical samples. Alcohol Health Res World 1998;22(1): 73–9.

53. Foster JH, Marshall EJ, Peters TJ. Application of a quality of life measure, the life situation survey (LSS), to alcohol-dependent subjects in relapse and remission. Alcohol Clin Exp Res 2000;24(11): 1687–92.

54. Drummond SP, Gillin JC, Smith TL, et al. The sleep of abstinent pure primary alcoholic patients: natural course and relationship to relapse. Alcohol Clin Exp Res 1998;22(8):1796–802.

55. Luyster FS, Buysse DJ, Strollo PJ. Comorbid insomnia and obstructive sleep apnea: challenges for clinical practice and research. J Clin Sleep Med 2010;6(2):196–204.

56. Chung KF. Insomnia subtypes and their relationships to daytime sleepiness in patients with obstructive sleep apnea. Respiration 2005;72(5): 460–5.

57. Krell SB, Kapur VK. Insomnia complaints in patients evaluated for obstructive sleep apnea. Sleep Breath 2005;9(3):104–10.

58. Krakow B, Melendrez D, Ferreira E, et al. Prevalence of insomnia symptoms in patients with

sleep-disordered breathing. Chest 2001;120(6): 1923–9.

59. Smith S, Sullivan K, Hopkins W, et al. Frequency of insomnia report in patients with obstructive sleep apnoea hypopnea syndrome (OSAHS). Sleep Med 2004;5(5):449–56.

60. Wickwire E, Smith M, Birnbaum S, et al. The relationship between insomnia complaints and CPAP use in a patient sample. Sleep 2009;32(Abstract Suppl):A227.

61. Aloia MS, Arnedt JT, Stanchina M, et al. How early in treatment is PAP adherence established? Revisiting night-to-night variability. Behav Sleep Med 2007;5(3):229–40.

62. Lichstein KL, Riedel BW, Lester KW, et al. Occult sleep apnea in a recruited sample of older adults with insomnia. J Consult Clin Psychol 1999;67(3): 405–10.

63. Lavigne G, Sessle BJ, editors. Sleep and pain. Seattle (WA): International Association for the Study of Pain; 2007. p. 473.

64. Lavigne G, McMillan D, Zucconi M. Pain and sleep. In: Kryger MH, Roth T, Dement WC, editors. Principles and practice of sleep medicine online. Philadelphia: W B Saunders Co; 2005.

65. Smith MT, Haythornthwaite JA. How do sleep disturbance and chronic pain inter-relate? Insights from the longitudinal and cognitive-behavioral clinical trials literature. Sleep Med Rev 2004;8(2): 119–32.

66. Smith MT, Quartana PJ, Okonkwo RM, et al. Mechanisms by which sleep disturbance contributes to osteoarthritis pain: a conceptual model. Curr Pain Headache Rep 2009;13(6):447–54.

67. Smith MT, Edwards RR, McCann UD, et al. The effects of sleep deprivation on pain inhibition and spontaneous pain in women. Sleep 2007;30(4):494–505.

68. Ong JC, Stepanski EJ, Gramling SE. Pain coping strategies for tension-type headache: possible implications for insomnia? J Clin Sleep Med 2009; 5(1):52–6.

69. Roehrs T, Hyde M, Blaisdell B, et al. Sleep loss and REM sleep loss are hyperalgesic. Sleep 2006; 29(2):145–51.

70. Smith MT, Wickwire EM, Grace EG, et al. Sleep disorders and their association with laboratory pain sensitivity in temporomandibular joint disorder. Sleep 2009;32(6):779–90.

71. Lineberger M, Means M, Edinger J. Sleep disturbance in fibromyalgia. Sleep Med Clin 2007;2:31–9.

72. Carney CE, Edinger JD, Manber R, et al. Beliefs about sleep in disorders characterized by sleep and mood disturbance. J Psychosom Res 2007; 62(2):179–88.

73. Burns JW, Crofford LJ, Chervin RD. Sleep stage dynamics in fibromyalgia patients and controls. Sleep Med 2008;9(6):689–96.

74. Landis CA, Lentz MJ, Rothermel J, et al. Decreased sleep spindles and spindle activity in midlife women with fibromyalgia and pain. Sleep 2004;27(4):741–50.

75. Hawker GA, French MR, Waugh EJ, et al. The multidimensionality of sleep quality and its relationship to fatigue in older adults with painful osteoarthritis. Osteoarthr Cartil 2010, in press. Available at: http:// dx.doi.org/10.1016/j.joca.2010.08.002. Accessed August 25, 2010.

76. Allen KD, Renner JB, Devellis B, et al. Osteoarthritis and sleep: the Johnston county osteoarthritis project. J Rheumatol 2008;35(6):1102–7.

77. Argoff CE. The coexistence of neuropathic pain, sleep, and psychiatric disorders: a novel treatment approach. Clin J Pain 2007;23(1):15–22.

78. Benoliel R, Eliav E, Sharav Y. Self-reports of pain-related awakenings in persistent orofacial pain patients. J Orofac Pain 2009;23(4):330–8.

79. Magnússon S, Gislason T. Chronic bronchitis in Icelandic males: prevalence, sleep disturbances and quality of life. Scand J Prim Health Care 1999;17(2):100–4.

80. Klink M, Quan SF. Prevalence of reported sleep disturbances in a general adult population and their relationship to obstructive airways diseases. Chest 1987;91(4):540–6.

81. Dodge R, Cline MG, Quan SF. The natural history of insomnia and its relationship to respiratory symptoms. Arch Intern Med 1995;155(16): 1797–800.

82. Mulloy E, McNicholas WT. Theophylline improves gas exchange during rest, exercise, and sleep in severe chronic obstructive pulmonary disease. Am Rev Respir Dis 1993;148(4 Pt 1):1030–6.

83. Martin RJ, Pak J. Overnight theophylline concentrations and effects on sleep and lung function in chronic obstructive pulmonary disease. Am Rev Respir Dis 1992;145(3):540–4.

84. Berry RB, Desa MM, Branum JP, et al. Effect of theophylline on sleep and sleep-disordered breathing in patients with chronic obstructive pulmonary disease. Am Rev Respir Dis 1991; 143(2):245–50.

85. Veale D, Cooper BG, Griffiths CJ, et al. The effect of controlled-release salbutamol on sleep and nocturnal oxygenation in patients with asthma and chronic obstructive pulmonary disease. Respir Med 1994;88(2):121–4.

86. McNicholas WT, Calverley PM, Lee A, et al. Long-acting inhaled anticholinergic therapy improves sleeping oxygen saturation in COPD. Eur Respir J 2004;23(6):825–31.

87. Martin RJ, Bartelson BL, Smith P, et al. Effect of ipratropium bromide treatment on oxygen saturation and sleep quality in COPD. Chest 1999; 115(5):1338–45.

88. Lo Coco D, Mattaliano A, Lo Coco A, et al. Increased frequency of restless legs syndrome in chronic obstructive pulmonary disease patients. Sleep Med 2009;10(5):572—6.

89. Charokopos N, Leotsinidis M, Pouli A, et al. Periodic limb movement during sleep and chronic obstructive pulmonary disease. Sleep Breath 2008;12(2):155—9.

90. Chen WC, Lim PS, Wu WC, et al. Sleep behavior disorders in a large cohort of Chinese (Taiwanese) patients maintained by long-term hemodialysis. Am J Kidney Dis 2006;48(2):277—84.

91. Koch BCP, Nagtegaal JE, Hagen EC, et al. Subjective sleep efficiency of hemodialysis patients. Clin Nephrol 2008;70(5):411—6.

92. Esposito MG, Cesare CM, De Santo RM, et al. Parathyroidectomy improves the quality of sleep in maintenance hemodialysis patients with severe hyperparathyroidism. J Nephrol 2008;21(Suppl 13): S92—6.

93. Zucker I, Yosipovitch G, David M, et al. Prevalence and characterization of uremic pruritus in patients undergoing hemodialysis: uremic pruritus is still a major problem for patients with end-stage renal disease. J Am Acad Dermatol 2003; 49(5):842—6.

94. Koch BCP, van der Putten K, Van Someren EJW, et al. Impairment of endogenous melatonin rhythm is related to the degree of chronic kidney disease (CREAM study). Nephrol Dial Transplant 2010; 25(2):513—9.

95. Koch BCP, Nagtegaal JE, Hagen EC, et al. The effects of melatonin on sleep-wake rhythm of daytime haemodialysis patients: a randomized, placebo-controlled, cross-over study (EMSCAP study). Br J Clin Pharmacol 2009;67(1):68—75.

96. Nordgren L, Sörensen S. Symptoms experienced in the last six months of life in patients with end-stage heart failure. Eur J Cardiovasc Nurs 2003; 2(3):213—7.

97. Skaug K, Eide GE, Gulsvik A. Prevalence and predictors of symptoms in the terminal stage of lung cancer: a community study. Chest 2007; 131(2):389—94.

98. Mandler RN, Anderson FA, Miller RG, et al. CARE Study Group. The ALS Patient Care Database: insights into end-of-life care in ALS. Amyotroph Lateral Scler Other Motor Neuron Disord 2001; 2(4):203—8.

99. Akechi T, Okuyama T, Akizuki N, et al. Associated and predictive factors of sleep disturbance in advanced cancer patients. Psychooncology 2007; 16(10):888—94.

100. Mystakidou K, Parpa E, Tsilika E, et al. How is sleep quality affected by the psychological and symptom distress of advanced cancer patients? Palliat Med 2009;23(1):46—53.

101. Jindal RD. Insomnia in patients with depression: some pathophysiological and treatment considerations. CNS Drugs 2009;23(4):309—29.

102. Krystal A, Fava M, Rubens R, et al. Evaluation of eszopiclone discontinuation after cotherapy with fluoxetine for insomnia with coexisting depression. J Clin Sleep Med 2007;3(1):48—55.

103. Asnis GM, Chakraburtty A, DuBoff EA, et al. Zolpidem for persistent insomnia in SSRI-treated depressed patients. J Clin Psychiatry 1999; 60(10):668—76.

104. Roth T, Workshop Participants. Does effective management of sleep disorders reduce substance dependence? Drugs 2009;69(Suppl 2):65—75.

105. Sutter K, Gache P. [The use of psychotropic drugs in alcoholism]. Rev Med Suisse 2005;1(26):1734—9 [in French].

106. Friedmann PD, Herman DS, Freedman S, et al. Treatment of sleep disturbance in alcohol recovery: a national survey of addiction medicine physicians. J Addict Dis 2003;22(2):91—103.

107. Johansson BA, Berglund M, Hanson M, et al. Dependence on legal psychotropic drugs among alcoholics. Alcohol Alcohol 2003;38(6):613—8.

108. Karam-Hage M, Brower KJ. Open pilot study of gabapentin versus trazodone to treat insomnia in alcoholic outpatients. Psychiatry Clin Neurosci 2003;57(5):542—4.

109. Jenkins CD, Stanton BA, Niemcryk SJ, et al. A scale for the estimation of sleep problems in clinical research. J Clin Epidemiol 1988;41(4): 313—21.

110. Smith MT, Huang MI, Manber R. Cognitive behavior therapy for chronic insomnia occurring within the context of medical and psychiatric disorders. Clin Psychol Rev 2005;25(5):559—92.

111. Arnedt JT, Conroy D, Rutt J, et al. An open trial of cognitive-behavioral treatment for insomnia comorbid with alcohol dependence. Sleep Med 2007; 8(2):176—80.

112. Currie SR, Clark S, Hodgins DC, et al. Randomized controlled trial of brief cognitive-behavioural interventions for insomnia in recovering alcoholics. Addiction 2004;99(9):1121—32.

113. Berry RB, Patel PB. Effect of zolpidem on the efficacy of continuous positive airway pressure as treatment for obstructive sleep apnea. Sleep 2006;29(8):1052—6.

114. Rosenberg R, Roach JM, Scharf M, et al. A pilot study evaluating acute use of eszopiclone in patients with mild to moderate obstructive sleep apnea syndrome. Sleep Med 2007;8(5):464—70.

115. Sériès F, Workshop Participants. Can improving sleep influence sleep-disordered breathing? Drugs 2009;69(Suppl 2):77—91.

116. Bradshaw DA, Ruff GA, Murphy DP. An oral hypnotic medication does not improve continuous

positive airway pressure compliance in men with obstructive sleep apnea. Chest 2006;130(5): 1369–76.

117. Engleman HM, Wild MR. Improving CPAP use by patients with the sleep apnoea/hypopnoea syndrome (SAHS). Sleep Med Rev 2003;7(1):81–99.

118. Olsen S, Smith S, Oei T, et al. Health belief model predicts adherence to CPAP before experience with CPAP. Eur Respir J 2008;32(3):710–7.

119. Weaver TE, Kribbs NB, Pack AI, et al. Night-to-night variability in CPAP use over the first three months of treatment. Sleep 1997;20(4):278–83.

120. Morphy H, Dunn KM, Lewis M, et al. Epidemiology of insomnia: a longitudinal study in a UK population. Sleep 2007;30(3):274–80.

121. Turk DC, Cohen MJM. Sleep as a marker in the effective management of chronic osteoarthritis pain with opioid analgesics. Semin Arthritis Rheum 2010;39(6):477–90.

122. Dimsdale JE, Norman D, DeJardin D, et al. The effect of opioids on sleep architecture. J Clin Sleep Med 2007;3(1):33–6.

123. Rosenthal M, Moore P, Groves E, et al. Sleep improves when patients with chronic OA pain are managed with morning dosing of once a day extended-release morphine sulfate (AVINZA): findings from a pilot study. J Opioid Manag 2007;3(3): 145–54.

124. Papaleontiou M, Henderson CR, Turner BJ, et al. Outcomes associated with opioid use in the treatment of chronic noncancer pain in older adults: a systematic review and meta-analysis. J Am Geriatr Soc 2010;58(7):1353–69.

125. James IGV, O'Brien CM, McDonald CJ. A randomized, double-blind, double-dummy comparison of the efficacy and tolerability of low-dose transdermal buprenorphine (BuTrans seven-day patches) with buprenorphine sublingual tablets (Temgesic) in patients with osteoarthritis pain. J Pain Symptom Manage 2010;40(2):266–78.

126. Gilron I. Gabapentin and pregabalin for chronic neuropathic and early postsurgical pain: current evidence and future directions. Curr Opin Anaesthesiol 2007;20(5):456–72.

127. Gordh TE, Stubhaug A, Jensen TS, et al. Gabapentin in traumatic nerve injury pain: a randomized, double-blind, placebo-controlled, cross-over, multi-center study. Pain 2008;138(2):255–66.

128. Straube S, Derry S, Moore RA, et al. Pregabalin in fibromyalgia—responder analysis from individual patient data. BMC Musculoskelet Disord 2010;11: 150.

129. Pick CG, Chernes Y, Rigai T, et al. The antinociceptive effect of zolpidem and zopiclone in mice. Pharmacol Biochem Behav 2005;81(3):417–23.

130. Moldofsky H, Lue FA, Mously C, et al. The effect of zolpidem in patients with fibromyalgia: a dose ranging, double blind, placebo controlled, modified crossover study. J Rheumatol 1996;23(3): 529–33.

131. Weschules DJ, Maxwell T, Reifsnyder J, et al. Are newer, more expensive pharmacotherapy options associated with superior symptom control compared to less costly agents used in a collaborative practice setting? Am J Hosp Palliat Care 2006; 23(2):135–49.

132. Roth T, Price JM, Amato DA, et al. The effect of eszopiclone in patients with insomnia and coexisting rheumatoid arthritis: a pilot study. Prim Care Companion J Clin Psychiatry 2009;11(6):292–301.

133. Roth T. Hypnotic use for insomnia management in chronic obstructive pulmonary disease. Sleep Med 2009;10(1):19–25.

134. Stege G, Vos PJE, van den Elshout FJJ, et al. Sleep, hypnotics and chronic obstructive pulmonary disease. Respir Med 2008;102(6):801–14.

135. Steens RD, Pouliot Z, Millar TW, et al. Effects of zolpidem and triazolam on sleep and respiration in mild to moderate chronic obstructive pulmonary disease. Sleep 1993;16(4):318–26.

136. Kryger M, Roth T, Wang-Weigand S, et al. The effects of ramelteon on respiration during sleep in subjects with moderate to severe chronic obstructive pulmonary disease. Sleep Breath 2009;13(1):79–84.

137. Sabbatini M, Crispo A, Pisani A, et al. Zaleplon improves sleep quality in maintenance hemodialysis patients. Nephron Clin Pract 2003;94(4): c99–103.

138. Durán JC, Greenspan A, Diago JI, et al. Evaluation of risperidone in the treatment of behavioral and psychological symptoms and sleep disturbances associated with dementia. Int Psychogeriatr 2005; 17(4):591–604.

139. Brusco LI, Fainstein I, Márquez M, et al. Effect of melatonin in selected populations of sleep-disturbed patients. Biol Signals Recept 1999; 8(1-2):126–31.

140. Singer C, Tractenberg RE, Kaye J, et al. Alzheimer's Disease Cooperative Study. A multicenter, placebo-controlled trial of melatonin for sleep disturbance in Alzheimer's disease. Sleep 2003; 26(7):893–901.

141. Matsuo N, Morita T. Efficacy, safety, and cost effectiveness of intravenous midazolam and flunitrazepam for primary insomnia in terminally ill patients with cancer: a retrospective multicenter audit study. J Palliat Med 2007;10(5):1054–62.

142. Matsuo N, Morita T. Intravenous infusion of midazolam and flunitrazepam for insomnia on Japanese palliative care units. J Pain Symptom Manage 2005;30(4):301–2.

143. Joffe H, Petrillo L, Viguera A, et al. Eszopiclone improves insomnia and depressive and anxious symptoms in perimenopausal and postmenopausal

women with hot flashes: a randomized, double-blinded, placebo-controlled crossover trial. Am J Obstet Gynecol 2010;202(2):171.e1–171.e11.

144. Eichling PS, Sahni J. Menopause related sleep disorders. J Clin Sleep Med 2005;1(3):291–300.

145. Spoormaker VI, Montgomery P. Disturbed sleep in post-traumatic stress disorder: secondary symptom or core feature? Sleep Med Rev 2008; 12(3):169–84.

146. Pollack M, Kinrys G, Krystal A, et al. Eszopiclone coadministered with escitalopram in patients with insomnia and comorbid generalized anxiety disorder. Arch Gen Psychiatry 2008;65(5):551–62.

147. O'Donnell JF. Insomnia in cancer patients. Clin Cornerstone 2004;6(Suppl 1D):S6–14.

148. Ranjbaran Z, Keefer L, Farhadi A, et al. Impact of sleep disturbances in inflammatory bowel disease. J Gastroenterol Hepatol 2007;22(11): 1748–53.

149. Orr WC. Sleep and gastroesophageal reflux disease: a wake-up call. Rev Gastroenterol Disord 2004;4(Suppl 4):S25–32.

150. Menza M, Dobkin RD, Marin H, et al. Treatment of insomnia in Parkinson's disease: a controlled trial of eszopiclone and placebo. Mov Disord 2010; 25(11):1708–14.

151. Gunn DG, Naismith SL, Lewis SJG. Sleep disturbances in Parkinson disease and their potential role in heterogeneity. J Geriatr Psychiatry Neurol 2010;23(2):131–7.

Therapeutics for Sleep-disordered Breathing

Francoise J. Roux, MD, PhD[a],*, Meir H. Kryger, MD[b,c]

KEYWORDS

- Obstructive sleep apnea • Pharmacotherapy
- Central apnea

Obstructive sleep apnea (OSA) is the most common sleep breathing disorder and its prevalence in the last decades has increased steadily in parallel to the obesity epidemic. An apnea is defined as cessation of airflow for at least 10 seconds in the presence of thoracoabdominal ventilatory efforts. A hypopnea is a reduction in airflow of at least 30% with a decrease in oxygen saturation of 2% or more for at least 10 seconds in the presence of thoracoabdominal ventilatory efforts.[1] The apnea-hypopnea index (AHI) is the sum of apneas and hypopneas per hour of sleep. An AHI of 5/h or greater establishes the diagnosis of OSA according to the criteria of the American Academy of Sleep Medicine. The evidence for the prevalence of OSA derives from large studies that estimated that, in Western countries, 24% of men and 15% of women have OSA, and 4% of men and 2% of women have OSA with symptoms of sleepiness.[2] It is now well established that OSA significantly increases the risk for developing hypertension,[3] coronary artery disease,[4] stroke,[5] and cardiac death,[6] and even all-cause mortality. Continuous positive airway pressure (CPAP) is considered the mainstay therapy for OSA. CPAP for OSA has been shown to improve sleep architecture,[7] decrease nocturnal desaturation events,[8] decrease daytime somnolence,[9] and improve neurocognitive function.[10] Treatment of OSAs with CPAP also plays an important role in improving cardiovascular outcomes such as hypertension[11]

and left ventricular function.[12] In addition, patients with OSAS who are treated with CPAP have decreased health care use and costs compared with untreated patients.[13,14] Despite these benefits, various studies have shown that compliance with CPAP therapy can vary dramatically[15,16] and may depend on multiple variables such as the degree of daytime hypersomnia. CPAP is not entirely free of pressure-related side effects. As a result, there has been an attempt to explore other therapeutic options such as pharmacologic therapy.

POTENTIAL BENEFICIAL DRUG TREATMENT OF OSA
Pharmacotherapy for Weight Loss

Sibutramine

Obesity is a chronic disease that has become an epidemic in the United States and worldwide. Approximately 127 million adults in the United States are overweight (body mass index [BMI], calculated as weight in kilograms divided by the square of height in meters of 25.0–29.9 kg/m^2) and 60 million are obese (BMI>30.0 kg/m^2).[17] Recent genetic studies suggest that shared susceptibility genes exist for obesity and OSA.[18] Swartz and colleagues[19] showed that upper airway collapsibility is higher among obese people compared with nonobese controls. Obesity can cause narrowing of the pharynx by the effect of

[a] Section of Pulmonary and Critical Care Medicine, Yale Center for Sleep Medicine, Yale University School of Medicine, 333 Cedar Street, PO Box 208057, New Haven, CT 06520-8057, USA
[b] Department of Medicine, University of Connecticut School of Medicine, 263 Farmington Avenue, Farmington, CT 06030, USA
[c] Gaylord Sleep Medicine, 400 Gaylord Farm Road, Wallingford, CT 06492, USA
* Corresponding author.
E-mail address: francoise.roux@yale.edu

Sleep Med Clin 5 (2010) 647–657
doi:10.1016/j.jsmc.2010.09.001

subcutaneous and periluminal fat deposits; obesity can also alter compliance of the airway wall secondary to increased fat deposition, thus promoting airway collapse.[20] Increasing weight has been associated with an increasing prevalence of OSA[2] and has also been shown to worsen OSA.[21] Weight loss has been shown to alleviate OSA,[21] thus strengthening a causal relationship between obesity and OSA. Dietary treatments have been disappointing, with an overall success rate of only 14% over long periods of time in the general population.[22] As a result, the American College has recommended pharmacologic therapy for patients with a BMI of 30 kg/m^2 or greater, or a BMI of 27 kg/m^2 or greater if comorbid conditions such as cardiovascular disease, OSA, or diabetes were present.[23] The medications used to promote weight loss act mostly on neurotransmitters of the central nervous system to reduce appetite. Sibutramine was initially developed as a potential antidepressant but was noted to have some weight-loss properties. It was approved by the US Food and Drug Administration (FDA) in 1997 as a long-term weight-loss agent and is commonly used. It is a serotonin and norepinephrine reuptake inhibitor that suppresses appetite, increases energy expenditure, and has been shown to be effective as a weight-loss agent. Sibutramine has been shown to decrease visceral fat in obese patients,[24] which would confer significant metabolic advantage because visceral adiposity could affect upper airway control in patients who have sleep-disordered breathing.[25] Many studies using sibutramine have been carried out in obese women. Among obese men with OSA the effect of combined sibutramine-dietary treatment was investigated in an uncontrolled cohort study. After 24 weeks of this combined regimen, the breathing disturbance index dropped from 46 to 30 per hour with a concomitant weight loss of about 8%.[26] However, only a minority of patients were cured from their OSA.

A 6-month study of the largest cohort of obese men (BMI 30–38 kg/m^2) with moderate to severe OSA examined the combined effect of sibutramine with 600-Kcal–deficit diet and exercise.[27] Intraabdominal, subcutaneous, and liver fat were assessed using computed tomography scans. At 6 months, there was only a 7.5% decrease in weight but a marked reduction in visceral, subcutaneous, and liver fat, with a small improvement in insulin sensitivity. Despite these decreases in weight and fat stores, there was only a partial improvement in sleep-disordered breathing, with the respiratory disturbance index dropping from 45.9 ($\pm$23) to 30.2 ($\pm$20.4)/h. Other studies have shown a modest decrease in weight loss in the order of

5% in patients on sibutramine compared with those on placebo.[28] Because of its noradrenergic activity, sibutramine has the potential to contribute to systemic arterial hypertension and cardiac arrhythmias. Thus, sibutramine might not be the optimal choice in patients with sleep-disordered breathing who are already at increased risk for adverse cardiovascular consequences, although the Sibutramine Cardiovascular Outcome (SCOUT) trial did not show any adverse cardiovascular complications in patients with preexisting cardiovascular disease, diabetes, or hypertension on sibutramine for 6 weeks.[29] In summary, there is still insufficient evidence to justify sibutramine as the main therapy in obese patients with sleep-disordered breathing.

Antidepressants

Paroxetine and fluoxetine

During breathing, various forces promote airway collapse and airway patency in the upper airways. The 2 primary forces tending to collapse the airway are the intraluminal negative pressure generated by the diaphragm during inspiration and the extraluminal tissue pressure (the pressure resulting from tissues and bony structures surrounding the airway). These forces are counterbalanced primarily by the action of pharyngeal dilator muscles. The hypoglossal muscle is the main dilator muscle of the upper airways, and serotoninergic mechanisms can increase hypoglossal nerve activity. Multiple serotonin (5HT) receptor subtypes have been identified in the motor neurons of the upper airways,[30] but serotonin delivery to these upper airway dilator motor neurons seems to be decreased during sleep in patients with OSA.[31] OSA has also been shown to be worse during rapid eye movement (REM) sleep and selective serotonin reuptake inhibitors (SSRI) are known to decrease REM sleep. As a result, various clinical studies in humans have focused on the potential beneficial effect of SSRI to improve sleep-disordered breathing. The efficacy of paroxetine was assessed in a double-blind, randomized, placebo-controlled trial in patients with severe OSA. Paroxetine could induce an increased genioglossal electromyogram activity but this increase was not sufficient to significantly alter the severity of the OSA.[32] Another randomized, double-blind, placebo-controlled, cross-over study investigated the effect of 6 weeks of paroxetine on OSA indices. Paroxetine reduced the apnea index by about 35% during non-REM sleep but had no effect during REM sleep. Paroxetine had no significant effect on the hypopnea indices or on the daytime sleepiness.[33] Protriptyline has also been shown to activate hypoglossal motor neurons. A prospective, cross-over, unblinded study compared the effect of 4 weeks of fluoxetine with protriptyline in patients with OSA. Fluoxetine was as effective as protriptyline in reducing sleep-disordered breathing, with a decrease in AHI from 57 ($\pm$9)/h to 34 ($\pm$6)/h and 33 ($\pm$8)/h, with fluoxetine and protriptyline, respectively. However, despite 4 weeks of treatment, most patients were still left with severe residual OSA.[34] Fluoxetine was better tolerated than protriptyline.

Mirtazapine
Mirtazapine is another antidepressant that can increase serotonergic and noradrenergic systems. Mirtazapine is a 5HT1 agonist with 5HT2 and 5HT3 antagonist activity. In rats, mirtazapine has been shown to increase genioglossus activity at a dose commonly used to treat depression.[35] In humans, the effect of mirtazapine was assessed for 3 consecutive 7-day treatments during a randomized, double-blind, placebo-controlled, 3-way, cross-over study in patients with moderate OSA.[36] Mirtazapine reduced the AHI by about 50% compared with placebo, but no concomitant significant improvement in oxygenation or sleep architecture was seen. However, most patients were not cured of their OSA despite the improvement in AHI. In contrast, another randomized, placebo-controlled trial showed that mirtazapine did not improve sleep-disordered breathing and was even associated with weight gain compared with placebo,[37] which has the potential to worsen OSA.

Protrityline
Protrityline is a nonsedating tricyclic antidepressant that has been used for many years and is a profound REM suppressant agent. It was believed that it could improve sleep-disordered breathing because of its REM suppressant activity but also through increasing dilator muscle tone in the upper airways. However, various randomized, placebo-controlled trials failed to show any clinically relevant efficacy as a treatment of OSA despite a decrease in REM sleep, even in patients with mild to moderate OSA.[38,39]

In summary, the antidepressants do not dramatically affect the severity of sleep-disordered breathing despite their potential to increase upper airway tone.

Cholinergic Medications
It has been suggested that decreased brainstem cholinergic projections could contribute to sleep-disordered breathing in multisystem atrophy.[40]

Acetylcholine might play a role in upper airway patency through both central and peripheral mechanisms.

Physostigmine
Physostigmine is an acetylcholinesterase inhibitor that increases muscle contraction through its action at the neuromuscular junction. Physostigmine was given as an overnight infusion to patients with moderate to severe OSA in a placebo-controlled, randomized trial. Overall physostigmine decreased the AHI by about 21% but had a more pronounced effect during REM sleep, with a decrease in AHI of 67.5% compared with placebo. However, despite these improvements with physostigmine, residual OSA was still evident in all but 1 patient.[41]

Donepezil
Donepezil is also an acetylcholinesterase inhibitor that has been approved to increase acetylcholine transmission in patients with Alzheimer disease. Donepezil was given for 3 months to patients with Alzheimer disease with mild to moderate OSA in a randomized, placebo-controlled trial. Most patients (81%) taking donepezil showed some improvement in sleep-disordered breathing compared with no change in the placebo group.[42] The donepezil group had a reduction in AHI from 20/h to 9.9/h with concomitant improvement in oxygenation.

Ventilatory Modulants
Various classes of medications have been tested for their ability to increase ventilatory drive.

Acetalozamide
Acetalozamide is a carbonic anhydrase inhibitor, an enzyme that was first discovered in the 1930s. This enzyme leads to renal excretion of bicarbonate, which produces a metabolic acidosis. This metabolic acidosis acts on peripheral and central chemoreceptors to increase ventilation.[43] Most of the studies on the efficacy of acetazolamide in patients with OSA involved small number of patients. Inoue and colleagues[44] recruited 75 patients with moderate to severe OSA, including some with central apneas, and found that 39 days of acetazolamide decreased the AHI from 27.1/h to 19.1/h and increased the oxygen saturation from a nadir of 71.9% to 79.5%. All types of apneas were reduced after acetazolamide use. Another small study found improvement in OSA after acetazolamide treatment.[45] The effect of 14 day of acetazolamide was investigated in a randomized, double-blind, placebo-controlled study in 10 patients with OSA. Acetazolamide

significantly reduced the AHI indices compared with placebo, but there was significant residual OSA, with an AHI of 26/h, and some patients experienced side effects in the form of paresthesias. Acetazolamide did not improve daytime somnolence.[38] Acetazolamide has also been shown to have some beneficial effect on central apneas,[46] most likely through its effect on chemoreceptors.

The methylxanthine derivatives

Theophylline and aminophylline are methylxanthine derivates and were traditionally used to treat chronic obstructive lung disease because they have bronchodilator properties. Theophylline seems also to induce a cAMP-mediated excitation of respiratory neurons.[47] There are few studies of the effect of theophylline on OSA. Mulloy and McNicholas[48] examined the effect of 4 weeks of theophylline in patients with OSA in a double-blind, placebo-controlled, cross-over trial. The AHI in the theophylline group improved in a small but significant fashion, from 49/h to 40/h, with fewer oxygen desaturations, but sleep efficiency was reduced. In contrast, another study showed that theophylline had no significant effect on sleep architecture and improved sleep-disordered breathing mainly in patients with moderate OSA.[49] Theophylline can also improve central apneas in patients with Cheyne-Stokes breathing and congestive heart failure.[50]

Progesterone and estrogen therapy

Progesterone has been shown in humans to increase the ventilatory response to hypercapnia and hypoxia. Progesterone seems to act through central mechanisms to achieve a stimulant ventilatory effect.[51] The incidence of OSA is increased among postmenopausal women and estrogen enhances chemosensitivity. A small pilot study examined the effect of estradiol with and without progesterone in postmenopausal women with OSA. Estradiol alone reduced the AHI from 22.7/h to 12.2/h, but the addition of progesterone had no additional beneficial effect.[52] In contrast, another pilot study found that 1 month of estrogen therapy could reduce the respiratory disturbance index by 25% in postmenopausal women with sleep apnea, and the addition of progesterone further reduced the index to 50%.[53] However, Cistulli and colleagues[54] found that short-term treatment with estrogen either alone or in combination with progesterone had no significant effect on sleep-disordered breathing in postmenopausal women with OSA. These results were confirmed in a larger, randomized, controlled, cross-over trial studying the effect of estrogen replacement therapy on postmenopausal women. Estrogen therapy for 3 months had minimal effect on upper airway resistance syndrome or apneas in these postmenopausal women.[55] A recent randomized placebo-controlled trial examined the potential benefit of 6 months of estrogen and progestin treatment in pre- and late-postmenopausal women. The investigators found no benefit of estrogen-progestin treatment on sleep quality using objective measures such as polysomnography.[56] A randomized, double-blind trial in men also failed to show any benefit of medroxyprogesterone acetate on the frequency or duration of sleep-disordered breathing.[57]

Nicotine

Nicotinic acetylcholine receptors are expressed in the brainstem and spinal cord. Nicotinic receptors can increase respiratory drive and modulate the hypoglossal nerve output and, as such, might play a therapeutic role in sleep-disordered breathing.[58] A study involving a small number of patients suggested that nicotine could improve sleep-disordered breathing in patients with OSA. Transdermal nicotine was given to nonsmoking patients with OSA in a randomized, placebo-controlled fashion. Nicotine reduced the intensity of snoring but had no effect on the apneas. Nicotine also had a detrimental effect on sleep architecture, with decreased sleep efficiency and prolonged sleep latency.[59] Another recent randomized, double-blind, cross-over trial examined the effect of transdermal nicotine in patients with OSA using polysomnography. Despite high levels of nicotine in the saliva, nicotine had no effect on the AHI indices in those patients.[60]

Opiate Antagonists

Naloxone and naltrexone

Endogenous opiates can depress the respiratory drive. An increase in opioid activity was noted in the cerebrospinal fluid of patients with OSA compared with controls,[61] suggesting that opioids might play a role in the pathogenesis of OSA. Naloxone and naltrexone are opiate antagonists, and have been proposed as a therapeutic option in patients with sleep-disordered breathing. A study involving 12 patients with OSA in the late 1980s showed that naltrexone could reduce apnea indices.[62] The same investigators showed that naltrexone could improve nocturnal oxygenation through its effect on the sleep architecture, decreasing REM sleep and increasing wake after sleep onset.[63] In patients with moderate to severe OSA, other reports have shown that naloxone shortened the duration of apneas but had no significant effect on their number.[64,65]

Antihypertensive Medications

Even mild OSA significantly increases the risk of developing hypertension.[3] Hypertension is common among patients with OSA. Animal models have shown that hypertension per se can worsen pharyngeal collapsibility and increase the severity of sleep apnea, whereas a decrease in blood pressure had the reverse effect.[66,67] A small, randomized, double-blind trial investigated the effect of 1 week of either metoprolol or cilazapril on sleep-disordered breathing in patients with OSA. The investigators found that metoprolol and cilazapril induced, respectively, only a small reduction in the AHI from 45/h to 34/h and 54 to 40/h.[68] A small study, using clonidine, and a large, randomized, double-blind trial of cilazapril failed to show any significant effect of these antihypertensive medications on sleep-disordered breathing in patients with OSA despite blood pressure reduction.[69,70] These studies do not show any significant effect of blood pressure reduction on sleep-disordered breathing.

Intranasal Medications

Nasal obstruction is common in the general population and rhinitis has been associated with an increased likelihood of habitual snoring.[71] Increased nasal resistance induces a more negative intrapharyngeal pressure, which might promote upper airway collapse. However, the role of nasal obstruction in the pathogenesis of OSA is still debated but might be a cofactor, especially among patients with mild OSA. Topical nasal steroids have been found to improve subjective parameters of sleep quality such as fatigue and daytime sleepiness, but had no effect on the apnea/hypopnea indices in patients with allergic rhinitis treated for 4 weeks.[72] In contrast, patients with OSA and associated rhinitis experienced some improvement in their sleep-disordered breathing after 4 weeks of intranasal corticosteroid therapy in a randomized, placebo-controlled, cross-over study.[73] There was no difference in snoring between the treatment and placebo groups. Randomized, controlled studies in patients with OSA and chronic nasal congestion treated with a nasal decongestant such as xylometazoline or oxymetazoline failed to show any clinically significant improvement in sleep-disordered breathing or sleep quality/daytime sleepiness[74] even when nasal resistance was reduced.[75] Those studies suggest that the nose is not a significant contributor to the pathogenesis of OSA, but the number of patients studied is small.

Domperidone

Domperidone is a selective dopaminergic antagonist with prokinetic properties. In patients with OSA, domperidone was shown to improve peripheral chemosensitivity and increase the hypercapnic ventilatory response.[76] The combination of domperidone and pseudoephedrine sulfate for 30 days was shown to significantly reduce snoring compared with placebo in habitual loud snorers.[77] In patients with snoring and witnessed apneas, a retrospective case series showed that the combination of pseudoephedrine and domperidone led to disappearance of severe snoring and apneas, with significant improvement in nocturnal oximetry and decreased daytime hypersomnia in most patients.[78] However, the safety of long-term use of pseudoephedrine is a concern because of its adverse cardiovascular effects.

MEDICATIONS WITH POSSIBLE DETRIMENTAL EFFECT ON SLEEP-DISORDERED BREATHING
Hypnotics

Benzodiazepines
Benzodiazepines are widely prescribed hypnotics. OSA can present with manifestations of insomnia, especially in women. The benzodiazepines bind nonselectively to the γ-aminobutyric acid A (GABA-A) receptor in the brain. GABA-A is the predominant central nervous system inhibitory neurotransmitter. This nonselective binding of the benzodiazepines is responsible for side effects such as muscle relaxation and sedation. These side effects might potentially worsen sleep-disordered breathing and cause hypoventilation and respiratory depression in predisposed hosts. A randomized, placebo-controlled trial examined the effect of flurazepam on sleep-disordered breathing and nocturnal oximetry in asymptomatic patients. Flurazepam taken before bedtime led to a significant increase in the number and duration of apneas compared with placebo, with a decrease in nocturnal oxygen saturation as determined by polysomnography.[79] A case report showed that flurazepam induced OSA in a patient with insomnia, which resolved after withdrawal of flurazepam.[80] Conversely, a small study showed that temazepam did not worsen sleep-disordered breathing in insomniac patients with underlying mild OSA.[81] In a group of normal patients and chronic snorers, a randomized trial showed no effect of triazolam and flunitrazepam on the respiratory disturbance and oxygen desaturation indices.[82] Other investigators have shown no significant effect of benzodiazepines on nocturnal breathing in normal subjects.[83] In summary, the effect of benzodiazepines on nocturnal breathing

is controversial and requires further studies involving a larger number of patients.

Nonbenzodiazepines

The nonbenzodiazepines (eg, zolpidem, eszopiclone) are structurally different from the benzodiazepines and bind more selectively to GABA-A receptor subtypes, leading to sedation but fewer side effects and no myorelaxant activity. A case report even described that zolpidem could improve idiopathic central apneas in a patient complaining of nocturnal sleep disruption.[84] A case series confirmed those findings and showed that 9 weeks of zolpidem significantly improved the central apnea indices without worsening the obstructive apneas or the oxygenation component in most of the patients with idiopathic central apneas. However, there was no randomization and no placebo control in that study; 3 patients experienced worsening of the obstructive events.[85] The effect of a single dose of zolpidem on breathing during sleep was also studied in a randomized, double-blind, cross-over trial in patients with OSA.[86] The investigators found that zolpidem did not worsen sleep-disordered breathing in these patients with OSA, but significantly decreased nocturnal oxygenation compared with placebo. Another study, using the same methodology, assessed the effect of eszopiclone for 2 nights in patients with mild to moderate OSA.[87] Eszopiclone did not worsen the sleep apnea parameters compared with placebo and was well tolerated. Limited data on the effect of nonbenzodiazepines on OSA are available and further studies are needed to ensure the safety of the nonbenzodiazepines in this patient population.

Ramelteon

Ramelteon is a novel synthetic analogue of melatonin that binds selectively to the melatonin MT1/MT2 receptors in the suprachiasmatic nucleus of the hypothalamus. Ramelteon is a novel chronohypnotic approved by the FDA for the treatment of insomnia. Unlike other hypnotics, ramelteon does not produce central nervous system depression and side effects such as daytime sedation that are associated with some of the classic hypnotics. Only 1 randomized, double-blind, placebo-controlled, cross-over study has examined the effect of 16 mg (twice the therapeutic dose indicated for insomnia) of ramelteon in patients with mild to moderate OSA, using polysomnography. Ramelteon had no significant effect on the AHI and on the nocturnal oxygen saturation compared with placebo.[88] In summary, ramelteon treatment seems to be safe in patients with mild to moderate OSA, but more studies are needed to ensure the safety of this novel hypnotic.

Antipsychotics

Quetiapine

Quetiapine is an atypical antipsychotic approved for the treatment of schizophrenia and bipolar disorder. It is a 5HT-2A, histamine, and dopamine D2 receptor antagonist and is usually well tolerated. However, some recent studies have raised the concern that quetiapine might have some detrimental respiratory effects even at normal doses. Some case reports highlighted that quetiapine, in addition to benzodiazepines, can lead to acute respiratory failure in patients with underlying OSA.[89] Rishi and colleagues[90] examined the effect of atypical antipsychotics on OSA, including quetiapine, compared with a control group. This retrospective study supported a possible weight-independent association between the intake of atypical antipsychotics and the severity of OSA; however, the sample size was small.

Muscle Relaxants

Baclofen

Baclofen is a GABA-B agonist with muscle relaxant and antispasmodic properties. It is commonly prescribed in patients with chronic neurologic disorders such as multiple sclerosis or spinal cord lesions. As a muscle relaxant, baclofen has the potential to promote upper airway collapse during sleep and worsen sleep-disordered breathing. Baclofen was given before sleep in patients with mild OSA in a double-blind, placebo-controlled, cross-over study. The polysomnographic parameters revealed that baclofen did not increase the apnea/hypopnea indices and produced only a mild decrease in nocturnal oxygen saturation in this OSA population.[91] However, considering the paucity of studies, baclofen should be used cautiously in patients with sleep-disordered breathing.

Opiates

The prescription of acute and chronic opiates has dramatically increased in the last decade. For example, the retail distribution of methadone has increased by more than 1000% in the last 10 years and is likely to be used by patients with undiagnosed OSA. However, data from Utah revealed that the unintentional death rate had also increased in relation to methadone and oxycodone treatment.[92] Opiates are well known to decrease the respiratory drive though their stimulation of the μ-opioid receptor in the brain and of the respiratory neurons. Given the known opiate effects on respiration, it is surprising that only in 2001 was it reported that patients in a methadone maintenance program experienced central apneas.[93] Later, a small study found that the prevalence of central apneas can reach up to 30% in patients on a methadone maintenance program.[94] A retrospective cohort study showed that chronic opioid use was associated with the development of central apneas with a dose response effect.[95] These central apneas are distinct from Cheyne-Stokes respiration, and are characterized by an irregular pattern of breathing during non-REM sleep called Biot respiration or ataxic breathing. It is less clear whether chronic opioid therapy is a risk factor for developing OSA. There have been anecdotal reports and small studies showing that patients on long-term opioid therapy experienced prolonged obstructive apneas during sleep.[96] Conversely, other studies, including one with 50 patients on long-term methadone therapy, did not report any increase in the occurrence of obstructive events compared with placebo.[94] Nonetheless, opioid therapy affects the control of breathing and has the potential for adverse effects. Opioid therapy should be prescribed under close clinical supervision in susceptible patients, especially those with underlying OSA.

Sodium Oxybate

OSA occurs more commonly in patients with narcolepsy than in the general population, affecting up to 24% of narcoleptic patients.[97] Sodium oxybate is approved by the FDA for treatment of cataplexy and excessive daytime sleepiness in narcoleptic patients. Sodium oxybate is a central nervous system depressant and has the potential to lead to respiratory depression if associated with alcohol or other central respiratory drive depressants. A case report found that narcoleptic patients treated with sodium oxybate experienced a significant worsening in their OSA, with an AHI increasing from a baseline of 11/h without sodium oxybate to 45/h after 2 nights on sodium oxybate.[98] In contrast, a randomized, cross-over study showed that 9 g of sodium oxybate, in patients with mild to moderate OSA not treated with CPAP, did not worsen the obstructive events compared with placebo. However, an increase in central apneas was noted in the sodium oxybate group compared with placebo.[99] After studying the acute effect of sodium oxybate intake, the same author examined the effect of 2 weeks of sodium oxybate administration (4.5 g for 13 nights, then 9 g for day 14) on patients with mild to moderate OSA. Sodium oxybate administration for 14 days did not worsen the obstructive or the

central events compared with placebo; however, concurrent CPAP therapy was not controlled in this study.[100] In summary, sodium oxybate, when prescribed at maximal dose, should be prescribed cautiously in patients with underlying OSA who are not compliant with CPAP therapy.

Phosphodiesterase-5 Inhibitors

Sildenafil

Sildenafil is commonly used to treat pulmonary hypertension and erectile dysfunction, the latter being a common complaint among patients with OSA. It is a specific phosphodiesterase-5 inhibitor that can increase NO availability with resulting smooth muscle relaxation and vasodilatation. This specific enzyme is expressed in the nasal cavity, tracheobronchial muscles, and pulmonary vasculature and could potentially worsen OSA by decreasing nasal patency and relaxing upper airway muscles. Roizenblatt and colleagues[101] studied the effect of a single dose of 50 mg of sildenafil in patients with severe OSA using a randomized, placebo-controlled trial. Sildenafil worsened OSA by increasing the AHI from 27/h at baseline to 43.5/h with sildenafil, and also increasing the duration of oxygen saturation less than 90%.

MEDICATIONS THAT DECREASE THE SYMPTOMS OF SLEEP-DISORDERED BREATHING
Modafinil and Armodafinil

Modafinil and armodafinil have been approved by the FDA to treat patients with sleep-disordered breathing with residual hypersomnia despite adequate treatment and compliance with CPAP. Amphetamines have been prescribed in the past for the same indication but have many drawbacks, including cardiovascular side effects. Armodafinil is the R-enantiomer of modafinil and has a much longer half-life of up to 14 hours. Modafinil was effective in reducing daytime hypersomnia measured by the Epworth Sleepiness Scale and Multiple Sleep Latency Tests in patients with OSA with residual hypersomnia despite treatment with CPAP. However, in a multicenter, double-blind, placebo-controlled study involving a large number of patients, the objective measures of daytime sleepiness improved but did not normalize.[102] Another multicenter randomized trial also found that modafinil could decrease daytime hypersomnia in patients with OSA and persistent sleepiness, but only to a certain extent.[103] Another study looked at the effect of armodafinil on sleepiness compared with placebo in patients with hypersomnia associated with OSA despite adequate treatment with CPAP. Armodafinil improved the ability to stay awake compared with placebo, as shown by an improvement in Maintenance Wakefulness Test sleep latency of about 2.3 minutes in comparison with placebo.[104] Armodafinil was also found to reduce fatigue and improve memory in those patients. This improvement in residual daytime sleepiness with armodafinil, despite effective treatment with CPAP, was also confirmed by a large multicenter trial and the improvement was maintained for a 12-week period.[105]

SUMMARY

Pharmacotherapy for OSA would be ideal because CPAP therapy is generally not well accepted by patients, especially by those who do not experience daytime hypersomnia.

Many trials have investigated the effect of various medications on sleep-disordered breathing but most studies have involved a small number of patients and/or inadequate duration of the pharmacologic treatment. The most promising of these medications, such as the serotonergic drugs, only moderately improved the apnea/hypopnea indices and failed to completely normalize sleep-disordered breathing. Cardiovascular complications may arise even in patients with mild OSA. Consequently, it is important to achieve nearly complete resolution of sleep-disordered breathing to prevent downstream diseases, but no single pharmacologic agent has been identified that can fulfill this treatment goal. An improved characterization of the different phenotypes of OSA, coupled with more selective neuropharmacologic therapy, is warranted to achieve this important goal. For the present, CPAP therapy remains the best therapeutic option despite its limitations.

REFERENCES

1. Sleep-related breathing disorders in adults: recommendations for syndrome definition and measurement techniques in clinical research. The Report of an American Academy of Sleep Medicine Task Force. Sleep 1999;22:667–89.
2. Young T, Palta M, Dempsey J, et al. The occurrence of sleep-disordered breathing among middle-aged adults. N Engl J Med 1993;328:1230–5.
3. Peppard PE, Young T, Palta M, et al. Prospective study of the association between sleep-disordered breathing and hypertension. N Engl J Med 2000;342:1378–84.
4. Peker Y, Kraiczi H, Hedner J, et al. An independent association between obstructive sleep apnoea and coronary artery disease. Eur Respir J 1999;14:179–84.
5. Yaggi HK, Concato J, Kernan WN, et al. Obstructive sleep apnea as a risk factor for stroke and death. N Engl J Med 2005;353:2034–41.
6. Gami AS, Howard DE, Olson EJ, et al. Day-night pattern of sudden death in obstructive sleep apnea. N Engl J Med 2005;352:1206–14.
7. McArdle N, Douglas NJ. Effect of continuous positive airway pressure on sleep architecture in the sleep apnea-hypopnea syndrome: a randomized controlled trial. Am J Respir Crit Care Med 2001;164:1459–63.
8. Iber C, O'Brien C, Schluter J, et al. Single night studies in obstructive sleep apnea. Sleep 1991;14:383–5.
9. Jenkinson C, Davies RJ, Mullins R, et al. Comparison of therapeutic and subtherapeutic nasal continuous positive airway pressure for obstructive sleep apnoea: a randomised prospective parallel trial. Lancet 1999;353:2100–5.
10. Bardwell WA, Ancoli-Israel S, Berry CC, et al. Neuropsychological effects of one-week continuous positive airway pressure treatment in patients with obstructive sleep apnea: a placebo-controlled study. Psychosom Med 2001;63:579–84.
11. Faccenda JF, Mackay TW, Boon NA, et al. Randomized placebo-controlled trial of continuous positive airway pressure on blood pressure in the sleep apnea-hypopnea syndrome. Am J Respir Crit Care Med 2001;163:344–8.
12. Parker JD, Brooks D, Kozar LF, et al. Acute and chronic effects of airway obstruction on canine left ventricular performance. Am J Respir Crit Care Med 1999;160:1888–96.
13. Bahammam A, Delaive K, Ronald J, et al. Health care utilization in males with obstructive sleep apnea syndrome two years after diagnosis and treatment. Sleep 1999;22:740–7.
14. Kapur VK, Redline S, Nieto FJ, et al. The relationship between chronically disrupted sleep and healthcare use. Sleep 2002;25:289–96.
15. Kribbs NB, Pack AI, Kline LR, et al. Objective measurement of patterns of nasal CPAP use by patients with obstructive sleep apnea. Am Rev Respir Dis 1993;147:887–95.
16. Meslier N, Lebrun T, Grillier-Lanoir V, et al. A French survey of 3,225 patients treated with CPAP for obstructive sleep apnoea: benefits, tolerance, compliance and quality of life. Eur Respir J 1998;12:185–92.
17. Bliwise DL, Feldman DE, Bliwise NG, et al. Risk factors for sleep disordered breathing in heterogeneous geriatric populations. J Am Geriatr Soc 1987;35:132–41.

18. Patel SR. Shared genetic risk factors for obstructive sleep apnea and obesity. J Appl Physiol 2005;99:1600–6.

19. Schwartz AR, Gold AR, Schubert N, et al. Effect of weight loss on upper airway collapsibility in obstructive sleep apnea. Am Rev Respir Dis 1991;144:494–8.

20. Strobel RJ, Rosen RC. Obesity and weight loss in obstructive sleep apnea: a critical review. Sleep 1996;19:104–15.

21. Peppard PE, Young T, Palta M, et al. Longitudinal study of moderate weight change and sleep-disordered breathing. JAMA 2000;284:3015–21.

22. Ayyad C, Andersen T. Long-term efficacy of dietary treatment of obesity: a systematic review of studies published between 1931 and 1999. Obes Rev 2000;1:113–9.

23. Snow V, Barry P, Fitterman N, et al. Pharmacologic and surgical management of obesity in primary care: a clinical practice guideline from the American College of Physicians. Ann Intern Med 2005;142:525–31.

24. Kim DM, Yoon SJ, Ahn CW, et al. Sibutramine improves fat distribution and insulin resistance, and increases serum adiponectin levels in Korean obese nondiabetic premenopausal women. Diabetes Res Clin Pract 2004;66(Suppl 1):S139–44.

25. Schwartz AR, Patil SP, Squier S, et al. Obesity and upper airway control during sleep. J Appl Physiol 2010;108:430–5.

26. Yee BJ, Phillips CL, Banerjee D, et al. The effect of sibutramine-assisted weight loss in men with obstructive sleep apnoea. Int J Obes (Lond) 2007;31:161–8.

27. Phillips CL, Yee BJ, Trenell MI, et al. Changes in regional adiposity and cardio-metabolic function following a weight loss program with sibutramine in obese men with obstructive sleep apnea. J Clin Sleep Med 2009;5:416–21.

28. Li Z, Maglione M, Tu W, et al. Meta-analysis: pharmacologic treatment of obesity. Ann Intern Med 2005;142:532–46.

29. Torp-Pedersen C, Caterson I, Coutinho W, et al. Cardiovascular responses to weight management and sibutramine in high-risk subjects: an analysis from the SCOUT trial. Eur Heart J 2007;28:2915–23.

30. Veasey SC. Pharmacotherapies for obstructive sleep apnea: how close are we? Curr Opin Pulm Med 2001;7:399–403.

31. Veasey SC. Serotonin agonists and antagonists in obstructive sleep apnea: therapeutic potential. Am J Respir Med 2003;2:21–9.

32. Berry RB, Yamaura EM, Gill K, et al. Acute effects of paroxetine on genioglossus activity in obstructive sleep apnea. Sleep 1999;22:1087–92.

33. Kraiczi H, Hedner J, Dahlof P, et al. Effect of serotonin uptake inhibition on breathing during sleep and daytime symptoms in obstructive sleep apnea. Sleep 1999;22:61–7.

34. Hanzel DA, Proia NG, Hudgel DW. Response of obstructive sleep apnea to fluoxetine and protriptyline. Chest 1991;100:416–21.

35. Berry RB, Koch GL, Hayward LF. Low-dose mirtazapine increases genioglossus activity in the anesthetized rat. Sleep 2005;28:78–84.

36. Carley DW, Olopade C, Ruigt GS, et al. Efficacy of mirtazapine in obstructive sleep apnea syndrome. Sleep 2007;30:35–41.

37. Marshall NS, Yee BJ, Desai AV, et al. Two randomized placebo-controlled trials to evaluate the efficacy and tolerability of mirtazapine for the treatment of obstructive sleep apnea. Sleep 2008;31:824–31.

38. Whyte KF, Gould GA, Airlie MA, et al. Role of protriptyline and acetazolamide in the sleep apnea/hypopnea syndrome. Sleep 1988;11:463–72.

39. Brownell LG, West P, Sweatman P, et al. Protriptyline in obstructive sleep apnea: a double-blind trial. N Engl J Med 1982;307:1037–42.

40. Gilman S, Chervin RD, Koeppe RA, et al. Obstructive sleep apnea is related to a thalamic cholinergic deficit in MSA. Neurology 2003;61:35–9.

41. Hedner J, Kraiczi H, Peker Y, et al. Reduction of sleep-disordered breathing after physostigmine. Am J Respir Crit Care Med 2003;168:1246–51.

42. Moraes W, Poyares D, Sukys-Claudino L, et al. Donepezil improves obstructive sleep apnea in Alzheimer disease: a double-blind, placebo-controlled study. Chest 2008;133:677–83.

43. Swenson ER. Carbonic anhydrase inhibitors and ventilation: a complex interplay of stimulation and suppression. Eur Respir J 1998;12:1242–7.

44. Inoue Y, Takata K, Sakamoto I, et al. Clinical efficacy and indication of acetazolamide treatment on sleep apnea syndrome. Psychiatry Clin Neurosci 1999;53:321–2.

45. Tojima H, Kunitomo F, Kimura H, et al. Effects of acetazolamide in patients with the sleep apnoea syndrome. Thorax 1988;43:113–9.

46. White DP, Zwillich CW, Pickett CK, et al. Central sleep apnea. Improvement with acetazolamide therapy. Arch Intern Med 1982;142:1816–9.

47. Pena F, Garcia O. Breathing generation and potential pharmacotherapeutic approaches to central respiratory disorders. Curr Med Chem 2006;13:2681–93.

48. Mulloy E, McNicholas WT. Theophylline in obstructive sleep apnea. A double-blind evaluation. Chest 1992;101:753–7.

49. Oberndorfer S, Saletu B, Gruber G, et al. Theophylline in snoring and sleep-related breathing disorders: sleep laboratory investigations on subjective

and objective sleep and awakening quality. Methods Find Exp Clin Pharmacol 2000;22:237–45.

50. Javaheri S, Parker TJ, Wexler L, et al. Effect of theophylline on sleep-disordered breathing in heart failure. N Engl J Med 1996;335:562–7.

51. Andersen ML, Bittencourt LR, Antunes IB, et al. Effects of progesterone on sleep: a possible pharmacological treatment for sleep-breathing disorders? Curr Med Chem 2006;13:3575–82.

52. Manber R, Kuo TF, Cataldo N, et al. The effects of hormone replacement therapy on sleep-disordered breathing in postmenopausal women: a pilot study. Sleep 2003;26:163–8.

53. Keefe DL, Watson R, Naftolin F. Hormone replacement therapy may alleviate sleep apnea in menopausal women: a pilot study. Menopause 1999;6:196–200.

54. Cistulli PA, Barnes DJ, Grunstein RR, et al. Effect of short-term hormone replacement in the treatment of obstructive sleep apnoea in postmenopausal women. Thorax 1994;49:699–702.

55. Polo-Kantola P, Rauhala E, Helenius H, et al. Breathing during sleep in menopause: a randomized, controlled, crossover trial with estrogen therapy. Obstet Gynecol 2003;102:68–75.

56. Kalleinen N, Polo O, Himanen SL, et al. The effect of estrogen plus progestin treatment on sleep: a randomized, placebo-controlled, double-blind trial in premenopausal and late postmenopausal women. Climacteric 2008;11:233–43.

57. Cook WR, Benich JJ, Wooten SA. Indices of severity of obstructive sleep apnea syndrome do not change during medroxyprogesterone acetate therapy. Chest 1989;96:262–6.

58. Shao XM, Feldman JL. Central cholinergic regulation of respiration: nicotinic receptors. Acta Pharmacol Sin 2009;30:761–70.

59. Davila DG, Hurt RD, Offord KP, et al. Acute effects of transdermal nicotine on sleep architecture, snoring, and sleep-disordered breathing in nonsmokers. Am J Respir Crit Care Med 1994;150:469–74.

60. Zevin S, Swed E, Cahan C. Clinical effects of locally delivered nicotine in obstructive sleep apnea syndrome. Am J Ther 2003;10:170–5.

61. Gislason T, Almqvist M, Boman G, et al. Increased CSF opioid activity in sleep apnea syndrome. Regression after successful treatment. Chest 1989;96:250–4.

62. Ferber C, Sanchez P, Lemoine P, et al. [Efficacy of the treatment of sleep apnea using naltrexone. A clinical, polygraphic and gasometric study]. C R Acad Sci III 1988;307:695–700 [in French].

63. Ferber C, Duclaux R, Mouret J. Naltrexone improves blood gas patterns in obstructive sleep apnoea syndrome through its influence on sleep. J Sleep Res 1993;2:149–55.

64. Greenberg HE, Rapoport DM, Rothenberg SA, et al. Endogenous opiates modulate the postapnea ventilatory response in the obstructive sleep apnea syndrome. Am Rev Respir Dis 1991;143:1282–7.

65. Sonka K, Roth B, Barvirova H, et al. Effect of naloxone on diurnal polysomnographic manifestations of hypersomnia with sleep apnoea. Physiol Bohemoslov 1989;38:477–9.

66. Schwartz AR, Rowley JA, O'Donnell C, et al. Effect of hypertension on upper airway function and sleep apnoea. J Sleep Res 1995;4:83–8.

67. Mayor AH, Schwartz AR, Rowley JA, et al. Effect of blood pressure changes on air flow dynamics in the upper airway of the decerebrate cat. Anesthesiology 1996;84:128–34.

68. Mayer J, Weichler U, Herres-Mayer B, et al. Influence of metoprolol and cilazapril on blood pressure and on sleep apnea activity. J Cardiovasc Pharmacol 1990;16:952–61.

69. Issa FG. Effect of clonidine in obstructive sleep apnea. Am Rev Respir Dis 1992;145:435–9.

70. Grote L, Wutkewicz K, Knaack L, et al. Association between blood pressure reduction with antihypertensive treatment and sleep apnea activity. Am J Hypertens 2000;13:1280–7.

71. Verse T, Pirsig W. Impact of impaired nasal breathing on sleep-disordered breathing. Sleep Breath 2003;7:63–76.

72. Craig TJ, Mende C, Hughes K, et al. The effect of topical nasal fluticasone on objective sleep testing and the symptoms of rhinitis, sleep, and daytime somnolence in perennial allergic rhinitis. Allergy Asthma Proc 2003;24:53–8.

73. Kiely JL, Nolan P, McNicholas WT. Intranasal corticosteroid therapy for obstructive sleep apnoea in patients with co-existing rhinitis. Thorax 2004;59:50–5.

74. Clarenbach CF, Kohler M, Senn O, et al. Does nasal decongestion improve obstructive sleep apnea? J Sleep Res 2008;17:444–9.

75. McLean HA, Urton AM, Driver HS, et al. Effect of treating severe nasal obstruction on the severity of obstructive sleep apnoea. Eur Respir J 2005;25:521–7.

76. Osanai S, Akiba Y, Fujiuchi S, et al. Depression of peripheral chemosensitivity by a dopaminergic mechanism in patients with obstructive sleep apnoea syndrome. Eur Respir J 1999;13:418–23.

77. Larrain A, Hudson M, Dominitz JA, et al. Treatment of severe snoring with a combination of pseudoephedrine sulfate and domperidone. J Clin Sleep Med 2006;2:21–5.

78. Larrain A, Kapur VK, Gooley TA, et al. Pharmacological treatment of obstructive sleep apnea with a combination of pseudoephedrine and domperidone. J Clin Sleep Med 2010;6:117–23.

79. Dolly FR, Block AJ. Effect of flurazepam on sleep-disordered breathing and nocturnal oxygen desaturation in asymptomatic subjects. Am J Med 1982;73:239–43.

80. Mendelson WB, Garnett D, Gillin JC. Flurazepam-induced sleep apnea syndrome in a patient with insomnia and mild sleep-related respiratory changes. J Nerv Ment Dis 1981;169:261–4.

81. Camacho ME, Morin CM. The effect of temazepam on respiration in elderly insomniacs with mild sleep apnea. Sleep 1995;18:644–5.

82. Schneider H, Grote L, Peter JH, et al. The effect of triazolam and flunitrazepam—two benzodiazepines with different half-lives—on breathing during sleep. Chest 1996;109:909–15.

83. Mak KH, Wang YT, Cheong TH, et al. The effect of oral midazolam and diazepam on respiration in normal subjects. Eur Respir J 1993;6:42–7.

84. Grimaldi D, Provini F, Vetrugno R, et al. Idiopathic central sleep apnoea syndrome treated with zolpidem. Neurol Sci 2008;29:355–7.

85. Quadri S, Drake C, Hudgel DW. Improvement of idiopathic central sleep apnea with zolpidem. J Clin Sleep Med 2009;5:122–9.

86. Cirignotta F, Mondini S, Zucconi M, et al. Zolpidem-polysomnographic study of the effect of a new hypnotic drug in sleep apnea syndrome. Pharmacol Biochem Behav 1988;29:807–9.

87. Rosenberg R, Roach JM, Scharf M, et al. A pilot study evaluating acute use of eszopiclone in patients with mild to moderate obstructive sleep apnea syndrome. Sleep Med 2007;8:464–70.

88. Kryger M, Wang-Weigand S, Roth T. Safety of ramelteon in individuals with mild to moderate obstructive sleep apnea. Sleep Breath 2007;11:159–64.

89. Freudenmann RW, Sussmuth SD, Wolf RC, et al. Respiratory dysfunction in sleep apnea associated with quetiapine. Pharmacopsychiatry 2008;41:119–21.

90. Rishi MA, Shetty M, Wolff A, et al. Atypical antipsychotic medications are independently associated with severe obstructive sleep apnea. Clin Neuropharmacol 2010;33:109–13.

91. Finnimore AJ, Roebuck M, Sajkov D, et al. The effects of the GABA agonist, baclofen, on sleep and breathing. Eur Respir J 1995;8:230–4.

92. Centers for Disease Control and Prevention (CDC). Increase in poisoning deaths caused by non-illicit drugs—Utah, 1991–2003. MMWR Morb Mortal Wkly Rep 2005;54:33–6.

93. Teichtahl H, Prodromidis A, Miller B, et al. Sleep-disordered breathing in stable methadone programme patients: a pilot study. Addiction 2001;96:395–403.

94. Wang D, Teichtahl H, Drummer O, et al. Central sleep apnea in stable methadone maintenance treatment patients. Chest 2005;128:1348–56.

95. Walker JM, Farney RJ, Rhondeau SM, et al. Chronic opioid use is a risk factor for the development of central sleep apnea and ataxic breathing. J Clin Sleep Med 2007;3:455–61.

96. Farney RJ, Walker JM, Cloward TV, et al. Sleep-disordered breathing associated with long-term opioid therapy. Chest 2003;123:632–9.

97. Sansa G, Iranzo A, Santamaria J. Obstructive sleep apnea in narcolepsy. Sleep Med 2010;11:93–5.

98. Seeck-Hirschner M, Baier PC, von Freier A, et al. Increase in sleep-related breathing disturbances after treatment with sodium oxybate in patients with narcolepsy and mild obstructive sleep apnea syndrome: two case reports. Sleep Med 2009;10:154–5.

99. George CF, Feldman N, Inhaber N, et al. A safety trial of sodium oxybate in patients with obstructive sleep apnea: acute effects on sleep-disordered breathing. Sleep Med 2010;11:38–42.

100. George CF, Feldman N, Zheng Y, et al. A 2-week, polysomnographic, safety study of sodium oxybate in obstructive sleep apnea syndrome. Sleep Breath 2010. [Epub ahead of print].

101. Roizenblatt S, Guilleminault C, Poyares D, et al. A double-blind, placebo-controlled, crossover study of sildenafil in obstructive sleep apnea. Arch Intern Med 2006;166:1763–7.

102. Pack AI, Black JE, Schwartz JR, et al. Modafinil as adjunct therapy for daytime sleepiness in obstructive sleep apnea. Am J Respir Crit Care Med 2001;164:1675–81.

103. Black JE, Hirshkowitz M. Modafinil for treatment of residual excessive sleepiness in nasal continuous positive airway pressure-treated obstructive sleep apnea/hypopnea syndrome. Sleep 2005;28:464–71.

104. Hirshkowitz M, Black JE, Wesnes K, et al. Adjunct armodafinil improves wakefulness and memory in obstructive sleep apnea/hypopnea syndrome. Respir Med 2007;101:616–27.

105. Roth T, White D, Schmidt-Nowara W, et al. Effects of armodafinil in the treatment of residual excessive sleepiness associated with obstructive sleep apnea/hypopnea syndrome: a 12-week, multicenter, double-blind, randomized, placebo-controlled study in nCPAP-adherent adults. Clin Ther 2006;28:689–706.

Therapeutics of Narcolepsy

Hashir Majid, MD[a], Max Hirshkowitz, PhD, D ABSM[b],*

KEYWORDS
- Narcolepsy • Excessive sleepiness
- Pharmacological treatment

Narcolepsy, an uncommon neurologic disorder with usual onset during adolescence, afflicts approximately 1 in 2000 individuals according to United States population estimates. Although its hallmark feature is excessive sleepiness, narcolepsy's other classic symptoms (cataplexy, sleep paralysis, and hypnagogic or hynapompic hallucinations) suggest rapid eye movement (REM) sleep intrusion into wakefulness.[1-7] In addition to this classic tetrad, individuals with narcolepsy may exhibit sleep disruption and fragmentation, report memory disturbances, and display automatisms.[8] Cataplexy is the most specific sign and is considered pathognomonic; the other symptoms accompany an assortment of sleep disorders and also occur in the general population.

The normal sleep-wake cycle is regulated by a complex interaction of neurohormones and chemicals. The monoaminergic and cholinergic systems are both involved in regulating sleep and wakefulness. Hypocretins (also known as orexins), peptides produced exclusively in the lateral hypothalamus, have recently been shown to play a major role in controlling the interplay between these two systems. Deficiency of hypocretins is now thought to be the underlying pathophysiology of narcolepsy.

Generally, the monoaminergic system has an excitatory role and promotes wakefulness and vigilance. The cholinergic system comprises two distinct neuronal populations that promote REM sleep (REM-on cells) and wakefulness (REM-on/ wake-on cells). A decrease in hypocretin levels is believed to cause an imbalance between the two systems and disrupt sleep state organization as well as maintenance of wakefulness.

The medications used in the treatment of narcolepsy are reviewed by the neurotransmitter system they predominantly affect (**Tables 1–3**).

MONOAMINERGIC SYSTEM
Overview

Norepinephrine, dopamine, serotonin, and histamine neurotransmitter pathways comprise the monoaminergic system. This system is primarily active during wakefulness and is responsible for alertness. It is less active during non-REM (NREM) sleep and is largely switched "off" during REM sleep.

Medications targeting the different pathways in the monoaminergic system alter neurotransmitter concentration at the synaptic level. They do so in a variety of ways, including: increasing precursors needed for synthesis, enhancing neurotransmitter release into the synaptic cleft, agonizing postsynaptic receptors, blocking presynaptic reuptake, or by inhibiting neurotransmitter. Most of these medications lack specificity to individual neurotransmitters and alter levels of multiple monoaminergic chemicals. Tricyclic antidepressants and monoamine oxidase inhibitors are probably the least specific.

Tricyclic Antidepressants

Tricyclic Antidepressants (TCAs) have long been used to treat mood disorders. These drugs predominantly increase norepinephrine and

[a] Section of Pulmonary, Critical Care and Sleep Medicine, Department of Medicine, Baylor College of Medicine, 1 Baylor Plaza, Houston, TX 77030, USA
[b] Sleep Disorders & Research Center, Michael E. DeBakey Veterans Affairs Medical Center (111i), 2002 Holcombe Boulevard, Building 100, Room 6C344, Houston, TX 77030, USA
* Corresponding author.
E-mail address: maxh@bcm.edu

Sleep Med Clin 5 (2010) 659–673
doi:10.1016/j.jsmc.2010.08.007
1556-407X/10/$ — see front matter. Published by Elsevier Inc.

Table 1
Neurotransmitters involved in sleep regulation

Neurotransmitter System	Brain Location	Sleep			Plausible Mode of Action of Narcolepsy Medication	Avoid
		Wake	NREM	REM		
Monoaminergic system						
Norepinephrine	Locus Ceruleus	Active	↓ activity	Off	NRIs, MAOIs, SNRIs, TCAs	α adrenergic blocker, Rapid TCA withdrawal
Dopamine	Striatum or ventral tegmental area[9,10,15]	Active	↓ activity	Off	Amphetamines or stimulants, MAOIs	Neuroleptics
Serotonin	Dorsal Raphe Nucleus	Active	↓ activity	Off	SSRIs, SNRIs, TCAs	Rapid SSRI withdrawal
Histamine	Tuberomammillary nucleus	Active	Off	Off	Histamine Uptake Inhibitor	Anti-histamines
Cholinergic system						
REM on	Lateral dorsal tegmental or pedunculopontine tegmental nuclei, basal forebrain	Off	Off	Active		
REM on or wake on		Active	Off	Very active		Cholinergic agonists
Hypocretin	Lateral hypothalamus	Active	? Off	? Subpopulation may be active	Hypocretin analogs	
GABA	Ventral lateral preoptic area	Off	Active	Reduced	GHB, BZD	Daytime GHB

Non-REM sleep is produced by neurons in the preoptic area and brainstem. VLPO is the best characterized of these locations.
Abbreviations: BZD, benzodiazepines; GHB, gamma hydroxybutyrate; MAOIs, monoamine oxidase inhibitors; NRIs, noradrenergic reuptake inhibitors; SNRIs, serotonin noradrenaline reuptake inhibitors; SSRIs, selective serotonin reuptake inhibitors; TCAs, tricyclic antidepressants.
Data from Carney RP, Berry RB, Geyer JD. Clinical sleep disorders. Philadelphia: Lippincott Williams and Wilkins; 2005.

Table 2
Medications used for narcolepsy

Medication Group	Commonly Used Medications	Usual Daily Dose	Half-life (hrs)	Side Effects and Special Issues
TCAs	Imipramine	10–100 mg	6–18	Anti-cholinergic effects (dry mouth, urinary retention, impotence, constipation, tachycardia), rebound cataplexy, with withdrawal
	Clomipramine	10–150 mg	32–69[a]	
	Desipramine	25–200 mg	7–60	
	Protriptyline	10 mg	54–92	Tolerance can occur
SSRIs	Fluoxetine	10–40 mg	1–9 d[b]	Gastrointestinal upset, CNS excitation, movement disorders, sexual dysfunction
	Fluvoxamine	50–300 mg	15 hrs	
SNRIs	Venlafaxine	75–375 mg	4	Nausea, insomnia, ejaculation disorder, tachycardia, hypertension
	Milnacipran	30–50 mg	8	
MAOIs	Selegiline	5–20 mg	3–21[c]	Hypertensive crisis, other sympathomimetic effects, interactions with other drugs (SSRIs, triptans), dietary precautions
	Phenelzine	60–90 mg	11	
NRIs	Atomoxetine	40–60 mg	5–8[d]	Atomoxetine: headache, xerostomia, insomnia or somnolence
	Reboxetine	8–10 mg	13	Reboxetine: anticholinergic effects
Amphetamines	Amphetamine	5–60 mg	13	Irritability, hyperactivity, headache, palpitations, sweating, tremors, insomnia
	Methamphetamine	20–60 mg	4–5	
	D-amphetamine	20–60 mg	16–30	Tolerance can occur
	Methylphenidate	20–40 mg	3	Abuse potential exists
Stimulants	Modafinil	100–400 mg in a split dose	11–14	Headache, nausea, rhinitis, induce metabolism of OCs
	Armodafinil	150–250 mg	15 (7 days in steady state)	
GHB	γ-hydroxybutyric acid	4.5–9 g/night	0.5–1.0	Nausea, nocturnal enuresis, confusional arousals, headache
				Possible abuse potential

Abbreviations: GHB, gamma hydroxybutyrate; MAOIs, monoamine oxidase inhibitors; NRIs, noradrenergic reuptake inhibitors; SNRIs, serotonin noradrenaline reuptake inhibitors; SSRIs, selective serotonin reuptake inhibitors; TCAs, tricyclic antidepressants.

[a] Clomipramine has an active metabolite (desmethylclomipramine) with a half life of 69 hours.

[b] Active metabolite of fluoxetine has a half life of 9.3 days.

[c] Selegiline is metabolically converted to three active compounds (desmethylselegeline, amphetamine and methamphetamine) with variable half-lives.

[d] Atomoxetine has active metabolites: 4-hydroxyatomoxetine and N-desmethylatomoxetine with longer half lives (8 hours); in poor metabolizers, half life can be prolonged to 40 hours.

Table 3
Indications for use of narcolepsy medications

Symptom	Suggested First-Line Therapy	Alternative
Excessive Daytime Somnolence/Sleep Attacks	**Modafinil** or **Sodium oxybate**	*Methylphenidate or amphetamines, scheduled naps* Ritanserin
Cataplexy	**Sodium oxybate**	*TCAs and SSRIs* *Venlafaxine* *Reboxetine* *Selegiline*
Sleep Paralysis and Hypnagogic Hallucinations	Sodium oxybate	TCAs and SSRIs *Venlafaxine*
Disturbed Nocturnal Sleep	Sodium oxybate	Benzodiazepines/hypnotics

Abbreviations: SSRIs, Selective Serotonin Reuptake Inhibitors; TCAs, Tricyclic Antidepressants.
Recommendations based on AASM 2007 guidelines.[14]
Bold type: strong recommendation (standard), *Italics*: moderate strength recommendation (guideline), Regular font: weak recommendation (option).

serotonin levels in the central nervous system (CNS) by inhibiting transporters for these chemicals; specifically, the serotonin transporter (SERT) and the norepinephrine transporter. They appear to have a negligible effect on the dopamine transporter.[9,10] The increased norepinephrine and serotonin levels effectively activate the "REM-off" system that would be expected to reduce cataplexy (on the assumption that cataplexy represents a feature of REM sleep intrusion into wakefulness). Thus, TCAs were, and continue to be, widely used to treat cataplexy in patients with narcolepsy.[11,12] Sleep paralysis and hypnagogic hallucinations are other symptoms for which TCAs are recommended.[13,14]

TCA side effects account for their diminishing popularity as medications with fewer adverse events became available. TCAs act as antagonists at the histaminic, muscarinic, and α_1 adrenergic receptors producing sedation, anticholinergic effects (eg, dry mouth, constipation, sweating, tachycardia), and orthostatic hypotension. Cardiac toxicity in overdose can also occur owing to inhibition of calcium and sodium channels. A recent meta-analysis focusing on quality of life outcome measures concluded that there is a lack of good quality evidence showing efficacy for TCAs in patients with narcolepsy.[15] Nonetheless, clinicians continue to use TCAs specifically to control cataplexy.

Monoamine Oxidase Inhibitors

This group of drugs—monoamine oxidase inhibitors (MAOIs)—inhibits the intracellular enzyme responsible for breaking down monoamine neurotransmitters. Monoamine oxidase has two isoforms: MAO-A and MAO-B. MAO-A deaminates dopamine, norepinephrine, epinephrine, melatonin, and serotonin. By contrast, MAO-B deaminates dopamine, phenylethylamine, and trace amines.

Nonselective MAOIs carry a high risk of side effects such as serotonin syndrome, hypertensive crisis, dietary interactions, and drug interactions. Therefore, they must be used with extreme caution in limited circumstances, usually as adjunctive therapy or when all other pharmacotherapeutics fail. Tranylcypromine is one such drug used for narcolepsy.[16,17]

Selective MAOIs, particularly MAO-B inhibitors (eg, selegiline), possess a safer side effect profile, particularly at low doses. A placebo-controlled trial using selegiline in a small group of patients with narcolepsy found dose-dependent nighttime REM sleep suppression with increased REM sleep latency. The trial also found improved daytime alertness, decreased sleep attacks, and diminished cataplexy symptoms.[18] Another study found selegiline-related daytime alertness improvement comparable to amphetamines.[19] These results suggest that selegiline can be considered as second line therapy for cataplexy and daytime sleepiness.[13] To the authors' knowledge, transdermal selegiline (Emsam patch) has not been studied systematically for treating narcolepsy.

Catecholaminergic Stimulants

Medications traditionally used to promote wakefulness primarily act via the catecholamine system (norepinephrine and dopamine). Medications acting through these mechanisms include amphetamines and its congeners (predominantly affecting the dopamine system), serotonin-noradrenergic reuptake inhibitors (NRIs), TCAs, serotoninin-noradrenergic reuptake inhibitors (usually affecting the norepinephrine system more than dopamine), and MAOIs (affecting both norepinephrine and dopamine).

Noradrenergic neurons are predominantly clustered in the locus ceruleus and lateral tegmental field. Their axons project to many structures in the cerebral cortex, hypothalamus, thalamus, and hippocampus. These neural pathways profoundly influence wakefulness and CNS arousal. Locus ceruleus activity peaks during wakefulness, progressively declines in NREM sleep, and virtual halts during REM sleep.[20] Norepinephrine is also thought to play a role in circadian regulation of the sleep-wake cycle; conversely, light is believed to be important in modulating the noradrenergic pathway activity.[21]

The alpha adrenergic receptor contributes significantly to the presentation of narcolepsy. Stimulation at the α_1 site appears to protect an individual from cataplexy,[22] whereas inhibition leads to cataplexy episodes.[23] Prazosin, an α_1 antagonist, can induce cataplexy[24–27] and is contraindicated in patients with narcolpsy.[28] Yohimbine, and other central α_2 agonists, have been shown to be protective for cataplexy in narcolepsy models.[29] The balance between the α_1 and α_2 receptor subtypes likely plays an important role in narcolepsy's pathophysiology.[30]

It has long been known that dopamine helps regulate behavior, particularly reward-seeking activities. In the past quarter century, dopamine's effect on wakefulness has been further elucidated. Although dopaminergic neurons' firing rates does not vary much between the wake and sleep states, CNS extracellular dopamine concentration is elevated during wakefulness.[31–34] The largest concentration of dopaminergic neurons are in the substantia nigra, ventral tegmental area and arcuate nucleus. Axonal projections from these areas innervate many parts of the brain—including the frontal cortex, striatum, and limbic areas—and influence cognition, reward, punishment, motivation, voluntary movement, behavior, attention, memory, and sleep-wake state.

The dopamine system promotes wakefulness. Agonists at the D_1, D_2, and D_3 CNS receptors increase alertness and reduce both REM and NREM sleep.[35–37] By contrast, dopamine receptor antagonists (eg, neuroleptics) and conditions marked by CNS dopamine depletion (eg, Parkinson's disease) are associated with sleepiness.[38–41] Interestingly, some dopamine receptor inhibitors (eg, clozapine) can produce cataplexy-like episodes.[42,43]

Amphetamines and amphetamine-like stimulants increase monoamine neurotransmitter levels. They achieve this by rupturing presynaptic vesicles thereby releasing monoamines and, then, by blocking presynaptic reuptake. They acutely increase levels of dopamine, norepinephrine, and serotonin in the CNS. In low doses, dopamine release predominates. Current evidence also suggests that the traditional stimulants' primary mechanism of action is via the dopamine system.[44,45]

Medications in this group include amphetamine, dextroamphetamine, methamphetamine (racemic mixture of levo- and dextroamphetamine isomers), and methylphenidate (the N-methyl derivative of amphetamine). These medications differ with respect to half-life, dosage frequency, central versus peripheral action, neurotransmitter specificity, and abuse potential. Methylphenidate has a shorter half-life (2–4 hours) compared with the moderately long half-life of the amphetamines (8–16 hours).[46,47] Therefore, it is administered in two to four times daily divided doses, in contrast to once or twice daily doses for the amphetamines. However, a sustained release form, used once daily, is also available. Methylphenidate reportedly has less abuse potential and releases less nondopamine monoamines compared with the other amphetamines. It also produces less peripheral effect than methamphetamine.

These medications increase levels of activity and wakefulness. Data to support their efficacy in narcolepsy patients comes from small studies and longstanding clinical experience.[12,48–53] Except for one study, effectiveness of these drugs has only been observed for a short-term duration (4 weeks or less). The only long-term data is from a retrospective self-report study[12] that showed decrease in improvement of daytime somnolence and cataplexy with dextroamphetamine. Nevertheless, the medications remain popular because of a long history of success in clinical practice.

Many of the side effects are related to activation of the sympathetic nervous system. CNS and gastrointestinal side effects are most frequent, although the cardiopulmonary system can also be affected. Headaches, irritability, nervousness, insomnia, anorexia, nausea, vomiting, sweating, tremors, palpitations, and, rarely, psychosis and orofacial dyskinesia can be seen. Disruption of sleep maintenance and architecture with decreased REM sleep[54,55] can occur. Tolerance develops in up to one-third of patients.[56] Abrupt discontinuation of amphetamines produces long periods of recovery sleep, disturbed sleep, and significant worsening of daytime somnolence. As mentioned, abuse potential exists and must be monitored clinically. In patients with narcolepsy, dependence is usually not a major issue.[57]

In an attempt to find alternatives to using amphetamines and their congeners to treat excessive sleepiness in narcolepsy, increased attention has focused on possibly using noradrenergic reuptake inhibitors (NRIs). These medications are commonly used to treat attention-deficit hyperactivity disorder in children. Atomoxetine is currently commercially available in the United States and raboxetine is available in Europe. NRIs reportedly can improve wakefulness and cataplexy in patients with narcolepsy.[58] Higher single neurotransmitter system specificity may help promote better tolerability and favorable side effect profiles (see **Table 2**). NRI use in narcolepsy appears to be emerging.[59] Caution should still be exercised when using atomoxetine because it can induce tachycardia and hypertension, especially at higher doses. Viloxazine, another NRI predominantly used for depression, also holds some promise in decreasing cataplexy and excessive daytime somnolence.[15,60]

Other Wake-Promoting Substances

Histamine is another major excitatory monoaminergic neurotransmitter. Histamine promotes alertness and wakefulness in the CNS, especially at the beginning of the wake cycle and possibly with behavior related arousal.[61] The tuberomammillary nucleus (TMN) in the posterior third of the hypothalamus is the only major source of histamine in the CNS. Projections from TMN innervate almost all structures of the brain. Histamine levels mirror those of norepinephrine; that is, they are highest during wakefulness and lowest during REM sleep, with intermediate levels during NREM sleep.[62,63]

Medications that inhibit stimulation of the postsynaptic histaminergic receptor in the CNS typically induce drowsiness. Central H_1 receptor antagonists (eg, diphenhydramine) and H_3 agonists (with their histaminergic neurons autoinhibitory effect) both cause sleepiness and should be avoided by patients with narcolepsy.[64–67] The soporific effects of many psychotropic medications stem (at least in part) from their antihistaminergic actions. This includes, but is not limited to, TCAs, trazodone, mirtazapine, and quetiapine. Conversely, H_1 agonists and H_3 antagonist enhance wakefulness with possible therapeutic implications for narcolepsy.[66,67] H_3 antagonists in particular appear to promise significant benefit in improving wakefulness in narcoleptics.[68,69]

Modafinil is currently the standard therapy for treating sleepiness associated with narcolepsy.[13,14,70] The exact mechanism by which it promotes wakefulness is not completely understood because it affects several neurotransmitter systems. Like other stimulant medications, it enhances release of catecholamines from synaptic terminals and activates norepinephrine and dopamine systems.[71–74] However, unlike the amphetamines and methylphenidate, it also appears to inhibit GABA transmission[73,75,76] and increases hypothalamic histamine levels.[77,78] It is now thought that modafinil's wake-promoting properties are largely due to its histaminergic mechanism. In addition to these pathways, modafinil also affects serotonergic circuitry[73] and increases levels of the excitatory neurotransmitter glutamate.[75,76,79]

Modafinil is the most studied drug among narcolepsy medications. At least four different randomized controlled trials demonstrated reduced excessive somnolence in patients diagnosed with narcolepsy according to standardized criteria.[80–83] Half-life estimates range from 10 to 12 hours and recommended dosing is 100 or 200 mg, once or twice daily. Generally well tolerated, modafinil's common side effects include nausea, diarrhea, nervousness, insomnia, and headache (which may remit with lower dosing, run-in titration, or after a few weeks). Hypertension and tachycardia may be seen with high doses. Surveillance data revealed a few rare cases in which patients developed serious, even life threatening, rash after beginning treated with modafinil. Clinicians should therefore monitor closely for rash. Caution should also be used when treating women of child bearing potential because modafinil can induce hepatic cytochrome P450 enzymes and enhance clearance of oral contraceptives. Therefore, in such cases, contraceptive ethinylestradiol doses of no lower than 50 mcg should be used or barrier method initiated to prevent pregnancy. Patients with narcolepsy seldom develop tolerance[82] and abuse potential appears to be low in this group.

Modafinil's right-handed or R enantiomer (armodafinil), also appears effective for treating excessive sleepiness associated with narcolepsy.[84] Like modafinil, armodafinil produces mostly mild-to-moderate side effects such as headaches, dizziness, insomnia, and nausea. More serious adverse events include tachycardia, hypertension, and elevation of liver function tests in a small percentage of patients with obstructive sleep apnea[85] in whom sleepiness persisted notwithstanding otherwise adequate treatment with positive airway pressure therapy.

Selective Serotonin and Norepinephrine Reuptake Inhibitors

The neurotransmitters serotonin and acetylcholine both assert major influence in regulating REM sleep. Serotonin inhibits REM sleep. It also increases periods of wakefulness.[86–88] Like other monoamines, its levels are highest during wakefulness and lowest during REM sleep.[89–91] The medial and dorsal raphe nuclei, centered around the reticular formation of the brainstem, represent the CNS's principal source of serotonin.[92,93] Neurons in this area act as REM-off cells that, along with REM-on cells in the cholinergic lateral dorsal tegmental/pedunculopontine tegmental nuclei (LDT/PPT) regulate REM sleep through reciprocal inhibition. Selective serotonin-reuptake inhibitors (SSRIs) predominantly exert their influence via the serotonergic system. Other narcolepsy medications that affect this system include TCAs and serotonin norepinephrine reuptake inhibitors (SNRIs).

These medicines are more selective in their action toward SERT than the TCAs and have a narrower side effect profile. In higher doses, however, they also affect other monoaminergic transporters. SSRIs reduce cataplexy.[11,94–98] To a lesser extent, they also reduce sleep paralysis.[94] However, SSRIs effects are considered less pronounced compared with TCAs and consequently higher doses are often used.[99] As a group, SNRIs' common side effects include anorexia, weight changes, nausea, and vomiting, CNS excitation, sexual dysfunction, and movement disorders.

Two small cases series showed reduced cataplexy symptoms with venlafaxine.[100–102] These studies also reported reduced daytime somnolence[101] and reduced hypnagogic hallucination.[100] Common side effects include gastrointestinal upset, hypertension, and tachycardia.

CHOLINERGIC SYSTEM

As previously mentioned, acetylcholine is crucially involved in regulating sleep and wakefulness. Cholinergic thalamocortical signaling shows high activity during both wakefulness and REM sleep but is relatively inactive during NREM sleep, especially during slow wave sleep.[103–105] In the wake state, acetylcholine mediates behavioral and memory processes. Cholinergic REM-on cells in the dorsal brainstem LDT/PPT areas modulate REM sleep in reciprocal inhibition with the REM-off cells in the dorsal raphe and locus ceruleus. Muscarinic receptors, particularly the M_2 and possibly M_3, appear to be more important in the pathophysiology of narcolepsy than the nicotinic receptor.[106]

Medications activating cholinergic receptors (ie, cholinergic agonists and acetylcholinesterase inhibitors) enhance REM sleep.[107–111] The clinician should avoid using these drugs in patients with narcolepsy because evidence suggests cholinergic agonists can induce cataplexy episodes.[112,113] Cholinergic antagonists suppress REM sleep[114–118]; however, significant and serious side effects associated with such compounds limit their therapeutic utility for treating narcolepsy.

GABAERGIC SYSTEM
Overview

γ-Aminobutyric acid (GABA) represents one of the major inhibitory neurotransmitters in mammalian CNS. The ventrolateral preoptic (VLPO) area of the hypothalamus is rich with GABA and galanin, another inhibitory neurotransmitter.[119,120] Neurons from this region innervate the wake-promoting histaminergic TMN and other monoaminergic areas[121,122] and produce both REM and NREM sleep by inhibition of these structures.[123]

Medications acting through the GABAergic system include benzodiazepines, barbiturates, alcohol, some steroids, and sodium oxybate. GABA agonists induce sleepiness and should be avoided during the daytime in patients with narcolepsy. Interestingly, nocturnal use of these medications reportedly can sometimes produce beneficial outcomes. Notwithstanding narcolepsy's classification as a disorder of excessive sleepiness, significantly abnormal and disturbed sleep remains a hallmark feature of the condition.[124] Sleep disturbances in narcolepsy include fragmented sleep patterns and abnormal sleep architecture. Patients with narcolepsy manifest frequent sleep-stage shifts, decreased sleep efficiency, prolonged wake after sleep onset, sleep-onset REM episodes, increased stage 1 sleep, and diminished slow wave sleep.[125–127] Current medications commonly prescribed to treat disturbed nocturnal sleep act via the GABA system.

Benzodiazepines

Benzodiazepines (BZDs) and benzodiazepine receptor agonists (BZRAs) represent sedative-hypnotics traditionally used to improve disturbed nocturnal sleep in narcolepsy. One small-scale, short-term study in 10 patients found improvements in sleep efficiency and quality.[128] To the authors' knowledge, no large-scale, randomized, controlled trials have documented safety and efficacy of BZDs or BZRAs to support their use in narcolepsy.

Sodium Oxybate

A naturally occurring metabolite of GABA, γ-hydroxybutyrate (GHB) is known to improve nocturnal sleep in patients with narcolepsy and control cataplexy.[129] It acts via GABA-B receptor activation and through its own receptor.[130,131]

GHB was classified as a schedule 1 controlled substance owing to abuse as a date-rape drug. It is colorless, odorless, and tasteless but produces rapid sedation. Other abuse includes self-dosing by body-builders and athletes for its metabolic effects. On the street it goes by many names including G, fantasy, liquid X, easy lay, and soap. The US Food and Drug Administration (FDA) recently approved GHB in its sodium salt form (sodium oxybate) for treating cataplexy, excessive daytime somnolence, and disturbed nocturnal sleep in narcolepsy but limited its distribution through a central pharmacy. Several randomized, double-blind, placebo-controlled trials reported reduced daytime sleepiness, sleep attacks, cataplexy episodes, and disrupted night-time sleep (ie, fewer nocturnal awakenings) with this compound.[132–135] Additionally, it efficacy for treating excessive sleepiness appears further improved when used in conjunction with modafinil.[136]

Owing to its short half-life of 30 to 60 minutes, patients take sodium oxybate in two divided doses at night. Patients take the first dose at bedtime and the second during a scheduled awakening 2.5 to 4 hours later. The second dose should be prepared and ready at bedside. Starting dose is 4.5 g/night, with a maximum dose of 9 g/night. Nausea is the main side effect. Other potential adverse events include enuresis, dizziness, sleep walking, and hallucinations. The monitored prescription program helps counteract the drug's high abuse potential, at least for drug obtained legally. Unlike antidepressants, rebound cataplexy does not characteristically accompany drug discontinuation.

OREXINS/HYPOCRETINS

These recently discovered neuropeptides[137,138] appear to be integral in the pathogenesis of narcolepsy. Discovery occurred in close temporal proximity in two different laboratories. Researchers at University Health Science Center in Dallas researching feeding behavior named these neuropeptides "orexins" because they altered appetite. By contrast, the group at Stanford University in California chose the name hypocretins to reflect their anatomic localization in lateral and posterior hypothalamus. Orexin/hypocretins consist of two compounds: orexin A and B or alternatively hypocretin 1 and 2. They affect both the monoaminergic and cholinergic neurotransmitter systems via widespread neuronal projections from the hypothalamus to other areas in the brain.[137,139,140]

Genetic mutations in hypocretin alleles and receptors are seen in narcolepsy. Studies also show animals and patients with narcolepsy have decreased hypocretin levels.[141,142] It is hypothesized that an autoimmune process may underlie degeneration of hypocretin neurons and thereby leads to narcolepsy.[143]

Hypocretins promote wakefulness and vigilance.[144–147] Hypocretin levels are elevated during wake state, especially in times of increased arousals and motor activity.[148,149] The decreased levels seen in narcolepsy presumably cause excessive sleepiness, inappropriate sleep onsets, and predisposition to sleep attacks. Exercise, low CNS glucose levels and periods of forced wakefulness appear to elevate hypocretin concentrations, possibly as a countermeasure to increased sleep propensity.[150–152] This may help explain why patients with narcolepsy often appear unable to fend off sleep for prolonged periods notwithstanding the presence of alerting stimuli.

To date, no commercial formulations are available to activate the hypocretin system. One difficulty in developing such a product stems from the inability of large peptides to cross the blood brain barrier. The short half lives of such molecules adds to the logistical complexity. Animal models using direct intracerebroventricular and intravenous injections verify hypocretins' somnolytic properties. Achieving significant CNS hypocretin levels requires large doses and confers associated peripheral side effects. These factors further limit the clinical utility of the drug when administered intravenously.

Intranasal administration holds some promise for hypocretin analogs. Drug administration via this route bypasses the blood brain barrier. The exact mechanism of drug delivery is unknown; however, suspected entry to CNS may occur through olfactory or trigeminal nerve paths or via nasal lymphatics or vasculature.[153] Successful intranasal hypocretin administration has been demonstrated in both laboratory animals and human subjects with narcolepsy.[8,154] In a small patient cohort, intranasal hypocretin improved olfactory function and cognitive disturbances associated with narcolepsy. Notwithstanding the difficulties administering already prepared compounds, hypocretin-based therapy could well revolutionize the treatment of narcolepsy in the future. Gene therapy and transplantation of hypocretin neurons represent potential therapeutic modalities.

OTHER CONSIDERATIONS
Children and Pregnant Women

Therapeutic approach in pediatric narcolepsy is similar to that of adults and is even more largely based on clinical experience than research findings. There is a great need for rigorously conducted treatment outcome trials in this population.

A similar paucity of data exists for pregnant patients. Most medications used in narcolepsy are FDA category C or D. Their use, therefore, is not recommended during pregnancy. Women who become pregnant while taking these medications are gradually withdrawn from the drugs. To compound difficulty, excessive sleepiness naturally accompanies the first trimester of pregnancy. Furthermore, the clinician must consider that rapid withdrawal from REM-suppressing antidepressants can lead to rebound cataplexy or status epilepticus.

Behavioral and Activity Modification

Regularizing and assuring an adequate sleep schedule and employing scheduled naps can improve alertness in patients with narcolepsy. These measures are recommended even in conjunction with stimulant therapy when treating patients with persistent somnolence.[155–159] Adequate duration of nightly sleep is essential because patients with narcolepsy poorly maintain concentration and vigilance in the presence of sleep deprivation (presumably due to diminished physiologically increased hypocretin tone with forced wakefulness). Patients should also receive career counseling; jobs involving professional driving, shift-work, overnight on-call schedules, and monotonous work requiring intense concentration for long periods are best avoided.

Persistent Sleepiness with Therapy

Stimulant medications significantly alleviate sleepiness symptoms in up to 80% of narcolepsy patients.[160] Persistent daytime somnolence in the face of adequate pharmacologic treatment should prompt evaluation for other pathologies such as obstructive sleep apnea, periodic limb movement disorder, depression, and so forth. Alternative diagnoses such as idiopathic hypersomnia and narcolepsy due to medical condition should also be considered.

REM Sleep Behavior Disorder

Theory attributes the cardinal symptoms of narcolepsy to dysfunctional REM sleep. Therefore, it comes as little surprise to find a high incidence of REM sleep behavior disorder (RBD) among patients with narcolepsy.[161–163] No trials exist to guide RBD therapeutics in such cases. Conventional therapy for RBD, usually with clonazepam, is generally used in these patients.

Immunosuppressive Therapy

Rationale for immunotherapy stems from the putative autoimmune nature of narcolepsy. Steroids, intravenous immunoglobulins, and plasmapheresis have been tried in a few patients.[164–169] Some authors have claimed success with use of such therapy early in the course of the disease. However, results, at best, have been mixed.

FUTURE DIRECTIONS AND SUMMARY

Cutaneous temperature manipulation and thyroid releasing hormone (TRH) may play a role in the treatment of narcolepsy. TRH and agonists improve wakefulness and decrease cataplexy episodes in canine narcolepsy models.[100,170] Skin temperature regulation is dysfunctional in narcoleptics, possibly due to hypocretin deficiency. Manipulating cutaneous temperature can alter vigilance, sleepiness, and sleep architecture in patients with narcolepsy.[171–173] This could have a potential role in improving disturbed nocturnal sleep in narcoleptics. Further work is required to establish the clinical utility of these modalities. Hypocretin-based gene therapy or hypocretin neural transplantation represent important areas for development.

Narcolepsy is a debilitating neurologic disorder of excessive sleepiness. Current therapeutic approaches are based on symptomatic relief and are often associated with undesirable side effects. Management has improved significantly over the past several decades, especially with use of modafinil and sodium oxybate. However, impairment of function and quality of life persists in a considerable number of patients. Further therapeutic options need to be developed. Hypocretin-based therapy appears to hold the most promise.

REFERENCES

1. NINDS. National Institute of Neurological Disorders and Stroke. [Internet]. Available at: http://www. ninds.nih.gov/disorders/narcolepsy/detail_narcolepsy. htm. Accessed March 31, 2010.

2. Longstreth WT Jr, Ton TG, Koepsell T, et al. Prevalence of narcolepsy in King County, Washington, USA. Sleep Med 2009;10:422–6.

3. Silber MH, Krahn LE, Olson EJ, et al. The epidemiology of narcolepsy in Olmsted County, Minnesota: a population-based study. Sleep 2002;25:197–202.

4. Dement WC, Zarcone V, Varner V, et al. The prevalence of narcolepsy [abstract]. Sleep Res 1972;1:148.

5. Dement WC, Carskadon MA, Ley R. The prevalence of narcolepsy II [abstract]. Sleep Res 1973;2:147.

6. Dauvilliers Y, Montplaisir J, Molinari N, et al. Age at onset of narcolepsy in two large populations of patients in France and Quebec. Neurology 2001;57:2029–33.

7. Hayes D Jr. Narcolepsy with cataplexy in early childhood. Clin Pediatr (Phila) 2006;45:361–3.

8. Baier PC, Weinhold SL, Huth V, et al. Olfactory dysfunction in patients with narcolepsy with cataplexy is restored by intranasal Orexin A (Hypocretin-1). Brain 2008;131:2734–41.

9. Wise MS, Arand DL, Auger RR, et al. Treatment of narcolepsy and other hypersomnias of central origin. Sleep 2007;30:1712–27.

10. Vignatelli L, D'Alessandro R, Candelise L. Antidepressant drugs for narcolepsy. Cochrane Database Syst Rev 2008;1:CD003724.

11. Tatsumi M, Groshan K, Blakely RD, et al. Pharmacological profile of antidepressants and related compounds at human monoamine transporters. Eur J Pharmacol 1997;340:249–58.

12. Gillman PK. Tricyclic antidepressant pharmacology and therapeutic drug interactions updated. Br J Pharmacol 2007;151:737–48.

13. Schachter M, Parkes JD. Fluvoxamine and clomipramine in the treatment of cataplexy. J Neurol Neurosurg Psychiatry 1980;43:171–4.

14. Chen SY, Clift SJ, Dahlitz MJ, et al. Treatment in the narcoleptic syndrome: self assessment of the action of dexamphetamine and clomipramine. J Sleep Res 1995;4:113–8.

15. Morgenthaler TI, Kapur VK, Brown T, et al. Standards of Practice Committee of the American Academy of Sleep Medicine. Practice parameters for the treatment of narcolepsy and other hypersomnias of central origin. Sleep 2007;30:1705–11.

16. Clemons WE, Makela E, Young J. Concomitant use of modafinil and tranylcypromine in a patient with narcolepsy: a case report. Sleep Med 2004;5:509–11.

17. Gernaat HB, Haffmans PM, Knegtering H, et al. Tranylcypromine in narcolepsy. Pharmacopsychiatry 1995;28:98–100.

18. Mayer G, Ewert Meier K, Hephata K. Selegeline hydrochloride treatment in narcolepsy. A double-blind, placebo-controlled study. Clin Neuropharmacol 1995;18:306–19.

19. Roselaar SE, Langdon N, Lock CB, et al. Selegiline in narcolepsy. Sleep 1987;10:491–5.

20. Aston-Jones G, Bloom FE. Activity of norepinephrine-containing locus coeruleus neurons in behaving rats anticipates fluctuations in the sleep-waking cycle. J Neurosci 1981;1:876–86.

21. González MM, Aston-Jones G. Circadian regulation of arousal: role of the noradrenergic locus coeruleus system and light exposure. Sleep 2006;29:1327–36.

22. Renaud A, Nishino S, Dement WC, et al. Effects of SDZ NVI-085, a putative subtype-selective alpha 1-agonist, on canine cataplexy, a disorder of rapid eye movement sleep. Eur J Pharmacol 1991;205:11–6.

23. Mignot E, Guilleminault C, Bowersox S, et al. Central alpha 1 adrenoceptor subtypes in narcolepsy-cataplexy: a disorder of REM sleep. Brain Res 1989;490:186–91.

24. Wu MF, Gulyani SA, Yau E, et al. Locus coeruleus neurons: cessation of activity during cataplexy. Neuroscience 1999;91:1389–99.

25. Aldrich MS, Rogers AE. Exacerbation of human cataplexy by prazosin. Sleep 1989;12(3):254–6.

26. Cortés MD, Arias-Montaño JA, Eguibar JR. Prazosin increases immobility episodes in taiep rats without changes in the properties of alpha1 receptors. Neurosci Lett 2007;412:159–62.

27. Mignot E, Guilleminault C, Bowersox S, et al. Effect of alpha 1-adrenoceptors blockade with prazosin in canine narcolepsy. Brain Res 1988;444:184–8.

28. Guilleminault C, Mignot E, Aldrich M, et al. Prazosin contraindicated in patients with narcolepsy. Lancet 1988;2:511.

29. Nishino S, Haak L, Shepherd H, et al. Effects of central alpha-2 adrenergic compounds on canine narcolepsy, a disorder of rapid eye movement sleep. J Pharmacol Exp Ther 1990;253:1145–52.

30. Aldrich MS, Prokopowicz G, Ockert K, et al. Neurochemical studies of human narcolepsy: alpha-adrenergic receptor autoradiography of human narcoleptic brain and brainstem. Sleep 1994;17:598–608.

31. Miller JD, Farber J, Gatz P, et al. Activity of mesencephalic dopamine and non-dopamine neurons across stages of sleep and walking in the rat. Brain Res 1983;273:133–41.

32. Steinfels GF, Heym J, Strecker RE, et al. Behavioral correlates of dopaminergic unit activity in freely moving cats. Brain Res 1983;258:217–28.

33. Feenstra MG, Botterblom MH, Mastenbroek S. Dopamine and noradrenaline efflux in the prefrontal cortex in the light and dark period: effects of novelty and handling and comparison to the

nucleus accumbens. Neuroscience 2000;100: 741–8.

34. Monti JM, Monti D. The involvement of dopamine in the modulation of sleep and waking. Sleep Med Rev 2007;11:113–33.

35. Monti JM, Fernandez M, Jantos H. Sleep during acute dopamine D1 agonist SKF 38393 or D1 antagonist SCH 23390 administration in rats. Neuropsychopharmacology 1990;3:153–62.

36. Trampus M, Ferri N, Monopoli A, et al. The dopamine D1 receptor is involved in the regulation of REM sleep in the rat. Eur J Pharmacol 1991;194:189–94.

37. Trampus M, Ferri N, Adami M, et al. The dopamine D1 receptor agonists, A68930 and SKF 38393, induce arousal and suppress REM sleep in the rat. Eur J Pharmacol 1993;235:83–7.

38. Ongini E, Bonizzoni E, Ferri N, et al. Differential effects of dopamine D-1 and D-2 receptor antagonist antipsychotics on sleep-wake patterns in the rat. J Pharmacol Exp Ther 1993;266:726–31.

39. Neylan TC, van Kammen DP, Kelley ME, et al. Sleep in schizophrenic patients on and off haloperidol therapy. Clinically stable vs relapsed patients. Arch Gen Psychiatry 1992;49:643–9.

40. Roth T, Rye DB, Borchert LD, et al. Assessment of sleepiness and unintended sleep in Parkinson's disease patients taking dopamine agonists. Sleep Med 2003;4:275–80.

41. Lu CY, Yi PL, Tsai CH, et al. TNF-NF-kappaB signaling mediates excessive somnolence in hemiparkinsonian rats. Behav Brain Res 2010;208: 484–96.

42. Desarkar P, Goyal N, Khess CR. Clozapine-induced cataplexy. J Neuropsychiatry Clin Neurosci 2007;19:87–8.

43. Chiles JA, Cohn S, McNaughton A. Dropping objects: possible mild cataplexy associated with clozapine. J Nerv Ment Dis 1990;178:663–4.

44. Koob GF, Sanna PP, Bloom FE. Neuroscience of addiction. Neuron 1998;21:467–76.

45. Koob GF. Drugs of abuse: anatomy, pharmacology and function of reward pathways. Trends Pharmacol Sci 1992;13:177–84.

46. Davis JM, Kopin IJ, Lemberger L, et al. Effects of urinary pH on amphetamine metabolism. Ann N Y Acad Sci 1971;179:493–501.

47. Faraj BA, Israili ZH, Perel JM, et al. Metabolism and disposition of methylphenidate-14C: studies in man and animals. J Pharmacol Exp Ther 1974;191:535–47.

48. Mitler MM, Hajdukovic R, Erman MK. Treatment of narcolepsy with methamphetamine. Sleep 1993; 16:306–17.

49. Mitler MM, Hajdukovic R, Erman M, et al. Narcolepsy. J Clin Neurophysiol 1990;7:93–118.

50. Shindler J, Schachter M, Brincat S, et al. Amphetamine, mazindol, and fencamfamin in narcolepsy. BMJ 1985;290:1167–70.

51. Daly DD, Yoss RE. The treatment of narcolepsy with methylphenylpiperidylacetate: a preliminary report. Mayo Clin Proc 1956;31:620–6.

52. Yoss RE, Daly D. Treatment of narcolepsy with Ritalin. Neurology 1959;9:171–3.

53. Mitler MM, Shafor R, Hajdukovich R, et al. Treatment of narcolepsy: objective studies on methylphenidate, pemoline, and protriptyline. Sleep 1986;9:260–4.

54. Nicholson AN, Stone BM. Heterocyclic amphetamine derivatives and caffeine on sleep in man. Br J Clin Pharmacol 1980;9:195–203.

55. Saletu B, Frey R, Krupka M, et al. Differential effects of a new central adrenergic agonist—modafinil—and D-amphetamine on sleep and early morning behavior in young healthy volunteers. Int J Clin Pharmacol Res 1989;9:183–95.

56. Mitler MM, Aldrich MS, Koob GF, et al. Narcolepsy and its treatment with stimulants. ASDA standards of practice. Sleep 1994;17:352–71.

57. Guilleminault C. Amphetamines and narcolepsy: use of the Stanford database. Sleep 1993;16: 199–201.

58. Larrosa O, de la Llave Y, Bario S, et al. Stimulant and anticataplectic effects of reboxetine in patients with narcolepsy: a pilot study. Sleep 2001;24: 282–5.

59. Mignot E, Nishino S. Emerging therapies in narcolepsy-cataplexy. Sleep 2005;28:754–63.

60. Guilleminault C, Mancuso J, Salva MA, et al. Viloxazine hydrochloride in narcolepsy: a preliminary report. Sleep 1986;9:275–9.

61. Parmentier R, Ohtsu H, Djebbara-Hannas Z, et al. Anatomical, physiological, and pharmacological characteristics of histidine decarboxylase knock-out mice: evidence for the role of brain histamine in behavioral and sleep-wake control. J Neurosci 2002;22:7695–711.

62. Steininger TL, Alam MN, Gong H, et al. Sleep-waking discharge of neurons in the posterior lateral hypothalamus of the albino rat. Brain Res 1999; 840:138–47.

63. Ko EM, Estabrooke IV, McCarthy M, et al. Wake-related activity of tuberomammillary neurons in rats. Brain Res 2003;992:220–6.

64. Roehrs TA, Tietz EI, Zorick FJ, et al. Daytime sleepiness and antihistamines. Sleep 1984;7:137–41.

65. Tasaka K, Chung YH, Sawada K, et al. Excitatory effect of histamine on the arousal system and its inhibition by H1 blockers. Brain Res Bull 1989;22: 271–5.

66. Monti JM, Pellejero T, Jantos H. Effects of H1- and H2-histamine receptor agonists and antagonists on sleep and wakefulness in the rat. J Neural Transm 1986;66:1–11.

67. Monti JM, Jantos H, Ponzoni A, et al. Sleep and waking during acute histamine H3 agonist BP

2.94 or H3 antagonist carboperamide (MR 16155) administration in rats. Neuropsychopharmacology 1996;15:31–5.

68. Lin JS, Dauvilliers Y, Arnulf I, et al. An inverse agonist of the histamine H(3) receptor improves wakefulness in narcolepsy: studies in orexin-/- mice and patients. Neurobiol Dis 2008;30:74–83.

69. Guo RX, Anaclet C, Roberts JC, et al. Differential effects of acute and repeat dosing with the H3 antagonist GSK189254 on the sleep-wake cycle and narcoleptic episodes in Ox-/- mice. Br J Pharmacol 2009;157:104–17.

70. Ursin R. The effects of 5-hydroxytryptophan and L-tryptophan on wakefulness and sleep patterns in the cat. Brain Res 1976;106:105–15.

71. Wojcik WJ, Fornal C, Radulovacki M. Effect of tryptophan on sleep in the rat. Neuropharmacology 1980;19:163–7.

72. Bjorvatn B, Ursin R. Effects of zimeldine, a selective 5-HT reuptake inhibitor, combined with ritanserin, a selective 5-HT2 antagonist, on waking and sleep stages in rats. Behav Brain Res 1990;40:239–46.

73. Trulson ME, Jacobs BL. Raphe unit activity in freely moving cats: correlation with level of behavioral arousal. Brain Res 1979;163:135–50.

74. Puizillout JJ, Gaudin-Chazal G, Daszuta A, et al. Release of endogenous serotonin from "encephale isole" cats. II - Correlations with raphe neuronal activity and sleep and wakefulness. J Physiol 1979;75:531–7.

75. Portas CM, Bjorvatn B, Fagerland S, et al. On-line detection of extracellular levels of serotonin in dorsal raphe nucleus and frontal cortex over the sleep/wake cycle in the freely moving rat. Neuroscience 1998;83:807–14.

76. Takahashi H, Nakashima S, Ohama E, et al. Distribution of serotonin-containing cell bodies in the brainstem of the human fetus determined with immunohistochemistry using antiserotonin serum. Brain Dev 1986;8:355–65.

77. Wu MF, John J, Boehmer LN, et al. Activity of dorsal raphe cells across the sleep-waking cycle and during cataplexy in narcoleptic dogs. J Physiol 2004;554:202–15.

78. Törk I. Anatomy of the serotonergic system. Ann N Y Acad Sci 1990;600:9–34.

79. Schrader H, Kayed K, Bendixen Markset AC, et al. The treatment of accessory symptoms in narcolepsy: a double-blind cross-over study of a selective serotonin re-uptake inhibitor (femoxetine) versus placebo. Acta Neurol Scand 1986;74:297–303.

80. Langdon N, Shindler J, Parkes JD, et al. Fluoxetine in the treatment of cataplexy. Sleep 1986;9:371–3.

81. Malamed Y, Daliahu Y, Paleacu D. Narcolepsy and psychotic states—a case report. Isr J Psychiatry Relat Sci 2009;46:70–3.

82. Frey J, Darbonne C. Fluoxetine suppresses human cataplexy: a pilot study. Neurology 1994;44:707–9.

83. Thirumalai SS, Shubin RA. The use of citalopram in resistant cataplexy. Sleep Med 2000;1:313–6.

84. Nishino S, Mignot E. Pharmacological aspects of human and canine narcolepsy. Prog Neurobiol 1997;52:27–78.

85. Møller LR, Østergaard JR. Treatment with venlafaxine in six cases of children with narcolepsy and with cataplexy and hypnagogic hallucinations. J Child Adolesc Psychopharmacol 2009;19:197–201.

86. Smith M, Parkes JD, Dahlitz M. Venlafaxine in the treatment of the narcoleptic syndrome. J Sleep Res 1996;5(Suppl):217.

87. Billiard M, Bassetti C, Dauvilliers Y, et al. EFNS Task Force. EFNS guidelines on management of narcolepsy. Eur J Neurol 2006;13:1035–48.

88. Lin JS, Roussel B, Akaoka H, et al. Role of catecholamines in modafinil and amphetamine induced wakefulness, a comparative pharmacological study. Brain Res 1992;591:319–26, 9.

89. Mignot E, Nishino S, Guilleminault C, et al. Modafinil binds to the dopamine uptake carrier site with low affinity. Sleep 1994;17:436–7.

90. Ferraro L, Tanganelli S, O'Connor WT, et al. The vigilance promoting drug modafinil increases dopamine release in the rat nucleus accumbens via the involvement of a local GABAergic mechanism. Eur J Pharmacol 1996;306:33–9.

91. Wisor JP, Nishino S, Sora I, et al. Dopaminergic role in stimulant-induced wakefulness. J Neurosci 2001;21:1787–94.

92. Ferraro L, Antonelli T, Tanganelli S, et al. The vigilance promoting drug modafinil increases extracellular glutamate levels in the medial preoptic area and the posterior hypothalamus of the conscious rat: prevention by local GABAA receptor blockade. Neuropsychopharmacology 1999;20:346–56.

93. Ferraro L, Antonelli T, O'Connor WT, et al. The effects of modafinil on striatal, pallidal and nigral GABA and glutamate release in the conscious rat: evidence for a preferential inhibition of striato-pallidal GABA transmission. Neurosci Lett 1998;253:135–8.

94. Ishizuka T, Murakami M, Yamatodani A. Involvement of central histaminergic systems in modafinil-induced but not methylphenidate-induced increases in locomotor activity in rats. Eur J Pharmacol 2008;578:209–15.

95. Ishizuka T, Sakamoto Y, Sakurai T, et al. Modafinil increases histamine release in the anterior hypothalamus of rats. Neurosci Lett 2003;339:143–6.

96. Ferraro L, Antonelli T, O'Connor WT, et al. The antinarcoleptic drug modafinil increases glutamate release in thalamic areas and hippocampus. Neuroreport 1997;8:2883–7.

97. Billiard M, Besset A, Montplaisir J, et al. Modafinil: a double-blind multicenter study. Sleep 1994; 17(Suppl):107–12.

98. Broughton RJ, Fleming JAE, George CFP, et al. Randomized, double-blind, placebo-controlled crossover trial of modafinil in the treatment of excessive daytime sleepiness in narcolepsy. Neurology 1997;49:444–51.

99. US Modafinil in Narcolepsy Multicenter Study Group. Randomized trial of modafinil for the treatment of pathological somnolence in narcolepsy. Ann Neurol 1998;43:88–97.

100. US Modafinil in Narcolepsy Multicenter Study Group. Randomized trial of modafinil as a treatment for the excessive daytime somnolence of narcolepsy. Neurology 2000;54:1166–75.

101. Harsh JR, Hayduk R, Rosenberg R, et al. The efficacy and safety of armodafinil as treatment for adults with excessive sleepiness associated with narcolepsy. Curr Med Res Opin 2006;22:761–74.

102. Roth T, White D, Schmidt-Nowara W, et al. Effects of armodafinil in the treatment of residual excessive sleepiness associated with obstructive sleep apnea/hypopnea syndrome: a 12-week, multicenter, double-blind, randomized, placebo-controlled study in nCPAP-adherent adults. Clin Ther 2006;28:689–706.

103. Steriade M, Datta S, Pare D, et al. Neuronal activities in brain-stem cholinergic nuclei related to tonic activation processes in thalamocortical systems. J Neurosci 1990;10:2541–59.

104. Williams JA, Comisarow J, Day J, et al. State dependent release of acetylcholine in rat thalamus measured by in vivo microdialysis. J Neurosci 1994;14:5236–42.

105. Marrosu F, Portas C, Mascia MS, et al. Microdialysis measurement of cortical and hippocampal acetylcholine release during sleep-wake cycle in freely moving cats. Brain Res 1995;671:329–32.

106. Reid MS, Tafti M, Nishino S, et al. Cholinergic regulation of cataplexy in canine narcolepsy in the pontine reticular formationis mediated by M2 muscarinic receptors. Sleep 1994;17:424–35.

107. Sitaram N, Moore AM, Gillin JC. The effect of physostigmine on normal human sleep and dreaming. Arch Gen Psychiatry 1978;35:1239–43.

108. Gillin JC, Sitaram N, Mendelson WB, et al. Physostigmine alters onset but not duration of REM sleep in man. Psychopharmacology (Berl) 1978;58: 111–4.

109. Holsboer-Trachsler E, Hatzinger M, Stohler R, et al. Effects of the novel acetylcholinesterase inhibitor SDZ ENA 713 on sleep in man. Neuropsychopharmacology 1993;8:87–92.

110. Nissen C, Nofzinger EA, Feige B, et al. Differential effects of the muscarinic M1 receptor agonist RS-86 and the acetylcholine-esterase inhibitor donepezil on REM sleep regulation in healthy volunteers. Neuropsychopharmacology 2006;31:1294–300.

111. Nissen C, Power AE, Nofzinger EA, et al. M1 muscarinic acetylcholine receptor agonism alters sleep without affecting memory consolidation. J Cogn Neurosci 2006;18:1799–807.

112. Nishino S, Tafti M, Reid MS, et al. Muscle atonia is triggered by cholinergic stimulation of the basal forebrain: implication for the pathophysiology of canine narcolepsy. J Neurosci 1995;15: 4806–14.

113. Reid MS, Tafti M, Geary JN, et al. Cholinergic mechanisms in canine narcolepsy–I. Modulation of cataplexy via local drug administration into the pontine reticular formation. Neuroscience 1994; 59:511–22.

114. Diefenbach K, Arold G, Wollny A, et al. Effects on sleep of anticholinergics used for overactive bladder treatment in healthy volunteers aged > or = 50 years. BJU Int 2005;95:346–9.

115. Hohagen F, Lis S, Riemann D, et al. Influence of biperiden and bornaprine on sleep in healthy subjects. Neuropsychopharmacology 1994;11: 29–32.

116. Salin-Pascual RJ, Granados-Fuentes D, Galicia-Polo L, et al. Biperiden administration in normal sleep and after rapid eye movement sleep deprivation in healthy volunteers. Neuropsychopharmacology 1991;5:97–102.

117. Gillin JC, Sutton L, Ruiz C, et al. Dose dependent inhibition of REM sleep in normal volunteers by biperiden, a muscarinic antagonist. Biol Psychiatry 1991;30:151–6.

118. Rauniar GP, Gitanjali B, Shashindran C. Comparative effects of hyoscine butylbromide and atropine sulphate on sleep architecture in healthy human volunteers. Indian J Physiol Pharmacol 1998;42: 395–400.

119. Gallopin T, Fort P, Eggermann E, et al. Identification of sleep-promoting neurons in vitro. Nature 2000; 404:992–5.

120. Gaus SE, Strecker RE, Tate BA, et al. Ventrolateral preoptic nucleus contains sleep-active, galaninergic neurons in multiple mammalian species. Neuroscience 2002;115:285–94.

121. Sherin JE, Elmquist JK, Torrealba F, et al. Innervation of histaminergic tuberomammillary neurons by GABAergic and galaninergic neurons in the ventrolateral preoptic nucleus of the rat. J Neurosci 1998;18:4705–21.

122. Steininger TL, Gong H, McGinty D, et al. Subregional organization of preoptic area/anterior hypothalamic projections to arousal-related monoaminergic cell groups. J Comp Neurol 2001;429: 638–53.

123. Koyama Y, Hayaishi O. Firing of neurons in the preoptic/anterior hypothalamic areas in rat: its

possible involvement in slow wave sleep and para-doxical sleep. Neurosci Res 1994;19:31–8.

124. Rechtschaffen A, Wolpert EA, Dement WC, et al. Nocturnal sleep of narcoleptics. Electroencephalogr Clin Neurophysiol 1963;15:599–609.

125. Montplaisir J, Billiard M, Takahashi S, et al. Twenty-four-hour recording in REM-narcoleptics with special reference to nocturnal sleep disruption. Biol Psychiatry 1978;13:73–89.

126. Baker TL, Guilleminault C, Nino-Murcia G, et al. Comparative polysomnographic study of narcolepsy and idiopathic central nervous system hypersomnia. Sleep 1986;9:232–42.

127. Folkerts M, Rosenthal L, Roehrs T, et al. The reliability of the diagnostic features in patients with narcolepsy. Biol Psychiatry 1996;40:208–14.

128. Thorpy MJ, Snyder M, Aloe FS, et al. Short-term triazolam use improves nocturnal sleep of narcoleptics. Sleep 1992;15:212–6.

129. Broughton R, Mamelak M. The treatment of narcolepsy-cataplexy with nocturnal gamma-hydroxybutyrate. Can J Neurol Sci 1979;6:1–6.

130. Maitre M. The gamma-hydroxybutyrate signalling system in brain: organization and functional implications. Prog Neurobiol 1997;51:337–61.

131. Pardi D, Black J. gamma-Hydroxybutyrate/sodium oxybate: neurobiology, and impact on sleep and wakefulness. CNS Drugs 2006;20:993–1018.

132. US Xyrem Multicenter Study Group. A randomized, double blind, placebo-controlled multicenter trial comparing the effects of three doses of orally administered sodium oxybate with placebo for the treatment of narcolepsy. Sleep 2002;25:42–9.

133. US Xyrem Multicenter Study Group. A 12-month, open-label, multicenter extension trial of orally administered sodium oxybate for the treatment of narcolepsy. Sleep 2003;26:31–5.

134. US Xyrem Multicenter Study Group. Sodium oxybate demonstrates long-term efficacy for the treatment of cataplexy in patients with narcolepsy. Sleep Med 2004;5:119–23.

135. Xyrem International Study Group. Further evidence supporting the use of sodium oxybate for the treatment of cataplexy: a double-blind, placebo-controlled study in 228 patients. Sleep Med 2005;6:415–21.

136. Black J, Houghton WC. Sodium oxybate improves excessive daytime sleepiness in narcolepsy. Sleep 2006;29:939–46.

137. Sakurai T, Amemiya A, Ishii M, et al. Orexins and orexin receptors: a family of hypothalamic neuropeptides and G protein-coupled receptors that regulate feeding behavior. Cell 1998;92:573–85.

138. de Lecea L, Kilduff TS, Peyron C, et al. The hypocretins: hypothalamus-specific peptides with neuroexcitatory activity. Proc Natl Acad Sci U S A 1998;95:322–7.

139. Lin L, Faraco J, Li R, et al. The sleep disorder canine narcolepsy is caused by a mutation in the hypocretin (orexin) receptor 2 gene. Cell 1999;98:365–76.

140. Chemelli RM, Willie JT, Sinton CM, et al. Narcolepsy in orexin knockout mice: molecular genetics of sleep regulation. Cell 1999;98:437–51.

141. Mignot E, Tafti M, Dement WC, et al. Narcolepsy and immunity. Adv Neuroimmunol 1995;5:23–37.

142. Peyron C, Tighe DK, van Den Pol AN, et al. Neurons containing hypocretin (orexin) project to multiple neuronal systems. J Neurosci 1998;18:9996–10015.

143. Nambu T, Sakurai T, Mizukami K, et al. Distribution of orexin neurons in the adult rat brain. Brain Res 1999;827:243–60.

144. Hagan JJ, Leslie RA, Patel S, et al. Orexin A activates locus coeruleus cell firing and increases arousal in the rat. Proc Natl Acad Sci U S A 1999;96:10911–6.

145. Methippara MM, Alam MN, Szymusiak R, et al. Effects of lateral preoptic area application of orexin-A on sleep- wakefulness. Neuroreport 2000;11:3423–6.

146. Bourgin P, Huitron-Resendiz S, Spier AD, et al. Hypocretin-1 modulates rapid eye movement sleep through activation of locus coeruleus neurons. J Neurosci 2000;20:7760–5.

147. España RA, Baldo BA, Kelley AE, et al. Wake-promoting and sleep-suppressing actions of hypocretin (orexin): basal forebrain sites of action. Neuroscience 2001;106:699–715.

148. Estabrooke IV, McCarthy MT, Ko E, et al. Fos expression in orexin neurons varies with behavioral state. J Neurosci 2001;21:1656–62.

149. Espana RA, Valentino RJ, Berridge CW. Fos immunoreactivity in hypocretin-synthesizing and hypocretin-1 receptor-expressing neurons: effects of diurnal and nocturnal spontaneous waking, stress and hypocretin-1 administration. Neuroscience 2003;121:201–17.

150. Wu MF, John J, Maidment N, et al. Hypocretin release in normal and narcoleptic dogs after food and sleep deprivation, eating, and movement. Am J Physiol Regul Integr Comp Physiol 2002;283:R1079–86.

151. Willie JT, Chemelli RM, Sinton CM, et al. To eat or to sleep? Orexin in the regulation of feeding and wakefulness. Annu Rev Neurosci 2001;24:429–58.

152. Yoshida Y, Fujiki N, Nakajima T, et al. Fluctuation of extracellular hypocretin-1 (orexin A) levels in the rat in relation to the light-dark cycle and sleep-wake activities. Eur J Neurosci 2001;14:1075–81.

153. Dhuria SV, Hanson LR, Frey WH 2nd. Intranasal drug targeting of hypocretin-1 (orexin-A) to the central nervous system. J Pharm Sci 2009;98:2501–15.

154. Deadwyler SA, Porrino L, Siegel JM, et al. Systemic and nasal delivery of orexin-A (Hypocretin-1) reduces the effects of sleep deprivation on cognitive performance in nonhuman primates. J Neurosci 2007;27:14239—47.

155. Godbout R, Montplaisir J. All-day performance variations in normal and narcoleptic subjects. Sleep 1986;9:200—4.

156. Mullington J, Broughton R. Scheduled naps in the management of daytime sleepiness in narcolepsy-cataplexy. Sleep 1993;16:444—56.

157. Helmus T, Rosenthal L, Bishop C, et al. The alerting effects of short and long naps in narcoleptic, sleep deprived, and alert individuals. Sleep 1997;20:251—7.

158. Rogers AE, Aldrich MS. The effect of regularly scheduled naps on sleep attacks and excessive daytime sleepiness associated with narcolepsy. Nurs Res 1993;42:111—7.

159. Rogers AE, Aldrich MS, Lin X. A comparison of three different sleep schedules for reducing daytime sleepiness in narcolepsy. Sleep 2001;24:385—91.

160. Billiard M. Narcolepsy: current treatment options and future approaches. Neuropsychiatr Dis Treat 2008;4:557—66.

161. Schenck CH, Mahowald MW. Motor dyscontrol in narcolepsy: rapid-eye-movement (REM) sleep without atonia and REM sleep behavior disorder. Ann Neurol 1992;32:3—10.

162. Nightingale S, Orgill JC, Ebrahim IO, et al. The association between narcolepsy and REM behavior disorder (RBD). Sleep Med 2005;6:253—8.

163. Billiard M. REM sleep behavior disorder and narcolepsy. CNS Neurol Disord Drug Targets 2009;8:264—70.

164. Boehmer LN, Wu MF, John J, et al. Treatment with immunosuppressive and anti-inflammatory agents delays onset of canine genetic narcolepsy and reduces symptom severity. Exp Neurol 2004;188:292—9.

165. Dauvilliers Y, Abril B, Mas E, et al. Normalization of hypocretin-1 in narcolepsy after intravenous immunoglobulin treatment. Neurology 2009;73:1333—4.

166. Hecht M, Lin L, Kushida CA, et al. Report of a case of immunosuppression with prednisone in an 8-year-old boy with an acute onset of hypocretin-deficiency narcolepsy. Sleep 2003;26:809—10.

167. Chen W, Black J, Call P, et al. Late-onset narcolepsy presenting as rapidly progressing muscle weakness: response to plasmapheresis. Ann Neurol 2005;58:489—90.

168. Lecendreux M, Maret S, Bassetti C, et al. Clinical efficacy of high-dose intravenous immunoglobulins near the onset of narcolepsy in a 10-year-old boy. J Sleep Res 2003;12:347—8.

169. Fronczek R, Verschuuren J, Lammers GJ. Response to intravenous immunoglobulins and placebo in a patient with narcolepsy with cataplexy. J Neurol 2007;254:1607—8.

170. Riehl J, Honda K, Kwan M, et al. Chronic oral administration of CG-3703, a thyrotropin releasing hormone analog, increases wake and decreases cataplexy in canine narcolepsy. Neuropsychopharmacology 2000;23:34—45.

171. Fronczek R, Raymann RJ, Overeem S, et al. Manipulation of skin temperature improves nocturnal sleep in narcolepsy. J Neurol Neurosurg Psychiatry 2008;79:1354—7.

172. Fronczek R, Raymann RJ, Romeijn N, et al. Manipulation of core body and skin temperature improves vigilance and maintenance of wakefulness in narcolepsy. Sleep 2008;31:233—40.

173. Fronczek R, Overeem S, Lammers GJ, et al. Altered skin-temperature regulation in narcolepsy relates to sleep propensity. Sleep 2006;29:1444—9.

The Pharmacologic Management of Restless Legs Syndrome and Periodic Leg Movement Disorder

Maryann C. Deak, MD[a],*, John W. Winkelman, MD, PhD[b]

KEYWORDS
- Restless legs syndrome • Periodic leg movement disorder
- Sleep • Movement disorder

Four essential diagnostic criteria must be present to make a diagnosis of restless legs syndrome (RLS).[1] These include: (1) an urge to move the legs, which may be accompanied by unpleasant sensations; (2) worsening of symptoms during periods of rest; (3) partial or total relief of symptoms with movement, such as walking, for at least as long as the activity continues; (4) worsening of symptoms in the evening or night. RLS is often accompanied by periodic limb movements of sleep (PLMS), which is a polysomnographic finding of recurrent movements of the legs during sleep. However, PLMS can occur independently of RLS either in asymptomatic individuals or in patients with periodic limb movement disorder (PLMD), diagnosis of which requires the presence of otherwise unexplained hypersomnia or insomnia.[2]

TREATMENT OF RESTLESS LEGS SYNDROME
Introduction

The paradox of restless legs syndrome (RLS) treatment is that its most clinically important consequence, sleeplessness, is not one of its diagnostic criteria.[3] This led, in years past, to the widespread use of hypnotic agents for RLS, without good evidence for their use. However, more recent treatments, and those that are approved by regulatory agencies, address the core sensorimotor symptoms, which then commonly lead to relief of the secondary sleep-related consequences. In addition to the sleep-related consequences of RLS, emerging evidence suggests that RLS may be associated with additional impairments, including reduced health-related quality of life, elevated rates of mood disorders and anxiety disorders, and potentially increased risk of cardiovascular disease.[4] However, a causal link between RLS and these additional features has not been established and thus these features are not currently the basis for treatment decisions.

To assess the full extent of RLS-related symptoms, both before and during the course of treatment, use of a structured RLS instrument may be of value. The International Restless Legs Syndrome (IRLS) rating scale is a validated instrument for assessing symptom severity and has also been used as a therapeutic outcome measure in clinical trials.[5,6] The scale gauges many RLS features, including sensory and restlessness intensity of RLS, symptom frequency, as well as the effect of

J.W.W. has had research support from GlaxoSmithKline and Sepracor and is a consultant to GlaxoSmithKline, Impax Pharmaceuticals, Pfizer, and UCB.
[a] Division of Sleep Medicine, Department of Medicine, Harvard School of Medicine, 1505 Commonwealth Avenue 5th Floor, Boston, MA 02135, USA
[b] Department of Psychiatry, Brigham and Women's Hospital, Harvard School of Medicine, 1505 Commonwealth Avenue 5th Floor, Boston, MA 02135, USA
* Corresponding author.
E-mail address: maryann_deak@sleephealth.com

Sleep Med Clin 5 (2010) 675–687
doi:10.1016/j.jsmc.2010.08.011

RLS on sleep, daytime fatigue/sleepiness, mood symptoms, and work/home life. Subjects included in clinical research trials usually fall into the category of moderate to severe RLS based on the IRLS rating scale.

Several essential principles should be considered in the treatment of RLS. Because current treatments for RLS can only provide relief of symptoms rather than resolution of the disorder, RLS treatments are often long-term and should be initiated only when the benefits are sufficient to outweigh potential, immediate, and long-term side effects. Before RLS-specific treatment is initiated, ample consideration must first be given to possible secondary causes of RLS. If identified, factors contributing to secondary RLS (such as iron deficiency) should be treated whenever possible because treatment may lead to resolution of RLS symptoms. When treating RLS symptoms, the frequency and timing of treatment should be carefully considered. Some patients may not require daily treatment and only require intervention on an as-needed basis. Also, patients without frequent symptoms are more likely to be treated effectively with nonpharmacologic therapy than those with frequent symptoms. Because RLS symptoms are activity dependent, adjustment in activity patterns may be an effective single or adjunctive approach to RLS. In addition to the presence of comorbidities, the quality of the patient's discomfort may also contribute to the choice of a pharmacologic agent. For example, patients who complain of a painful quality to their symptoms or who have RLS symptoms compounded by arthritic or neuropathic pain may benefit from alpha(2)delta agents such as gabapentin or pregabalin as a first line agent rather than from a dopamine agonist.[7] Finally, and most importantly, in distinction to most other medical disorders, RLS is time dependent in that it has a relatively predictable time of onset for an individual patient, usually in the evening. The provider must attempt to obtain an accurate idea of this time because the administration of pharmacologic therapies should be timed accordingly.

Primary RLS

Although RLS was depicted as early as the 1670s, it was not until the 1940s that Ekbom extensively described the syndrome and coined the term restless legs syndrome.[8,9] Similarly, various treatment modalities were described beginning as early as the 1680s. The effectiveness of levodopa (in combination with benserazide) for the treatment of RLS was first described in 1982.[10] Today, dopaminergic agents are the best-studied pharmacologic options and have become the first line treatment of RLS.[11,12] Alternatives to dopaminergic medications include antiepileptic medications, opioids, benzodiazepines, and iron therapy, each with their own advantages and disadvantages.

Dopaminergic agents

Levodopa Levodopa is a short-acting medication and reaches peak plasma concentration between 0.5 and 2 hours of administration and has a half-life of 1 to 3 hours. It is metabolized by the gastrointestinal tract, kidneys, and liver and is primarily renally excreted. The range of doses of levodopa in combination with carbidopa or benserazide used for the treatment of RLS is between 100/25 mg and 200/50 mg. Levodopa is usually administered about 30 minutes before symptom onset. If immediate-release levodopa is used, dosing may need to be repeated during the night.

Although levodopa was the first dopaminergic agent used for the treatment of RLS, there are few double-blind placebo-controlled trials that examine its effectiveness in the treatment of primary RLS.[13–15] Such studies noted improvements in sleep duration[14] and quality,[14,15] quality of life,[14] severity of RLS symptoms,[14] and periodic limb movements during sleep[13–15] when compared with placebo. Levodopa was well tolerated during short-term studies of levodopa and benserazide or levodopa and carbidopa.[14,16] In fact, given its reliable efficacy, levodopa has been proposed as the gold standard treatment of RLS. Common side effects in short-term studies included gastrointestinal symptoms, muscle weakness, somnolence, and headache.[16]

Although the dyskinetic characteristics of levodopa treatment of Parkinson disease have never been observed in RLS, long-term use of levodopa is associated with a worsening of symptoms, including early morning rebound and, most problematically, augmentation, which is discussed in greater detail later. Because of these side effects, use of levodopa has fallen out of favor for daily long-term treatment of RLS. However, levodopa may still be useful for intermittent use on an as-needed basis in patients with occasional RLS symptoms[7] or as an as-needed rescue when rapid relief of RLS symptoms is required.

Nonergot-derived dopamine agonists Nonergot dopamine agonists, including ropinirole, pramipexole, and rotigotine, have become the mainstay of RLS treatment because of their efficacy, intermediate half-life, as well as the reduced incidence of augmentation compared with levodopa. In addition, they are the only medications approved by the Food and Drug Administration (FDA) for the treatment of RLS. The nonergot dopamine agonists have been tested in a large number of randomized placebo-controlled trials, which, unlike levodopa trials, used the IRLS rating scale as the primary outcome measure.

Ropinirole Ropinirole demonstrated efficacy in several double-blind, placebo-controlled, randomized trials in primary moderate to severe RLS.[17–20] In addition, in one polysomnographic study, there were significant improvements in periodic limb movements during wake and sleep, as well as in several sleep parameters, including sleep-onset latency.[21] Ropinirole has a fairly rapid onset of action, reaching peak plasma levels in 1.5 hours and it has a half-life of 6 hours. Metabolized by the liver, it has some potential for drug interactions through the P450 1A2 pathway. In flexible-dose titration clinical trials, the mean effective dosage has often been between 1.5 and 2 mg/d.[17,18] If dosed according to the approved titration schedule, such target doses are reached in approximately 3 weeks. The FDA-approved dosing schedule calls for administration 1 to 3 hours before bedtime. In practice, ropinirole is sometimes dosed in the evening 1 to 3 hours before symptom onset and, in some cases, twice daily in the early evening and before bed.

Pramipexole There have been several randomized, double-blind, placebo-controlled trials using pramipexole, which have established its efficacy in RLS.[22–24] Other studies have noted improvements in periodic limb movements of sleep (PLMS)[22,25,26] and sleep parameters such as sleep-onset latency and total sleep time.[26]

Compared with ropinirole, pramipexole has a slower onset of action (1 to 3 hours) and a longer elimination half-life (10 hours). Pramipexole undergoes very little metabolism; it is excreted almost entirely in the urine, mostly in the form of unaltered drug. Pramipexole is generally administered at doses between 0.25 and 1 mg and like ropinirole, it can be dosed on-label 1 to 3 hours before bedtime or off-label 1 to 3 hours before symptom onset. The longer half-life of pramipexole allows it to be dosed once in the early evening, whereas ropinirole may require dosing twice per night when it is used to control early evening symptoms. Absorption of pramipexole, and thus onset of efficacy, is substantially slowed when taken with food.

Rotigotine Rotigotine is a short-acting dopamine agonist, and when administered via a transdermal patch, it can be applied once daily with a recommended dosage for RLS ranging between 1

to 3 mg/24 h.[27] For RLS, providing a steady concentration of the drug has the theoretic potential to reduce augmentation and rebound. On the other hand, the biologic value of 24-hour blood levels of the drug for a disorder that is usually present 8 to 12 hours per day remains to be established. Rotigotine is metabolized by the liver, involving several P450 enzymes; it is primarily excreted in the urine. The half-life is from 5 to 7 hours.

The rotigotine patch is a newer agent compared with ropinirole and pramipexole. There have been fewer placebo-controlled trials in RLS using rotigotine, although these trials have clearly established its efficacy in RLS.

Safety and tolerability With some important caveats (see section on Augmentation), dopamine agonists have been well tolerated during short- and long-term clinical trials in the treatment of RLS. The total daily dosage of dopamine agonists used for treatment of RLS is roughly 10% of that used for Parkinson disease. In addition, dopamine agonists are administered once a day in the evening for RLS as opposed to 3 times a day for Parkinson disease. The most common side effects for this class of drugs have generally been mild and include nausea, somnolence/fatigue, and dizziness. For rotigotine, skin reactions from the transdermal system were present in nearly half of all patients.

Patients taking dopamine agonists for Parkinson disease have experienced additional side effects, including sleep attacks. This symptom has not been noted in short- or long-term studies of dopamine agonists in RLS. Other side effects described with the use of dopamine agonists for Parkinson disease include gambling, excess spending and eating, and increased sexual desire. Recent evidence suggests that patients with RLS who intake dopamine agonists may also be susceptible to such impulse control symptoms.[28–30] Thus, it is reasonable to warn patients about these side effects when initiating therapy with a dopamine agonist.

Ergot-derived dopamine agonists The ergot dopamine agonists include pergolide and cabergoline. Although these medications initially showed promise in the treatment of RLS, they are no longer used in the United States for the treatment of RLS. In fact, sale of pergolide was withdrawn from the market because of 2 studies that demonstrated an increased frequency of clinically important heart valve regurgitation in patients taking pergolide and cabergoline compared with control subjects.[31,32] Thus, the risks of ergot-derived dopamine agonists outweigh the benefits in the treatment of RLS.

One trial comparing the efficacy of levodopa and cabergoline is the only randomized, double-blind, head-to-head study comparing levodopa and a dopamine agonist for the treatment of RLS.[33] Patients taking cabergoline had significantly greater improvement in IRLS rating scale scores compared with patients on levodopa. Rates of augmentation and tolerance were less in the cabergoline group than the levodopa group.

Augmentation Augmentation is a worsening of RLS symptoms due to medication treatment. It is most commonly manifested by a shift of symptom onset to an earlier time of the day than that was typical before treatment was initiated. Other manifestations include an increased intensity of symptoms, extension of RLS symptoms to additional parts of the body, a shorter period of rest resulting in symptoms, a reduced period of symptom relief with treatment, or the appearance or worsening of periodic leg movements while awake.

Although augmentation is a potential consequence of the use of any dopaminergic agent, it occurs more frequently with the use of levodopa than with dopamine agonists. However, because few studies have been specifically designed to examine rates of augmentation, the incidence of this treatment complication for particular drugs remains uncertain. Long-term trials of 2 to 24 months on use of levodopa in RLS were associated with augmentation incidence rates ranging from 18.6% to 82%. In one study, augmentation occurred more frequently in patients with more severe pretreatment RLS symptoms and those on higher doses of carbidopa with levodopa ($\geq$200/50 mg) and was severe enough to warrant a change in medication in 50% of patients with RLS.[34] In the same study, 20% of patients with RLS treated with levodopa experienced early morning rebound, in which symptoms worsened at a time consistent with withdrawal effects of the medication. With pramipexole, a retrospective study with a mean follow-up of 27 months demonstrated maintained effectiveness over time with generally mild side effects. However, augmentation developed in 33% of patients.[35] Another retrospective study found a similar rate, with 32% of patients experiencing augmentation, as well as 46% requiring increasing doses to maintain efficacy.[36] Nevertheless, in this study, augmentation was generally easily managed by dose adjustment, and few patients discontinued the drug use for this reason.

Management of augmentation is an important aspect of treating patients with RLS. First, it is useful to determine which patients with augmentation require modification of treatment of this complication. The World Association of Sleep Medicine recently devised a definition of clinically significant augmentation.[37] Symptoms are considered clinically relevant when they affect any of the following: quality of life, daily activities/behavior, treatment dose or timing of treatment, treatment dosing of concomitant medications such an analgesics, or any other specific aspect as judged by the evaluator.

Before augmentation is definitively identified in a patient treated for RLS, several factors that can produce worsening of RLS but are not treatment related (augmentation mimics) must be distinguished from true augmentation. These factors include a change in activity levels (eg, more sedentary during the day), addition of medications that worsen RLS (eg, serotonergic antidepressants, antihistamines, dopamine agonists), or iron depletion. In such cases, modification of such processes is indicated, if possible. For instance, because low ferritin levels have been associated with augmentation,[38,39] an initial approach to augmentation treatment should involve evaluation of a patient's ferritin level, and iron should be supplemented in patients with serum ferritin levels less than 50 μg/L.

If an underlying factor cannot be identified for the clinically significant worsening of RLS, a change in medication regimen may be necessary.[40] One approach is to administer the patient's current dopaminergic medication earlier, by either adding an additional dose or dividing the current dose. Alternatively, a dopaminergic drug can be switched from a shorter- to a longer-acting agent (eg, from levodopa to a dopamine agonist). If this is not effective or feasible, a change from a dopamine agonist to an opioid or an antiepileptic medication, such as gabapentin or pregabalin, may be effective.[40] Of note, a reduction in dopaminergic dose often ameliorates the augmentation, returning symptoms to near-pretreatment levels, although it may initially lead to a temporary worsening of symptoms. For this reason, using combination therapy with a low-dose dopaminergic medication and an alternative medication, such as an opioid, may help reduce burden of RLS symptoms. Finally, in some cases, a drug holiday can clarify the difference between the natural progressive worsening of RLS and the development of augmentation.[40] Overall, augmentation is a common side effect of the use of dopaminergic medications in the treatment of RLS. It is important for physicians managing patients with RLS to closely monitor these symptoms and treat them when appropriate.

Nondopaminergic agents

Compared with dopaminergic drugs, there is less evidence to support the use of nondopaminergic agents in the treatment of RLS. In addition, the FDA has not approved these medications for the treatment of RLS. For these reasons, nondopaminergic agents are usually not used in the first line therapy for RLS, although these drugs are useful in clinical practice, especially (1) as an alternative agent if there is a contraindication to the use of dopaminergic drugs, (2) as a dual purpose agent if the drug can be used to treat a comorbidity and RLS symptoms concomitantly, (3) if dopaminergic agents are poorly tolerated or only partially effective, or (4) as an alternative or an adjunctive agent in the setting of augmentation.

Antiepileptic drugs Several antiepileptic medications have been used in the treatment of RLS. The alpha 2 delta calcium channel ligands gabapentin and pregabalin are the most commonly used medication for RLS in this class. Less commonly used antiepileptics include carbamazepine and valproic acid. Gabapentin enacarbil is an extended-release prodrug of gabapentin and is not yet FDA approved but is undergoing investigation for the treatment of RLS.

Gabapentin Gabapentin is primarily used as an adjunctive agent for seizures and for the treatment of pain syndromes, such as postherpetic neuralgia and diabetic peripheral neuropathy. It is not metabolized and is renally excreted as an unchanged drug. It has a half-life of 5 to 7 hours. Gabapentin has a favorable side effect profile, with common side effects including dizziness, somnolence, and, more rarely, weight gain, nausea, and peripheral edema.

Although the evidence is less abundant than that for dopaminergic medications, gabapentin seems to be effective for both core symptoms and sleep-related symptoms of primary RLS. Unlike dopaminergic agents, twice-a-day dosing has been used in clinical trials of gabapentin for the treatment of RLS. Mean effective doses have ranged from 800 mg every night to 1800 mg every day, with one-third of the total dose given at 12 PM and two-thirds given at 8 PM.[41] Another study compared gabapentin (mean of 800 mg QHS) and ropinirole for the treatment of idiopathic RLS.[42] Compared with baseline, both gabapentin and ropinirole groups experienced significant improvements in RLS severity and PLMS index. Patients on gabapentin had a better sleep efficiency than patients on ropinirole.

Pregabalin Pregabalin, like gabapentin, is not hepatically metabolized but rather renally excreted as an unchanged drug. In distinction to gabapentin, it has linear dose pharmacokinetics. Two recent studies have demonstrated the efficacy of pregabalin in primary RLS.[43,44] The former was a flexible-dose crossover study and found efficacy between 300 and 450 mg, whereas the latter used fixed doses and efficacy was established on the IRLS rating scale at or greater than 150 mg. Using polysomnography, multiple measures of sleep, including slow wave sleep, showed improvement after 12 weeks of treatment.

Gabapentin enacarbil Gabapentin enacarbil, a promising investigational drug for RLS, was designed to overcome limitations of gabapentin, including variability in absorption that is related to a saturable transport mechanism.[45] Thus, in distinction to gabapentin, dose of gabapentin enacarbil is directly proportional to gabapentin plasma levels.[46] Several double-blind placebo-controlled trials have demonstrated the efficacy of gabapentin enacarbil in the treatment of RLS at doses of 600 to 1200 mg administered 5 hours before bed. Like gabapentin, the most common side effects of gabapentin enacarbil include dizziness and somnolence.[47,48]

Carbamazepine Carbamazepine is rarely used in the treatment of RLS, and there is considerably less evidence to support its use compared with dopaminergic medications or the alpha 2 delta agents. Randomized, double-blind, placebo-controlled studies that show improvement of RLS symptoms with carbamazepine treatment[49,50] have very high placebo response rates and do not use standard definitions of RLS or its severity.

Carbamazepine is hepatically metabolized and not only interacts with multiple other medications but also induces its own metabolism, thus its half-life decreases with continued use. There is a risk of potentially serious side effects such as Stevens-Johnson syndrome, aplastic anemia or agranulocytosis, and hepatic failure. Patients must be monitored closely.

Opioids Although opioids were used with good effect for the treatment of RLS as early as the 1600s,[8] today they are typically used in clinical practice only when patients have failed alternative therapy. The primary reason for their limited use in RLS is because of their stigma as addictive, associated with tolerance, abuse, and difficulty with discontinuation even after short-term use. In fact, although such concerns have not generally been observed in those using opioids for RLS, they must be carefully assessed in each patient for whom opioids are prescribed. Potential side effects with this class of medication include dizziness, somnolence, nausea, constipation, respiratory suppression, and urinary retention. However, opioids can be a very useful medication in patients with RLS who have failed multiple other medications or developed augmentation with dopaminergic medications.

Oxycodone Oxycodone is extensively metabolized by the liver and it has the potential to interact with other medications. It has a half-life of 3 to 4 hours. Based on one double-blind, placebo-controlled, crossover study oxycodone is likely effective for the treatment of RLS, with an average effective dose of approximately 15 mg.[51]

Methadone Methadone is a potent and long-acting opioid, is hepatically metabolized, and has a half-life of 22 hours. Although methadone has not been examined in a placebo-controlled trial in RLS, positive results were reported in a long-term open-label case series of patients who failed multiple other medications for the treatment of RLS.[52] Average dose of methadone was 15.5 ± 7.7 mg/d, which is a small fraction of that used for treatment of opioid addiction and chronic pain, the 2 conditions for which methadone is most commonly used. As a potent opioid, any provider prescribing methadone must be aware of the risk of respiratory depression. Thus, as with other opioids, use of methadone in the treatment of RLS should be limited to patients for whom previously attempted courses of therapy have been unsuccessful.

Tramadol Tramadol is a centrally acting analgesic that is closely related to codeine and morphine in structure. In addition to being a relatively weak opioid agonist, it inhibits the reuptake of norepinephrine and serotonin. The half-life is 6 hours and it is excreted through the kidneys. The risk of constipation and dependence may be less with tramadol compared with other opioids.[53] Tramadol was efficacious in the treatment of RLS in one open trial.[54] Tramadol may have the potential to induce augmentation.[55]

Benzodiazepines Benzodiazepines, in particular clonazepam, were among the first drugs used for the treatment of RLS, although there is limited evidence to support their specific efficacy for this indication.

Clonazepam Clonazepam is a long-acting benzodiazepine with a half-life of 30 to 40 hours. It is metabolized by the liver and excreted in the urine. Because of its long half-life, clonazepam accumulates with daily dosing and thus daytime drowsiness, cognitive impairment, and impaired coordination may be apparent over time, particularly in the elderly. Two controlled crossover studies found opposing results. One study demonstrated no significant difference in the improvement of RLS symptoms with clonazepam administration when compared with placebo,[56] and the other study showed improvement in RLS symptoms and quality of sleep with clonazepam compared with vibration.[57] Studies on polysomnographic recordings also have conflicting results, with one study showing improvement in the PLMS index[58] and another showing no change in the PLMS index but improved sleep efficiency.[59] Benzodiazepines, like clonazepam, likely have some efficacy in the treatment of RLS, although the evidence to support their use is limited. The logic of using this agent with long half-life for a disorder that is usually only present for less than 8 hours per day is unclear. Thus, if a benzodiazepine is desired for RLS treatment, although less extensively studied in the treatment of RLS, use of an intermediate-acting agent may lead to decreased likelihood of daytime somnolence.

Iron therapy Iron deficiency is a potential cause for secondary RLS and, in fact, may underlie other secondary RLS cases (eg, pregnancy, end-stage renal failure [ESRD]). Even in the absence of serum iron deficiency, brain iron insufficiency has been implicated in the pathophysiology of idiopathic RLS.[60] Both oral and intravenous (IV) iron preparations have been studied as therapeutic interventions for the treatment of both idiopathic and secondary RLS, with mixed results.

Oral iron therapy The efficacy of oral iron therapy is closely tied to a patient's baseline ferritin level. Patients with low-normal ferritin levels seem to derive the most benefit from oral iron therapy, probably because of the greater absorption of the mineral. The most commonly used oral iron formulation for the treatment of RLS is iron sulfate, often with a dosing of 2 to 3 times a day. Potential side effects of iron therapy include constipation, nausea, and abdominal pain.

One placebo-controlled case series found improvement in RLS symptoms with oral iron therapy, with the degree of improvement closely tied to baseline ferritin levels.[61] All the patients with RLS who had baseline ferritin levels less than 100 μg/L were treated with oral iron and showed an increase in ferritin levels, with a median change of 34 μg/L. The largest improvement in RLS symptoms was seen in patients with ferritin levels less than 45 μg/L. A randomized, double-blind, placebo-controlled study found no improvement in RLS symptoms with oral iron supplementation.[62] It is notable that baseline ferritin levels were higher in this study, suggesting that oral iron therapy is not effective in patients with sufficient iron stores. Interestingly, only the patients who reported improvement in RLS symptoms in this study had a statistically significant increase in their iron saturation. A more recent double-blind placebo-controlled study found significant improvement in IRLS rating scale score with oral iron therapy when compared with placebo.[63] Patients in this study again had low-normal iron levels, with mean baseline ferritin levels between 36 and 40 ng/mL. Ferritin levels also increased significantly more in the treatment group compared with the placebo group.

Oral iron supplementation is an effective means of reducing RLS symptoms in patients with low-normal ferritin levels. Thus, ferritin levels should be checked in all patients with RLS, and oral iron supplementation should be considered when appropriate.

IV iron therapy Several studies have used IV iron formulations for the treatment of RLS, particularly iron dextran and iron sucrose. IV iron supplementation has a smaller risk of inducing gastrointestinal side effects that are seen with oral iron formulations. However, the risk of iron overload may be greater. In addition, there is a risk of an anaphylactic reaction, particularly with the use of the iron dextran formulation.

As early as the 1950s and 1960s, open-label studies suggested the therapeutic benefit of iron dextran in the treatment of RLS.[64] A recent open-label study supported the efficacy of a single dose of iron dextran in improving RLS symptom severity and PLMS at 2 weeks postinfusion.[65] After a single dose of iron dextran, 5 patients received one or more supplemental iron gluconate infusions over 6 months to 2 years for symptom recurrence.[66] However, posttreatment ferritin levels declined at a more rapid rate than predicted. The rate of decline of ferritin level seemed to decrease with repeated infusions in this small number of patients, and slower rates of decline of ferritin level seemed to correlate with longer symptom improvements. A follow-up, double-blind, placebo-controlled study by the same group using iron sucrose found no significant benefit compared with placebo.[67] A randomized, double-blind, placebo-controlled study comparing iron sucrose with placebo in patients with RLS with baseline serum ferritin levels of 45 μg/L or less demonstrated benefit of treatment at week 7 but not at weeks 11 or 52 after treatment.[68] Mean ferritin levels increased from 20.1 μg/L (SD 11.9) to 118.4 μg/L (SD 74.5) with treatment, although ferritin levels did not correlate with improvement in RLS. Thus, although a promising therapy, the efficacy of IV iron infusion in the treatment of primary RLS needs to be further examined in controlled studies.

Miscellaneous pharmacologic treatment options Several open-label studies demonstrating the efficacy of additional miscellaneous medications in the treatment of RLS exist. However, given the large placebo response observed with RLS treatment trials, such studies must be interpreted with great caution. Folic acid may be an effective therapeutic option in folate-deficient individuals.[69] Oral magnesium oxide may be beneficial for the treatment of RLS, as suggested by an open-label case series.[70] A small open-label study suggested that the benzodiazepine receptor agonist zolpidem may provide some benefit in the treatment of RLS.[71]

Secondary RLS

Renal failure, pregnancy, iron deficiency (with or without anemia), and certain medications are all associated with increased rates of RLS. Each potential cause of secondary RLS is treated differently, although the evidence guiding treatment in these cases is less abundant than in primary RLS.

Renal failure

Approximately 20% to 40% of patients with ESRD have RLS.[72] Several pharmacologic therapies for RLS have been studied in patients with ESRD who are on dialysis. A randomized, crossover, open-label study found ropinirole to be more effective than levodopa in patients on long-term hemodialysis.[73] Ropinirole at a mean dose of 1.45 mg daily was used during the study. Ropinirole is hepatically metabolized and thus effectively cleared in the setting of renal failure. On the other hand, pramipexole is renally excreted and not well dialyzed, thus it should be used with caution in ESRD.

Gabapentin has also demonstrated efficacy for ESRD-related RLS in a placebo-controlled crossover study.[74] At a dose of 200 to 300 mg after each dialysis session, gabapentin reduced RLS symptoms compared with placebo based on a nonvalidated scale. In another study, gabapentin was superior to levodopa in symptom control and sleep parameters in patients undergoing hemodialysis.[75] Although likely effective in treating RLS, gabapentin is excreted by the kidney as an unchanged drug and can accumulate in patients with renal failure, leading to a higher risk of side effects. It is thus recommended that gabapentin be administered only on the night of dialysis.

IV iron dextran infusion improved RLS symptoms in patients with ESRD in a double-blind placebo-controlled trial.[76] The improvement in symptom severity was only statistically significant at 4 weeks postinfusion, despite adequate serum levels of iron and ferritin, although benefits were clearly evident at subsequent time points. Although IV iron therapy may be effective for RLS in patients with ESRD, the treatment frequency remains to be determined.

Pregnancy

RLS symptoms affect 19% to 26% of pregnant women, most commonly in the third trimester.[77,78] RLS in pregnancy is associated with lower hemoglobin levels and mean corpuscular volume, suggesting that low iron concentration may be related to the development of RLS during pregnancy.[77] Most medications that are used to treat RLS are pregnancy category C (adequate well-controlled human studies are lacking, and animal studies either have shown a risk to the fetus or are lacking) or D (studies in humans have demonstrated fetal risk). As a result, nonpharmacologic approaches should be attempted, whenever possible. Physicians should measure ferritin levels and prescribe adequate iron supplementation when appropriate, before other pharmacologic therapies are considered.[79] If use of other medications becomes necessary, medications with the lowest potential risk to the developing fetus, such as low-potency opioids, should be tried first. Such medications can potentially be delayed until late in the pregnancy when RLS is most prevalent.

Iron deficiency

See section on Iron Therapy in RLS.

Medications

Medications have the potential to induce or aggravate RLS symptoms. The most commonly prescribed medications associated with RLS are antidepressants, particularly selective serotonin reuptake inhibitors (SSRIs), although the incidence and persistence of this effect is unclear.[80–82] Other medications that can potentially result in RLS symptoms include lithium,[83] antihistamines, and dopamine antagonists including antipsychotics and antiemetics.[84,85] In the latter case, RLS symptoms can be difficult to distinguish from akathisia. However, patients with akathisia experience more diffuse inner restlessness, as opposed to leg paresthesias leading to motor restlessness as in RLS.[86] Also, akathisia does not generally have the clear circadian rhythm characteristic of RLS.[86]

There are no clear guidelines for how to treat patients with medication-induced RLS. In cases in which the RLS is bothersome and persistent and the psychiatric disease is not severe or refractory, a change in medication regimen may be made judiciously. For example, a switch from an SSRI to a nonserotonergic antidepressant, such as bupropion or desipramine, may be appropriate. However, in other cases in which medications cannot be changed, RLS can be treated as described earlier for primary RLS. In patients with RLS secondary to dopamine antagonists for psychosis, dopamine agonists should only be used after other approaches have been used, because of the risk of exacerbating the underlying psychiatric illness.

TREATMENT OF PERIODIC LIMB MOVEMENT DISORDER
Introduction

PLMS are a polysomnographic finding of stereotyped repetitive movements of the legs during sleep. They have a prevalence of 7.6% in the general population[87] and greater than 40% in community-dwelling individuals aged 65 years or older.[88] PLMS are present in more than 80% of patients with RLS. However, the clinical relevance of PLMS in the absence of RLS or subjective sleep complaints continues to be debated. The number of periodic limb movements of sleep index (PLMSI) does not generally correlate with polysomnographic sleep quality in healthy middle-aged individuals without sleep complaints, although, in one study, there was a small but significant association with subjective sleep quality in men.[89] A retrospective study found that there was no association between subjective sleep quality and PLMS in insomniac patients.[90] Periodic limb movements associated with arousal are more likely to be clinically significant than total PLMS.[2]

Periodic limb movement disorder (PLMD) is defined as the presence of PLMS in patients with otherwise unexplained hypersomnia or insomnia.[2] The diagnosis of PLMD can only be made after other sleep disorders have been excluded. Because the diagnosis of PLMD and the significance of PLMS remain controversial, few controlled trials on the treatment of PLMD have been undertaken. In addition, the inclusion criteria and end points in studies on PLMD or PLMS are variable, complicating the interpretation and comparison of the results. In practice, many clinicians use medications that have been studied for use in RLS for the treatment of PLMD. Further clinical studies are needed to delineate specific therapies for PLMD.

Pharmacologic Treatment of PLMD

Dopaminergic medications

Based on their benefit for treatment of core symptoms in RLS and for reduction of PLMS in RLS, dopaminergic agents are commonly used for treatment of PLMD. However, few studies have examined their efficacy in this disorder. Levodopa was compared with propoxyphene in a double-blind, placebo-controlled, crossover study in 6 patients with PLMD, although 3 of the 6 patients reported RLS-type symptoms.[91] Levodopa improved the PLMSI and several objective and subjective sleep parameters and had a more robust effect than propoxyphene. Another study found that levodopa and exercise were equally effective at reducing the PLMSI in patients with spinal cord injury.[92] Ropinirole was effective in improving the PLMSI, arousals related to PLMS, and morning cognitive performance in a placebo-controlled study in a group of patients diagnosed with PLMD based on the International Classification of Sleep Disorders.[93]

The efficacy of dopaminergic drugs in PLMD is still uncertain. However, because dopaminergic agents, particularly dopamine agonists, are generally well tolerated, a trial for the treatment of PLMD at doses similar to those used in RLS is a reasonable treatment approach. However, it should be noted that cases of PLMD (in which RLS was initially absent) evolving into RLS have been described with the use of dopaminergic agents, in a process similar to that of augmentation.

Benzodiazepines
Clonazepam at a dose of 1 mg has been shown to improve objective sleep efficiency and subjective sleep quality in PLMD, but the same study did not demonstrate improvement in the PLMSI.[59] Other studies have shown that clonazepam, 0.5 to 2 mg, improved subjective sleep complaints and the number of PLMS.[94,95] In a group of patients with insomnia symptoms and PLMD, clonazepam and cognitive behavioral therapy were equally effective.[96] Clonazepam is likely effective for the treatment of PLMD, although potential side effects as indicated earlier should also be considered.

Miscellaneous
Several other medications have been tried with some efficacy in the treatment of PLMD, generally in open uncontrolled studies. These medications include opioids,[91,97] magnesium,[70] valproic acid,[98] and melatonin.[99] Bupropion sustained release was efficacious in a case series of depressed patients with PLMD.[100] Specific treatment options for PLMD are limited, and more experimental work needs to be completed in treating PLMD.

SUMMARY

Pharmacological treatment of RLS has seen important advances over the past decade, with dopamine agonists being extensively studied in large trials. Investigation of alpha 2 delta calcium

channel ligands, such as gabapentin and pregabalin, has also yielded important results in recent years; and these medications remain viable alternatives to dopamine agonists for treatment of RLS. Although other medications have not been as thoroughly studied in clinical trials, there are several possible alternatives to the above, which may be useful in the setting of side effects to the above medications or co-morbidities. In contrast, pharmacological therapies for PLMD have not been studied in large trials, and further clinical studies are necessary to delineate effective therapies for PLMD.

REFERENCES

1. Allen RP, Picchietti D, Hening WA, et al. Restless legs syndrome: diagnostic criteria, special considerations, and epidemiology. A report from the restless legs syndrome diagnosis and epidemiology workshop at the National Institutes of Health. Sleep Med 2003;4(2):101–19.
2. Hornyak M, Feige B, Riemann D, et al. Periodic leg movements in sleep and periodic limb movement disorder: prevalence, clinical significance and treatment. Sleep Med Rev 2006;10(3):169–77.
3. Hening W, Walters AS, Allen RP, et al. Impact, diagnosis and treatment of restless legs syndrome (RLS) in a primary care population: the REST (RLS epidemiology, symptoms, and treatment) primary care study. Sleep Med 2004;5(3):237–46.
4. Winkelman JW, Finn L, Young T. Prevalence and correlates of restless legs syndrome symptoms in the Wisconsin Sleep Cohort. Sleep Med 2006; 7(7):545–52.
5. Abetz L, Arbuckle R, Allen RP, et al. The reliability, validity and responsiveness of the International Restless Legs Syndrome Study Group rating scale and subscales in a clinical-trial setting. Sleep Med 2006;7(4):340–9.
6. Walters AS, LeBrocq C, Dhar A, et al. Validation of the International Restless Legs Syndrome Study Group rating scale for restless legs syndrome. Sleep Med 2003;4(2):121–32.
7. Earley CJ. Clinical practice. Restless legs syndrome. N Engl J Med 2003;348(21):2103–9.
8. Winkelmann J. Restless legs syndrome. Arch Neurol 1999;56(12):1526–7.
9. Ekbom K, Ulfberg J. Restless legs syndrome. J Intern Med 2009;266(5):419–31.
10. Akpinar S. Treatment of restless legs syndrome with levodopa plus benserazide. Arch Neurol 1982;39(11):739.
11. Chesson AL Jr, Wise M, Davila D, et al. Practice parameters for the treatment of restless legs syndrome and periodic limb movement disorder. An American Academy of Sleep Medicine Report.

Standards of Practice Committee of the American Academy of Sleep Medicine. Sleep 1999;22(7): 961–8.

12. Littner MR, Kushida C, Anderson WM, et al. Practice parameters for the dopaminergic treatment of restless legs syndrome and periodic limb movement disorder. Sleep 2004;27(3):557–9.

13. Brodeur C, Montplaisir J, Godbout R, et al. Treatment of restless legs syndrome and periodic movements during sleep with L-dopa: a double-blind, controlled study. Neurology 1988;38(12): 1845–8.

14. Trenkwalder C, Stiasny K, Pollmacher T, et al. L-dopa therapy of uremic and idiopathic restless legs syndrome: a double-blind, crossover trial. Sleep 1995;18(8):681–8.

15. Benes H, Kurella B, Kummer J, et al. Rapid onset of action of levodopa in restless legs syndrome: a double-blind, randomized, multicenter, crossover trial. Sleep 1999;22(8):1073–81.

16. Vignatelli L, Billiard M, Clarenbach P, et al. EFNS guidelines on management of restless legs syndrome and periodic limb movement disorder in sleep. Eur J Neurol 2006;13(10):1049–65.

17. Trenkwalder C, Garcia-Borreguero D, Montagna P, et al. Ropinirole in the treatment of restless legs syndrome: results from the TREAT RLS 1 study, a 12 week, randomised, placebo controlled study in 10 European countries. J Neurol Neurosurg Psychiatr 2004;75(1):92–7.

18. Walters AS, Ondo WG, Dreykluft T, et al. Ropinirole is effective in the treatment of restless legs syndrome. TREAT RLS 2: a 12-week, double-blind, randomized, parallel-group, placebo-controlled study. Mov Disord 2004;19(12): 1414–23.

19. Bogan RK, Fry JM, Schmidt MH, et al. Ropinirole in the treatment of patients with restless legs syndrome: a US-based randomized, double-blind, placebo-controlled clinical trial. Mayo Clin Proc 2006;81(1):17–27.

20. Adler CH, Hauser RA, Sethi K, et al. Ropinirole for restless legs syndrome: a placebo-controlled crossover trial. Neurology 2004;62(8):1405–7.

21. Allen R, Becker PM, Bogan R, et al. Ropinirole decreases periodic leg movements and improves sleep parameters in patients with restless legs syndrome. Sleep 2004;27(5):907–14.

22. Partinen M, Hirvonen K, Jama L, et al. Efficacy and safety of pramipexole in idiopathic restless legs syndrome: a polysomnographic dose-finding study—the PRELUDE study. Sleep Med 2006;7(5): 407–17.

23. Winkelman JW, Sethi KD, Kushida CA, et al. Efficacy and safety of pramipexole in restless legs syndrome. Neurology 2006;67(6):1034–9.

24. Oertel WH, Stiasny-Kolster K, Bergtholdt B, et al. Efficacy of pramipexole in restless legs syndrome: a six-week, multicenter, randomized, double-blind study (effect-RLS study). Mov Disord 2007;22(2): 213–9.

25. Montplaisir J, Nicolas A, Denesle R, et al. Restless legs syndrome improved by pramipexole: a double-blind randomized trial. Neurology 1999; 52(5):938–43.

26. Jama L, Hirvonen K, Partinen M, et al. A dose-ranging study of pramipexole for the symptomatic treatment of restless legs syndrome: polysomnographic evaluation of periodic leg movements and sleep disturbance. Sleep Med 2009;10(6): 630–6.

27. Baldwin CM, Keating GM. Rotigotine transdermal patch: in restless legs syndrome. CNS Drugs 2008;22(10):797–806.

28. Driver-Dunckley ED, Noble BN, Hentz JG, et al. Gambling and increased sexual desire with dopaminergic medications in restless legs syndrome. Clin Neuropharmacol 2007;30(5):249–55.

29. Abler B, Hahlbrock R, Unrath A, et al. At-risk for pathological gambling: imaging neural reward processing under chronic dopamine agonists. Brain 2009;132(Pt 9):2396–402.

30. Cornelius JR, Tippmann-Peikert M, Slocumb NL, et al. Impulse control disorders with the use of dopaminergic agents in restless legs syndrome: a case-control study. Sleep 2010;33(1):81–7.

31. Zanettini R, Antonini A, Gatto G, et al. Valvular heart disease and the use of dopamine agonists for Parkinson's disease. N Engl J Med 2007; 356(1):39–46.

32. Schade R, Andersohn F, Suissa S, et al. Dopamine agonists and the risk of cardiac-valve regurgitation. N Engl J Med 2007;356(1):29–38.

33. Trenkwalder C, Benes H, Grote L, et al. Cabergoline compared to levodopa in the treatment of patients with severe restless legs syndrome: results from a multi-center, randomized, active controlled trial. Mov Disord 2007;22(5):696–703.

34. Allen RP, Earley CJ. Augmentation of the restless legs syndrome with carbidopa/levodopa. Sleep 1996;19(3):205–13.

35. Silber MH, Girish M, Izurieta R. Pramipexole in the management of restless legs syndrome: an extended study. Sleep 2003;26(7):819–21.

36. Winkelman JW, Johnston L. Augmentation and tolerance with long-term pramipexole treatment of restless legs syndrome (RLS). Sleep Med 2004; 5(1):9–14.

37. Garcia-Borreguero D, Allen RP, Kohnen R, et al. Diagnostic standards for dopaminergic augmentation of restless legs syndrome: report from a world association of sleep medicine-international restless

legs syndrome study group consensus conference at the Max Planck Institute. Sleep Med 2007;8(5): 520–30.

38. Frauscher B, Gschliesser V, Brandauer E, et al. The severity range of restless legs syndrome (RLS) and augmentation in a prospective patient cohort: association with ferritin levels. Sleep Med 2009; 10(6):611–5.

39. Trenkwalder C, Hogl B, Benes H, et al. Augmentation in restless legs syndrome is associated with low ferritin. Sleep Med 2008;9(5):572–4.

40. Garcia-Borreguero D, Allen RP, Benes H, et al. Augmentation as a treatment complication of restless legs syndrome: concept and management. Mov Disord 2007;22(Suppl 18):S476–84.

41. Garcia-Borreguero D, Larrosa O, de la Llave Y, et al. Treatment of restless legs syndrome with gabapentin: a double-blind, cross-over study. Neurology 2002;59(10):1573–9.

42. Happe S, Sauter C, Klosch G, et al. Gabapentin versus ropinirole in the treatment of idiopathic restless legs syndrome. Neuropsychobiology 2003; 48(2):82–6.

43. Garcia-Borreguero D, Larrosa O, Williams AM, et al. Treatment of restless legs syndrome with pregabalin: a double-blind, placebo-controlled study. Neurology 2010;74(23):1897–904.

44. Allen R, Chen C, Soaita A, et al. A randomized, double-blind, 6-week, dose-ranging study of pregabalin in patients with restless legs syndrome. Sleep Med 2010;11(6):512–9.

45. Stewart BH, Kugler AR, Thompson PR, et al. A saturable transport mechanism in the intestinal absorption of gabapentin is the underlying cause of the lack of proportionality between increasing dose and drug levels in plasma. Pharm Res 1993;10(2):276–81.

46. Lal R, Sukbuntherng J, Luo W, et al. Pharmacokinetics and tolerability of single escalating doses of gabapentin enacarbil: a randomized-sequence, double-blind, placebo-controlled crossover study in healthy volunteers. Clin Ther 2009;31(8): 1776–86.

47. Kushida CA, Becker PM, Ellenbogen AL, et al. Randomized, double-blind, placebo-controlled study of XP13512/GSK1838262 in patients with RLS. Neurology 2009;72(5):439–46.

48. Kushida CA, Walters AS, Becker P, et al. A randomized, double-blind, placebo-controlled, crossover study of XP13512/GSK1838262 in the treatment of patients with primary restless legs syndrome. Sleep 2009;32(2):159–68.

49. Telstad W, Sorensen O, Larsen S, et al. Treatment of the restless legs syndrome with carbamazepine: a double blind study. Br Med J (Clin Res Ed) 1984; 288(6415):444–6.

50. Lundvall O, Abom PE, Holm R. Carbamazepine in restless legs. A controlled pilot study. Eur J Clin Pharmacol 1983;25(3):323–4.

51. Walters AS, Wagner ML, Hening WA, et al. Successful treatment of the idiopathic restless legs syndrome in a randomized double-blind trial of oxycodone versus placebo. Sleep 1993;16(4):327–32.

52. Ondo WG. Methadone for refractory restless legs syndrome. Mov Disord 2005;20(3):345–8.

53. Grond S, Sablotzki A. Clinical pharmacology of tramadol. Clin Pharmacokinet 2004;43(13):879–923.

54. Lauerma H, Markkula J. Treatment of restless legs syndrome with tramadol: an open study. J Clin Psychiatry 1999;60(4):241–4.

55. Earley CJ, Allen RP. Restless legs syndrome augmentation associated with tramadol. Sleep Med 2006;7(7):592–3.

56. Boghen D, Lamothe L, Elie R, et al. The treatment of the restless legs syndrome with clonazepam: a prospective controlled study. Can J Neurol Sci 1986;13(3):245–7.

57. Montagna P, Sassoli de Bianchi L, Zucconi M, et al. Clonazepam and vibration in restless legs syndrome. Acta Neurol Scand 1984;69(6):428–30.

58. Horiguchi J, Inami Y, Sasaki A, et al. Periodic leg movements in sleep with restless legs syndrome: effect of clonazepam treatment. Jpn J Psychiatry Neurol 1992;46(3):727–32.

59. Saletu M, Anderer P, Saletu-Zyhlarz G, et al. Restless legs syndrome (RLS) and periodic limb movement disorder (PLMD): acute placebo-controlled sleep laboratory studies with clonazepam. Eur Neuropsychopharmacol 2001;11(2):153–61.

60. Allen RP, Barker PB, Wehrl F, et al. MRI measurement of brain iron in patients with restless legs syndrome. Neurology 2001;56(2):263–5.

61. O'Keeffe ST, Gavin K, Lavan JN. Iron status and restless legs syndrome in the elderly. Age Ageing 1994;23(3):200–3.

62. Davis BJ, Rajput A, Rajput ML, et al. A randomized, double-blind placebo-controlled trial of iron in restless legs syndrome. Eur Neurol 2000;43(2):70–5.

63. Wang J, O'Reilly B, Venkataraman R, et al. Efficacy of oral iron in patients with restless legs syndrome and a low-normal ferritin: a randomized, double-blind, placebo-controlled study. Sleep Med 2009;10(9): 973–5.

64. Parrow A, Werner I. The treatment of restless legs. Acta Med Scand 1966;180(4):401–6.

65. Earley CJ, Heckler D, Allen RP. The treatment of restless legs syndrome with intravenous iron dextran. Sleep Med 2004;5(3):231–5.

66. Earley CJ, Heckler D, Allen RP. Repeated IV doses of iron provides effective supplemental treatment of restless legs syndrome. Sleep Med 2005;6(4): 301–5.

67. Earley CJ, Horska A, Mohamed MA, et al. A randomized, double-blind, placebo-controlled trial of intravenous iron sucrose in restless legs syndrome. Sleep Med 2009;10(2):206–11.
68. Grote L, Leissner L, Hedner J, et al. A randomized, double-blind, placebo controlled, multi-center study of intravenous iron sucrose and placebo in the treatment of restless legs syndrome. Mov Disord 2009;24(10):1445–52.
69. Botez MI, Fontaine F, Botez T, et al. Folate-responsive neurological and mental disorders: report of 16 cases. Neuropsychological correlates of computerized transaxial tomography and radionuclide cisternography in folic acid deficiencies. Eur Neurol 1977;16(1–6):230–46.
70. Hornyak M, Voderholzer U, Hohagen F, et al. Magnesium therapy for periodic leg movements-related insomnia and restless legs syndrome: an open pilot study. Sleep 1998;21(5):501–5.
71. Bezerra ML, Martinez JV. Zolpidem in restless legs syndrome. Eur Neurol 2002;48(3):180–1.
72. Winkelman JW, Chertow GM, Lazarus JM. Restless legs syndrome in end-stage renal disease. Am J Kidney Dis 1996;28(3):372–8.
73. Pellecchia MT, Vitale C, Sabatini M, et al. Ropinirole as a treatment of restless legs syndrome in patients on chronic hemodialysis: an open randomized crossover trial versus levodopa sustained release. Clin Neuropharmacol 2004;27(4):178–81.
74. Thorp ML, Morris CD, Bagby SP. A crossover study of gabapentin in treatment of restless legs syndrome among hemodialysis patients. Am J Kidney Dis 2001;38(1):104–8.
75. Micozkadioglu H, Ozdemir FN, Kut A, et al. Gabapentin versus levodopa for the treatment of restless legs syndrome in hemodialysis patients: an open-label study. Ren Fail 2004;26(4):393–7.
76. Sloand JA, Shelly MA, Feigin A, et al. A double-blind, placebo-controlled trial of intravenous iron dextran therapy in patients with ESRD and restless legs syndrome. Am J Kidney Dis 2004;43(4):663–70.
77. Manconi M, Govoni V, De Vito A, et al. Restless legs syndrome and pregnancy. Neurology 2004;63(6):1065–9.
78. Suzuki K, Ohida T, Sone T, et al. The prevalence of restless legs syndrome among pregnant women in Japan and the relationship between restless legs syndrome and sleep problems. Sleep 2003;26(6):673–7.
79. Djokanovic N, Garcia-Bournissen F, Koren G. Medications for restless legs syndrome in pregnancy. J Obstet Gynaecol Can 2008;30(6):505–7.
80. Baughman KR, Bourguet CC, Ober SK. Gender differences in the association between antidepressant use and restless legs syndrome. Mov Disord 2009;24(7):1054–9.
81. Rottach KG, Schaner BM, Kirch MH, et al. Restless legs syndrome as side effect of second generation antidepressants. J Psychiatr Res 2008;43(1):70–5.
82. Page RL 2nd, Ruscin JM, Bainbridge JL, et al. Restless legs syndrome induced by escitalopram: case report and review of the literature. Pharmacotherapy 2008;28(2):271–80.
83. Terao T, Terao M, Yoshimura R, et al. Restless legs syndrome induced by lithium. Biol Psychiatry 1991;30(11):1167–70.
84. Kang SG, Lee HJ, Kim L. Restless legs syndrome and periodic limb movements during sleep probably associated with olanzapine. J Psychopharmacol 2009;23(5):597–601.
85. Khalid I, Rana L, Khalid TJ, et al. Refractory restless legs syndrome likely caused by olanzapine. J Clin Sleep Med 2009;5(1):68–9.
86. Walters AS, Hening W, Rubinstein M, et al. A clinical and polysomnographic comparison of neuroleptic-induced akathisia and the idiopathic restless legs syndrome. Sleep 1991;14(4):339–45.
87. Scofield H, Roth T, Drake C. Periodic limb movements during sleep: population prevalence, clinical correlates, and racial differences. Sleep 2008;31(9):1221–7.
88. Ancoli-Israel S, Kripke DF, Klauber MR, et al. Periodic limb movements in sleep in community-dwelling elderly. Sleep 1991;14(6):496–500.
89. Carrier J, Frenette S, Montplaisir J, et al. Effects of periodic leg movements during sleep in middle-aged subjects without sleep complaints. Mov Disord 2005;20(9):1127–32.
90. Hornyak M, Riemann D, Voderholzer U. Do periodic leg movements influence patients' perception of sleep quality? Sleep Med 2004;5(6):597–600.
91. Kaplan PW, Allen RP, Buchholz DW, et al. A double-blind, placebo-controlled study of the treatment of periodic limb movements in sleep using carbidopa/levodopa and propoxyphene. Sleep 1993;16(8):717–23.
92. de Mello MT, Poyares DL, Tufik S. Treatment of periodic leg movements with a dopaminergic agonist in subjects with total spinal cord lesions. Spinal Cord 1999;37(9):634–7.
93. Saletu M, Anderer P, Saletu B, et al. Sleep laboratory studies in periodic limb movement disorder (PLMD) patients as compared with normals and acute effects of ropinirole. Hum Psychopharmacol 2001;16(2):177–87.
94. Ohanna N, Peled R, Rubin AH, et al. Periodic leg movements in sleep: effect of clonazepam treatment. Neurology 1985;35(3):408–11.
95. Peled R, Lavie P. Double-blind evaluation of clonazepam on periodic leg movements in sleep. J Neurol Neurosurg Psychiatr 1987;50(12):1679–81.

96. Edinger JD, Fins AI, Sullivan RJ, et al. Comparison of cognitive-behavioral therapy and clonazepam for treating periodic limb movement disorder. Sleep 1996;19(5):442–4.

97. Kavey N, Walters AS, Hening W, et al. Opioid treatment of periodic movements in sleep in patients without restless legs. Neuropeptides 1988;11(4): 181–4.

98. Ehrenberg BL, Eisensehr I, Corbett KE, et al. Valproate for sleep consolidation in periodic limb movement disorder. J Clin Psychopharmacol 2000;20(5):574–8.

99. Kunz D, Bes F. Exogenous melatonin in periodic limb movement disorder: an open clinical trial and a hypothesis. Sleep 2001;24(2):183–7.

100. Nofzinger EA, Fasiczka A, Berman S, et al. Bupropion SR reduces periodic limb movements associated with arousals from sleep in depressed patients with periodic limb movement disorder. J Clin Psychiatry 2000;61(11):858–62.

Therapeutics for Parasomnias in Adults

Carlos H. Schenck, MD[a,b,*], Mark W. Mahowald, MD[b,c]

KEYWORDS

• Parasomnias • Therapeutics • Adults

Parasomnias encompass the undesirable physical events or experiences that occur during entry into sleep, within sleep, or during arousals from sleep.[1] Parasomnias are manifestations of central nervous system activation with outflows through skeletal muscle, autonomic nervous system, and emotional-experiential channels. Basic drive states emerge pathologically with the parasomnias, as seen with sleep-related aggression and locomotion, sleep-related eating disorder (SRED), and sleep-related abnormal sexual behaviors (sexsomnia). The last 2 states reflect intense (driven), recurrent, appetitive behaviors, with sleep itself considered to be an appetitive behavior. Complications from parasomnias include injuries, sleep disruption, adverse health effects, and adverse psychosocial effects. These complications can affect the patient, the bed partner (or both of them), roommates, and other members of a household or dormitory.

Parasomnias often involve complex, seemingly purposeful, and goal-directed behaviors, which presumably are performed with some personal meaning to the individual at the time, despite the illogical and risky nature of the behaviors that are enacted outside the realm of conscious experience. This feature highlights the core problem with parasomnias: dissociated states of experience and behavioral expression[2]; our bodies are moving and doing things while our brains remain largely asleep. To become activated and interact with the external world without concomitant wakeful awareness and sound judgment is a highly dangerous state of existence. This article describes the therapeutics for the parasomnias that carry the greatest health risks in adults: rapid-eye movement (REM) sleep behavior disorder (RBD), disorders of arousal from non-REM (NREM) sleep (confusional arousals, sleepwalking, sleep terrors), sexsomnia, and SRED.

RBD

RBD is a behavioral and dream disorder of REM sleep.[1,3,4] It is also a treatable disorder that predominantly affects pleasant, middle-aged and older men who usually enact distinctly altered dreams that feature confrontation, aggression, and violence.[1] These altered dreams are also commonly reported to be vivid and action packed. Recently there has been increased recognition of RBD in women, who may present with milder symptoms.[5] The vigorous and violent behaviors of RBD (enacted with the eyes closed and without awareness of the bedside environment) commonly result in injury, which at times can be severe and even life threatening.[6,7] There is often a compelling need to promptly and effectively control RBD. The potential for injury to oneself or the bed partner raises difficult forensic medicine questions.[8] There is an experimental animal model of RBD produced by brainstem lesions in cats (and more recently in rats), and the categories of RBD behaviors

[a] Department of Psychiatry, Minnesota Regional Sleep Disorders Center, Hennepin County Medical Center, 701 Park Avenue South, Minneapolis, MN 55415, USA
[b] University of Minnesota Medical School, Department of Psychiatry (CHS) and Neurology (MWM), Minneapolis, MN, USA
[c] Department of Neurology, Minnesota Regional Sleep Disorders Center, Hennepin County Medical Center, 701 Park Avenue South, Minneapolis, MN 55415, USA
* Corresponding author. Department of Psychiatry (CHS), Minnesota Regional Sleep Disorders Center, Hennepin County Medical Center, 701 Park Avenue South, Minneapolis, MN 55415.
E-mail address: schen010@umn.edu

Sleep Med Clin 5 (2010) 689–700
doi:10.1016/j.jsmc.2010.08.005
1556-407X/10/$ — see front matter © 2010 Published by Elsevier Inc.

found in the lesioned animals closely match the categories of clinical RBD behaviors in humans.[3]

RBD is the only parasomnia in the *International Classification of Sleep Disorders, 2nd Edition* (ICSD-2) that requires polysomnographic (PSG) confirmation.[1] There are 3 reasons for this requirement: first, the core electromyographic (EMG) abnormalities of RBD are present every night (given a sufficient amount of REM sleep, ie, >10% of total sleep time); second, RBD is not the only dream-enacting disorder in adults, and so objective confirmation is highly desirable; third, given the strong probability of future parkinsonism in men 50 years of age and older initially diagnosed with idiopathic RBD,[9] it is imperative to objectively diagnose RBD so that affected men (and their families) can be properly informed and be encouraged to plan for the future accordingly. The core EMG abnormalities of RBD are listed with the diagnostic criteria in **Box 1**. A point to emphasize is that dream-enacting behaviors are not required for diagnosing RBD, because some patients with RBD do not recall any dreams. Periodic limb movements and nonperiodic twitching during NREM sleep are common (often without arousals), indicating generalized REM/NREM sleep motor dyscontrol in RBD.[3]

RBD is most often a chronic condition that may be preceded by a lengthy prodrome consisting of new-onset (or intensified) sleeptalking, and prominent limb and body movements in sleep.[3] Although irregular jerking of the limbs may occur nightly (comprising the minimal RBD syndrome),

the major behavioral episodes appear intermittently with a frequency minimum of usually once in 2 weeks up to multiple times nightly for many consecutive nights. Sleeptalking runs the spectrum from short and garbled to long-winded and clearly articulated speech. Angry speech with shouting and profanity, and also humorous speech with laughter, can emerge. Aggressive and violent behavior manifests with punching and kicking. Nonviolent activity involves sitting up, looking around, searching for objects, laughing, singing, whistling, dancing, clapping, and so forth.[10] Prevalence of RBD is not yet reliably known (at least 0.4%),[1] but it is probably more common in middle-aged and elderly people than is currently appreciated. **Box 2** lists the causes associated with chronic RBD.

For patients with RBD, arousal from a dream-enacting episode typically results in rapid alertness, orientation, and detailed dream recall, which is typical of most awakenings from REM sleep, including those associated with nightmares.[1] This situation is different from the confusional arousals from slow-wave sleep found with sleepwalking and sleep terrors.

Any patient suspected of having RBD should undergo a systematic evaluation consisting of:

1. Review of sleep/wake complaints (from patient and/or bed partner)
2. Neurologic and psychiatric examinations
3. Sleep laboratory study that includes continuous videotaping of behavior during standard polysomnogram (PSG) monitoring of the electro-oculogram, electroencephalogram, electromyogram (submental, lower/upper extremity muscles), electrocardiogram, oral-nasal air flow, respiratory effort. A certified technician makes written notations of observed behaviors. Because of the association between RBD and

---

Box 1
Diagnostic criteria for RBD[1]

Presence of REM sleep without atonia: the EMG finding of excessive amounts of sustained or intermittent elevation of submental EMG tone and/or excessive phasic submental or (upper or lower) limb EMG twitching

At least one of the following is present:

Sleep-related injurious, potentially injurious, or disruptive behaviors by history

Abnormal REM sleep behaviors documented during PSG monitoring

Absence of electroencephalography (EEG) epileptiform activity during REM sleep unless RBD can be clearly distinguished from any concurrent REM sleep-related seizure disorder

The sleep disturbance is not better explained by another sleep disorder, medical or neurologic disorder, mental disorder, medication use, or substance use disorder

---

Box 2
Causes associated with chronic RBD

1. Idiopathic (cryptogenic?)
2. Neurologic disorders
3. Medication-induced:

    Selective serotonin reuptake inhibitors (SSRIs), venlafaxine, mirtazapine, tricyclic antidepressants (TCAs), monoamine oxidase inhibitors (MAOIs) (but not bupropion)

    β-Blockers (bisoprolol, atenolol)

    Anticholinesterase inhibitors

    Selegiline

4. Caffeine, chocolate: excessive consumption

narcolepsy, serious consideration should be given to administering a multiple sleep latency test the day after the overnight PSG study to document the presence or absence of objective hypersomnia and sleep-onset REM episodes.

More extensive neurologic testing, including magnetic resonance brain imaging and comprehensive neuropsychological testing, should also be considered. **Box 3** lists the neurologic disorders most commonly linked with chronic RBD.

RBD and Parkinsonism

As more patients with idiopathic RBD are carefully followed over time, it is becoming clear that most eventually develop neurodegenerative disorders, most notably the synucleinopathies (Parkinson disease, multiple system atrophy, dementia with Lewy bodies).[9,11] RBD may be the first manifestation of these conditions, and may precede any other manifestation of the underlying neurodegenerative process by more than 10 years, and for even as long as 50 years.[12-15]

Combined animal and human studies have identified physiologic and anatomic links between RBD and neurodegenerative disorders, leading to the proposal that neurodegeneration can begin in either the rostroventral midbrain or the ventral mesopontine junction and progressively extend to the rostral or caudal part of the brainstem. When the lesion starts in the ventral mesopontine region, RBD develops first, but when the lesion initially involves the rostroventral midbrain, Parkinson disease is the initial manifestation.[16]

RBD and Narcolepsy

RBD is present in more than half of patients with narcolepsy, and may be a presenting symptom in narcolepsy, including childhood narcolepsy.[17] Furthermore, TCAs, SSRIs and venlafaxine, prescribed to treat cataplexy, can trigger or

---

> **Box 3**
> **Neurologic disorders most commonly linked with chronic RBD**
>
> 1. Neurodegenerative disorders (especially parkinsonian disorders)
> 2. Narcolepsy-cataplexy
> 3. Cerebrovascular disorders
> 4. (NB Virtually all categories of neurologic disorders can trigger RBD: toxic-metabolic, vascular, neoplastic, infectious, postinfectious, autoimmune, degenerative, developmental, congenital, familial)

---

exacerbate RBD in narcoleptics.[17] The demographics (age and sex) of RBD in narcolepsy conform to those of narcolepsy (ie, younger adults, and nonmale predominant), indicating that RBD in these patients is yet another manifestation of state boundary dyscontrol (primarily REM sleep-wakefulness boundaries) seen in narcolepsy.

Pathophysiology

The generalized atonia of REM sleep results from active inhibition of motor activity by pontine centers of the perilocus coeruleus region that exert an excitatory influence on the reticularis magnocellularis nucleus of the medulla via the lateral tegmentoreticular tract. The reticularis magnocellularis nucleus, in turn, hyperpolarizes spinal motoneuron postsynaptic membranes via the ventrolateral reticulospinal tract.[3,11] Loss of muscle tone during REM sleep is complex, and has been shown to be caused by a combination of activation of brainstem motor inhibitory systems and deactivation of brainstem motor facilitatory systems.

The overwhelming male predominance in RBD begs the question of hormonal influences, as suggested in male-aggression studies in both animals and humans. However, serum sex hormone levels are normal in idiopathic RBD or in RBD associated with Parkinson disease, as reviewed.[17] Another possible explanation for the male predominance is sex differences in brain development and aging.

Treatment of RBD

The safety of the sleeping environment should always be maximized. Sharp objects should be removed from the bedside area, and the bed should not be placed near a window. Clonazepam is the cornerstone for the pharmacotherapy for RBD in most cases, with the usual dose range being 0.25 mg to 2.0 mg at bedtime, extending up to 4 mg. Several large case series in the world literature, totaling more than 250 patients with RBD, have reported a response rate to clonazepam therapy for 87% to 90%.[3] Clonazepam is not usually associated with dosage tolerance (habituation effect), despite years of nightly therapy.[18] The mechanism of action seems to be suppression of the excessive phasic motor-behavioral activity rather than restoration of REM atonia. Nevertheless, the literature is devoid of any double-blind, controlled, randomized trials of clonazepam (or other) therapy for RBD.[19,20] However, given the recurrent injuries usually associated with RBD (with major morbidity and potential lethality), it is doubtful that an ethical treatment trial can be devised with the approval of an Institutional Review Board.

Clonazepam side effects at times can occur with RBD, and include morning sedation, memory dysfunction, depression and personality changes (emerging at the outset of therapy), erectile dysfunction, hair loss, gastroesophageal reflux, and aggravation of obstructive sleep apnea. Underlying obstructive sleep apnea should be ruled out before prescribing clonazepam.[21]

A recognized second-line (or co-first-line) therapy for RBD is bedtime melatonin at robust pharmacologic doses ranging from 3 to 15 mg (or higher). The mechanism of action seems to be partial restoration (about 50%) of REM atonia. Therefore, combined melatonin-clonazepam therapy holds the appeal of using complementary mechanisms of action on the tonic and phasic motor systems disturbed during REM sleep in RBD. Melatonin efficacy has been reported in 3 case series of idiopathic and symptomatic RBD totaling 35 patients.[22–24] Side effects can include morning sedation and headaches.

Pramipexole, a dopamine receptor agonist, in 2 case series has been shown to be effective in 63% to 89% of patients with idiopathic RBD or RBD associated with mild cognitive impairment or mild Parkinson disease.[25,26] On the other hand, a prospective study of patients with combined RBD-Parkinson disease found no benefit when pramipexole was added to a stable levodopa regimen.[27] When used to treat RBD, the starting dose of pramipexole should be 0.125 mg at bedtime, with gradual increments by 0.125 mg up to a maximum of 2 to 4 mg at bedtime. Levodopa therapy for RBD has also been reported but also with mixed results in patients with Parkinson disease or dementia with Lewy bodies.

Acetylcholinesterase inhibitors, which can also trigger RBD,[17] have been reported in small numbers of patients to be effective as therapy for idiopathic RBD, including donepezil in the 10- to 20-mg dose range,[28,29] and rivastigmine in doses up to 6 mg at bedtime. As reviewed, other therapies of RBD reported to be beneficial in case reports and small case series include clonidine (a potent suppressor of REM sleep), desipramine/imipramine (TCAs that can also trigger or aggravate RBD), paroxetine (in Japanese patients), MAOIs, carbamazepine, gabapentin, zopiclone, temazepam, and sodium oxybate (which is an effective anticataplectic agent).[30] Immunosuppressive therapy (cycles of intravenous immunoglobulin and corticosteroids for >1 year) induced complete resolution of RBD in tandem with remission of autoimmune limbic encephalitis in 3 patients with potassium channel

antibody-associated limbic encephalitis.[31] In contrast, RBD persisted in 2 patients with partial resolution of the limbic syndrome. Pallidotomy has been effective in one case of RBD associated with Parkinson disease.[32]

Successful control of RBD with appropriate pharmacotherapy, or other somatic therapy, usually then also controls the environmental sleep disorder,[1] involving chronic, recurrent sleep disruption, in the spouse (typically the wife).

DISORDERS OF AROUSAL FROM NREM SLEEP (CONFUSIONAL AROUSALS, SLEEPWALKING, SLEEP TERRORS)

The hallmark of these 3 conditions is that they typically arise during abrupt, partial arousals from deep NREM sleep (ie, slow-wave sleep), and presumably they share a common pathophysiology.[1] This situation is also reflected in their comparable response to the same pharmacotherapies. They all share a strong familial-genetic predisposition. Although NREM parasomnias peak in childhood, they are nevertheless not uncommon in adults, with a prevalence range between 1% and 4%.[1,33,34] Most adult sleepwalkers claimed that they also sleepwalked as a child.[33]

Confusional Arousals

Confusional arousals are characterized by disoriented behavior and inappropriate vocalizations, which at times can lead to aggressive, violent, or sexual manifestations, during an arousal from slow-wave sleep. The episodes are usually not recalled the following day. Although typically lasting less than 5 minutes (including less than a minute), episodes can occasionally be prolonged. Precipitating factors include sedative-hypnotic medications, recovery from sleep deprivation, forced awakenings, periodic leg movements, and untreated sleep disorders such as sleep-disordered breathing.[1]

Sleepwalking

Sleepwalking is the combination of ambulation with the persistence of impaired consciousness following an abrupt arousal from slow-wave sleep. Amnesia for the sleepwalking is typical and the behaviors are frequently described as routine but inappropriate, such as placing a head of lettuce in a bathroom sink, or rearranging furniture in peculiar ways. Attempting to arouse the patient is often difficult and may worsen confusion, disorientation, and aggressiveness. Precipitating factors for sleepwalking include those noted earlier for confusional arousals, particularly sleep deprivation, untreated comorbid sleep disorders, and psychotropic medications.[1]

Sleep Terrors

Sleep terrors are episodes of intense fear initiated by a sudden cry or loud scream accompanied by increased autonomic nervous system activity. In adults, sleep terrors can involve impulsively bolting out of bed, without proper judgment, in response to an imminent threatening image or dream fragment. Severe injury or death may result from running into furniture or walls, falling down stairs, or jumping through a window. Complete amnesia for the events is typical, albeit with notable exceptions in some adults. Sleep terrors can last for many minutes and attempts to abort an episode commonly provoke greater agitation.

Treatment of NREM Parasomnias

The first steps in the therapeutic process include an assessment of the level of severity; a consideration of eliminating any presumed inducing medication; identification and treatment of any comorbid sleep disorder(s); and attention to maximizing environmental safety. This process also includes removal of firearms, knives, and other weapons from the bedroom. Use of a bedroom door alarm is a helpful and cheap way to fully awaken a sleepwalker and/or to signal to others that the sleepwalker is about to wander.

Most patients may be given reassurance and advised to avoid an irregular sleep schedule and sleep deprivation, and to learn how to properly manage stress. Situations that deserve consideration of pharmacotherapy include violent/potentially injurious behavior, or nonviolent dangerous behavior (eg, leaving the house during the winter, walking into a lake during the summer, opening an upper floor window).

Many violent parasomnia cases are related to physical proximity of the sleeping person, and could potentially be avoided. One report reviewed the nature of 32 medical and legal cases involving violent, sleep-related behavior. In most of the examples, the victim either was in passive close proximity to, or provoked, the parasomniac (100% of confusional arousal cases, 81% of sleep terror cases, 40%–90% of sleepwalking cases). The provocation was typically mild compared with the violent response, and the victims were not sought out by the sleepwalker.[35] These results strongly suggest that patients with a history of violent nocturnal behaviors should not sleep with a bed partner (at least until successful therapy

has been achieved) and contact should be avoided during episodes.

The primary pharmacologic intervention involves use of benzodiazepines (BZDs) at bedtime. However, the evidence for all therapies, pharmacologic and nonpharmacologic, is currently based on methodologically weak studies, typically case reports and case series.[36] Only rarely have there been more rigorous clinical investigations, but sample size in these controlled studies was typically small. The mechanism by which BZDs suppress NREM parasomnias is apparently through the suppression of cortical arousals.

Clonazepam,[6,18,37] at a dose of 0.5 to 1.0 mg at bedtime is usually effective; also, alprazolam,[18] 0.25 to 1.0 mg at bedtime; flurazepam,[37] 15 to 45 mg at bedtime; diazepam, 2 to 10 mg at bedtime; or triazolam, 0.125 to 0.5 mg at bedtime (triazolam has the advantage of a short half-life with minimal risk of carryover morning sedation). Patients should be instructed to take a BZD 30 to 60 minutes before anticipated sleep onset to ensure that the medication has sufficient time to be absorbed and distributed to key brain sites, because an NREM parasomnia episode can emerge as soon as 15 minutes after falling asleep.

Antidepressant medications with serotonergic activity (eg, the commonly prescribed SSRI antidepressants along with some TCAs) may also be effective in the treatment of NREM parasomnias. These medications include imipramine [38] and paroxetine,[39,40] with the latter agent (and SSRIs in general) being suggested to be uniquely effective for sleep terrors through serotonin effects on terror centers in the brainstem.[40] In particular, the periaquaductal gray matter in the midbrain has been implicated. More research, in particular a randomized controlled trial, is needed.[36] Hypnotherapy may be beneficial as primary or adjunctive therapy for NREM parasomnias,[41] although there are conflicting reports of efficacy.[42]

SEXSOMNIA

The first classification of sleep-related disorders associated with abnormal sexual behaviors and experiences has recently been published.[43] Several factors prompted the development of this classification. There has been growing awareness that abnormal sexual behaviors can emerge during sleep, described as "sleepsex," "atypical sexual behavior during sleep," and "sexsomnia."[44–46] The ICSD-2 formally recognized this phenomenon by classifying it as a parasomnia, that is, a variant of confusional arousals (and sleepwalking).[1] The cause of sleepsex can often be identified after clinical and PSG evaluations, and then effectively treated. Furthermore, there is an expanding set of sleep disorders and other nocturnal disorders known to be associated with abnormal sexual behaviors, or the misperception of sexual behaviors. The forensic aspects of abnormal sleep-related sexual behavior have commanded increasing attention, and so a formal classification of the clinical features was desirable from this perspective. This article focuses on the clinical and therapeutic aspects of parasomnias with abnormal sleep-related sexual behaviors (sexsomnia), and of sleep-related sexual seizures (epileptic sexsomnia).

Table 1 contains data on 31 published cases of parasomnias and 7 published cases of epilepsy with abnormal sleep-related sexual behaviors and experiences that were reported in the review mentioned earlier.[43] The parasomnia group is strongly male predominant. Age of onset of sleepsex in both groups is during early adulthood. Sleepsex was a long-standing problem in 8 patients with parasomnia and in 4 patients with epilepsy before clinical intervention.

Four categories of sleepsex behaviors were found in the parasomnia group, and 5 categories of sleepsex behaviors and/or experiences were found in the sleep epilepsy group. In the parasomnia group, women almost exclusively engaged in masturbation and sexual vocalizations, whereas men commonly engaged in sexual fondling and sexual intercourse with women. All 31 patients with parasomnia had full amnesia for their sleepsex episodes, whereas there was recall of sleepsex episodes in 5 of 7 patients with sleep-related seizures. Aggressive and assaultive sleepsex behaviors, sleepsex with minors, and legal consequences affected a substantial number of patients with parasomnia. Sleepsex was more frequently injurious to the bed partner than to the affected sexsomniac. Adverse psychosocial consequences were common in both the patients and their bed partners. Pleasurable experiences from the sleepsex were reported by 3 patients with sleep-related seizures, by the bed partners of 4 patients with parasomnia, and by one patient with sleep-related seizure.

In the parasomnia group, histories of multiple NREM sleep parasomnias were common, with confusional arousals being predominant. Sleepsex was rarely the only parasomnia behavior in the longitudinal histories of these patients. Two cases also involved sleepwalking with sleep driving and one case also involved SRED. Besides a clinical evaluation, PSG monitoring (without penile tumescence monitoring) took place in the preponderance of cases. Obstructive sleep apnea (OSA)

comorbidity that promoted sleepsex was present in 3 cases, with snoring during sleepsex being a prominent feature. Although 26 patients with parasomnia with sexsomnia had PSG studies, sometimes on multiple nights, sexual behaviors during sleep rarely occurred, and usually it was sexual moaning arising from slow-wave sleep. A total of 8 patients had identified psychiatric disorders, but without any presumed link with the sexsomnia.

Parasomnias, OSA, and seizure-induced sleepsex appeared readily amenable to therapy. The BZD clonazepam was effective in almost all treated parasomnia patients, continuous positive airway pressure (CPAP) was effective in all 3 treated OSA patients, and anticonvulsant medication was effective in all 5 treated seizure patients.

Adverse physical and psychosocial consequences were common with sexsomnia. In the parasomnia group, the bed partners often experienced physical injuries (ecchymoses, lacerations) from the sexual assaults, and to a lesser extent the patients were also physically injured (bruised penis; fractured digits). Moreover, both the patients and bed partners often experienced an array of adverse psychosocial consequences involving bewilderment, embarrassment, shame, guilt, despair, shock, alarm, anger, worry, annoyance, denial, feelings of inadequacy/low self-esteem, and reactive emotional distancing that led to some marital estrangement, with marriage counseling sometimes being sought. On the other hand, in 4 parasomnia cases, pleasurable aspects of the sleepsex were reported by the bed partners. Likewise, in 4 epilepsy cases, pleasurable aspects of sleep-related sexual seizures were reported by 3 patients and a bed partner.

In the parasomnia and epilepsy cases just described, psychopathology was uncommonly present and was not identified as a contributing factor to the abnormal, sleep-related sexual behaviors. Also, neither sexual deprivation or frustration, nor a prior history of paraphilia or criminal sexual misconduct was reported.

Since the original sleep and sex review article was published in 2007,[43] additional cases of sexsomnia have been reported that have expanded awareness and raised intriguing questions concerning contributing factors, comorbidities, and therapeutic responsivities related to sexsomnia. One report from Italy described 3 men (32–46 years old) who had unremarkable medical, neurologic, and psychiatric histories.[47] They each underwent PSG evaluation. A 42-year-old man had OSA (apnea/hypopnea index 38.5/h), without any sexual or other parasomnia behavior during the PSG study. CPAP therapy controlled the OSA and also induced a marked reduction of sexsomnia activity at home. A 32-year-old man had a prior sleepwalking (NREM parasomnia) history. During his PSG evaluation, he had 3 minor (nonsexual) motor events from slow-wave sleep. He was diagnosed to have an NREM parasomnia with sexsomnia. However, therapy was not mentioned. A 46-year-old man reported sexsomnia without any history of childhood parasomnia or family history of parasomnia. He presented with a history, provided by his wife, of aggressive/violent sleep behaviors and sexual behaviors during sleep (involving full intercourse), which were at times associated with sexual dreams. These events occurred during the second half of the night and early morning hours, when REM sleep is most predominant. PSG evaluation revealed REM sleep without atonia, but without any RBD behaviors. He was diagnosed to have RBD with sexsomnia. However, therapy with clonazepam (2 mg at bedtime) was not effective, nor were dopamine agonists or carbamazepine effective.

Another report from France presented two 36- and 40-year-old married women with sexsomnia.[48] Both women had histories of traumatic and sexual psychological stress during childhood. They both presented with sexsomnia, manifesting with sexual moaning, dirty talk, masturbation, and forced sexual intercourse with the bed partner. PSG evaluation in both patients identified multiple, abrupt, spontaneous arousals from slow-wave sleep, without any associated behaviors. Therapy with the SSRI escitalopram, 10 mg daily, in both patients (one with and one without clinical depression), induced complete control of sexsomnia, which was maintained at 9-month and 2-year follow-up, respectively. No rationale was given for the SSRI therapy for the sexsomnia. In contrast, a 30-year-old man from Holland without parasomnia history developed a de novo sexsomnia on a nightly basis for 3 weeks on starting therapy for major depression with the SSRI escitalopram, 10 mg daily.[49] His sexsomnia involved full intercourse with his bed partner. The sexsomnia immediately ceased on discontinuation of escitalopram. There was no recurrence of sexsomnia with duloxetine (serotonin-norepinephrine reuptake inhibitor) therapy for major depression. Another case of OSA-sexsomnia responsive to CPAP therapy has been reported.[50]

SRED

SRED is characterized by a disruption of the nocturnal fast with episodes of feeding after an arousal from nighttime sleep.[1,51] The disorder resembles sleepwalking, especially in the setting of sedative-hypnotic medication-induced amnesia. The most commonly cited agents associated with SRED are the BZD receptor agonists, in particular zolpidem. Like other NREM parasomnias, SRED is often associated with other sleep disorders, such as other NREM parasomnias, restless legs syndrome (RLS) and sleep-disordered breathing.[1,51] SRED may be more common than currently realized. A preliminary study found a prevalence of 5% in an unselected group of university students, and also 17% in eating-disordered inpatients, and 9% in eating-disordered outpatients.[52] Adverse consequences include weight gain, ingestion of nonfood or toxic substances, as well as aggravation of associated medical conditions such as diabetes mellitus and obesity.[1] **Box 4** contains the ICSD-2 diagnostic criteria for SRED.

Treatment of SRED

The first goal in treating dysfunctional nocturnal eating is to identify and correct any comorbid sleep disorders and eliminate suspected inducing agents. Dopaminergics, opioids, and BZDs are agents typically used in the treatment of RLS. In the original case series of 38 patients with SRED, combinations of these medications effectively eliminated nocturnal eating associated with RLS and periodic limb movement disorder (PLMD).[53] Dopaminergic therapy also appeared to be helpful in patients with SRED with comorbid sleepwalking and no RLS. In the original case series just described, 8 sleepwalking patients with SRED were effectively treated with bromocriptine, levodopa, and/or clonazepam.[53] BZDs, commonly used in the treatment of other NREM parasomnias, are typically ineffective as monotherapy for SRED.[54] SRED associated with OSA may be effectively treated with CPAP. In 2 cases of SRED with OSA, CPAP eliminated the nocturnal eating.[54]

Discontinuing the offending medication is the best treatment of drug-induced SRED.[55–59] Currently, 2 classes of pharmacotherapies seem to be the most effective in treating SRED: dopaminergics and the anticonvulsant topiramate. Serotonergic agents may also show promise. However, research on the therapy for SRED is still inchoate, and further investigations, in particular randomized controlled trials, are necessary.

In regards to dopaminergic agents, the original case series noted that either bedtime levodopa or bromocriptine was effective in eliminating nocturnal eating, especially in patients with associated RLS.[51] Two follow-up preliminary reports from the same investigators also indicated improved control of nocturnal eating with

Table 1
Data from 31 published cases of parasomnias and 7 published cases of epilepsy with abnormal sleep-related sexual behaviors and experiences

Category	Parasomnias (n = 31)	Sleep-related Epilepsy (n = 7)
Gender, % (n)		
Male	80.6% (25)	57.1% (4)
Female	19.4% (6)	42.9% (3)
Age, years, mean ± SD (n)		
Total	31.9 ± 8.0 (30)[a]	37.7 ± 8.5
Male	32.1 ± 8.5 (24)	34.0 ± 3.5
Female	30.8 ± 6.4 (6)	42.7 ± 11.6
Age, sleepsex onset, years, mean ± SD (n)		
Total	25.9 ± 8.7 (17)[b]	32.0 ± 9.6
Male	27.4 ± 7.9 (15)	27.0 ± 9.1
Female	14.5 ± 3.5 (2)	38.7 ± 5.6
Duration, sleepsex, years, mean ± SD (n)		
Total	9.5 ± 6.1 (8)[c]	12–16 (n = 3), brief (n = 4)
Male	8.3 ± 6.5 (6)	12,16 (n = 2)
Female	13.0 ± 4.2 (2)	12 (n = 1)
Sleepsex behaviors, % of patients (n)		
Masturbation	22.6 % (7) (4 male, 3 female)	14.3% (n=1) (1 male)
Sexual vocalizations, talking, shouting	19.3% (6) (n = 2 moaning; n = 4 talking) (2 male, 4 female)	28.6% (2) (n = 1 moaning; n = 1 shouting) (2 male)
Fondling another person (13 male, 1 female)	45.2% (14)	0%
Sexual intercourse	41.9% (13) (13 male, 0 female)	0%
Sexual hyperarousal (experiential)	0%	28.6% (n = 2) (male, female)
Ictal orgasm	N/A	42.9% (n = 3) (1 man, 2 women)
Ictal sexual automatisms	N/A	14.3% (n = 1) (male)
Total number of sleepsex behaviors	40	9
Amnesia for sleepsex, % (n)	100% (31)	28.6% (2)
Recall of sleepsex, % (n)	0% (0)	71.4% (5)
Agitated/assaultive sleep-related sexual behaviors, % (n)	45.2% (14)	14.3% (1)
Sleepsex with minors, % (n)	29.0% (9)	0%
Legal consequences from sleepsex, % (n) (2 with adults; 9 with minors[d])	35.5% (11)	0%
Other consequences, % (n)		
Adverse: physical		
Self	6.4% (2)	71.4% (5)
Other	61.3% (19)	0.0%

(continued on next page)

Table 1
(continued)

Category	Parasomnias (n = 31)	Sleep-related Epilepsy (n = 7)
Psychosocial		
Self	67.7% (21)	57.1% (4)
Other	80.6% (25)	14.3% (1)
Total	100% (31)	100% (7)
Positive, self/other (with or without adverse consequences)	12.9% (4)	57.1% (4)
PSG, % (n)	83.9% (26)	28.6% (2)
Sleep EEG (without PSG)	0%	14.3% (1)
No PSG or sleep EEG	16.1% (5)	57.1% (4)
Total number of parasomnias[e]	71	N/A (not reported)
Mean number (±SD) per patient (range, 1–4)	2.2 ± 1.0	
Final diagnosis, sleepsex cause,[f] % (n)		
DOA (confusional arousals, n = 26; sleepwalking, n = 2) (OSA comorbidity, n = 4)	90.3% (28)	N/A
RBD	9.7% (3)	N/A
Sleep-related seizures	N/A	100% (7)
Treatment efficacy[g] (controlling sleepsex), % (n)		
Clonazepam at bedtime	90.0% (9/10): (6/7 DOA; 3/3 RBD)	
Nasal CPAP at bedtime	100% (3/3 OSA)	N/A
Control of nocturnal seizures[h]	N/A	100% (5)

Abbreviations: DOA, disorder of arousal; N/A, not applicable; SD, standard deviation.
[a] N = 1, age not reported.
[b] Age of sleepsex onset was known in 54.8% (17/31) of patients, and was unknown or not reported in 45.2% (14/31) of patients.
[c] Duration of sleepsex reported on n = 8 patients; n = 8 had only one reported episode of sleepsex and n = 1 had 2 reported episodes within 1 month, so duration is not applicable; n = 14, duration not known.
[d] Adult men assaulted 9 girls (8–15 years old [n = 8], and a teenage girl [n = 1]).
[e] Confusional arousals (n = 24); sleepwalking (n = 21); sleeptalking and vocalizations, sexual and nonsexual (n = 15); sleep terrors (n = 7); RBD (n = 3); SRED (n = 1). (A history of enuresis was not included in these data).
[f] In all 3 patients with RBD, no behaviors (sexual or nonsexual) were documented in REM sleep.
[g] An additional patient with a DOA responded to clonazepam, but with remission maintained after clonazepam was discontinued. Another patient with a DOA did not respond to limited therapy consisting of low-dose (25 mg) clomipramine at bedtime. Therefore, these 2 cases were kept separate from the treatment outcome data. For the remaining n = 17, treatment was not mentioned.
[h] Control of nocturnal seizures was achieved with anticonvulsant medications. N = 2, treatment outcome was not mentioned.
Data from Schenck CH, Arnulf I, Mahowald MW. Sleep and sex: what can go wrong? A review of the literature on sleep related disorders and abnormal sexual behaviors and experiences. Sleep 2007;30:683–702.

dopaminergic and opioid therapy.[60,61] The mechanism by which dopamine agents may suppress nocturnal eating is unknown, although direct appetite suppression is a possibility.[53] Recently, pramipexole, a dopamine receptor agonist, was investigated in a small double-blind, placebo-controlled crossover trial. Pramipexole was well tolerated in all patients, including those without known RLS or PLMD. Patients on pramipexole noted improved sleep, and reduced nighttime activity was documented with actigraphy. There was no improvement in the number or duration of awakenings.[62] The main side effects of dopamine agonists include sedation, orthostasis, nausea, manic episodes, paranoia, psychosis, and hallucinations.

In regards to topiramate, an open-label trial of topiramate in 4 patients with nocturnal eating (2 with SRED) had positive results. The agent was well tolerated, nocturnal eating diminished, and

> **Box 4**
> **ICSD-2 diagnostic criteria for SRED**
>
> Recurrent episodes of involuntary eating and drinking occur during the main sleep period
>
> One or more of the following must be present with the recurrent episodes of involuntary eating and drinking:
>
> 1. Consumption of peculiar forms or combinations of food or inedible or toxic substances
> 2. Insomnia related to sleep disruption from repeated episodes of eating, with a complaint of nonrestorative sleep, daytime fatigue or somnolence
> 3. Sleep-related injury
> 4. Dangerous behaviors while in pursuit of food or while cooking with food
> 5. Morning anorexia
> 6. Adverse health consequences from recurrent binge eating of high-calorie foods
>
> The disturbance is not better explained by another sleep disorder, medical or neurologic disorder, mental disorder, or substance use disorder

weight loss (mean of 11.1 kg) was noted in all 4 individuals over 8.5 months.[63] A case report with similar results was recently published. This 28-year-old obese man had a 10-year history of nocturnal eating episodes that were eliminated with topiramate. It was also reported that the agent was well tolerated over a 2-year follow-up.[64] In a case series published as an abstract, of 17 patients with SRED treated with topiramate, 12 responded to treatment. The agent was well tolerated, and over 1.8 years there was a mean weight loss of 9.2 kg among the treatment responders.[65] Another chart review of 25 patients with SRED who were followed up reported that 68% of patients with SRED responded to treatment. However, over 1 year, only 28% of patients lost more than 10% of their body weight and 41% of patients discontinued the medication because of adverse effects.[66] The main side effects of topiramate were weight loss, paresthesias, renal calculus, cognitive dysfunction, and orthostasis.

Serotonergic acting drugs may also be effective in treating SRED. Fluoxetine was reported to effectively resolve nocturnal eating in 2 of 3 patients with SRED.[67] Further, other cases of nocturnal eating have also been responsive to serotonergic medications. However, conclusions regarding SRED treatment are difficult to draw from these reports because these patients had diagnoses other than SRED, most commonly the night eating syndrome.[68–70]

A DVD documentary film, *Sleep Runners: The Stories Behind Everyday Parasomnias*, has been produced in which patients with RBD, sleepwalking, sleep terrors, SRED, and other parasomnias (along with their spouses and family) describe their personal experiences with these abnormal, recurrent nocturnal events, and the gratifying response to treatment.[71]

SUMMARY

Parasomnias comprise a set of sleep disorders (often with prominent gender and age predilections) that is generally amenable to effective and safe therapies, usually pharmacologic. This situation is gratifying for the treating clinician, as there often are major, long-standing complications from parasomnias, including injuries, sleep disruption, and various adverse health and psychosocial consequences. Also, parasomnias not uncommonly have comorbidities with other sleep disorders, particularly sleep-disordered breathing, RLS, and narcolepsy, and so an increasingly accepted therapeutic strategy for managing parasomnias is first to treat any comorbid condition(s) and then to reassess if additional, specific therapy is warranted to fully control the parasomnia. Furthermore, there is increasing awareness of medication-induced or aggravated parasomnias, such as with RBD and SRED (and perhaps sexsomnia), and so eliminating a presumed offending agent needs to be carefully considered. Ensuring the safety of the sleeping environment must always be emphasized during discussions with patients afflicted with parasomnias.

REFERENCES

1. American Academy of Sleep Medicine. International classification of sleep disorders: diagnostic and coding manual. 2nd edition. Westchester (IL): American Academy of Sleep Medicine; 2005.
2. Mahowald MW, Schenck CH. Evolving concepts of human state dissociation. Arch Ital Biol 2001;139:269–300.
3. Schenck CH, Mahowald MW. REM sleep behavior disorder: clinical, developmental, and neuroscience perspectives 16 years after its formal identification in SLEEP. Sleep 2002;25:120–38.
4. Mahowald MW, Schenck CH. The REM sleep behavior disorder odyssey [editorial]. Sleep Med Rev 2009;13:381–4.
5. Bodkin CL, Schenck CH. Rapid eye movement sleep behavior disorder affecting females: relevance to general and specialty medical practice. J Women's Health 2009;18(12):1955–63.

6. Schenck CH, Hurwitz TD, Bundlie SR, et al. Sleep-related injury in 100 adult patients: a polysomnographic and clinical report. Am J Psychiatry 1989; 146:1166–73.
7. Schenck CH, Lee SA, Cramer Bornemann MA, et al. Potentially lethal behaviors associated with rapid eye movement sleep behavior disorder (RBD): review of the literature and forensic implications. J Forensic Sci 2009;54:6.
8. Cramer Bornemann MA, Mahowald MW, SchenckParasomnias CH. Clinical features and forensic implications. Chest 2006;130:605–10.
9. Boeve BF. REM sleep behavior disorder: updated review of the core features, the REM sleep behavior disorder-neurodegenerative disease connection, evolving concepts, controversies, and future directions. Ann N Y Acad Sci 2010;1184:17–56.
10. Oudiette D, De Cock VC, Lavault S, et al. Nonviolent elaborate behaviors may also occur in REM sleep behavior disorder. Neurology 2009;72:551–7.
11. Boeve BF, Silber MH, Saper CB, et al. Pathophysiology of REM sleep behavior disorder and relevance to neurodegenerative disease. Brain 2007;130:2770–88.
12. Schenck CH, Bundlie SR, Mahowald MW. Delayed emergence of a parkinsonian disorder in 38% of 29 older males initially diagnosed with idiopathic REM sleep behavior disorder. Neurology 1996;46: 388–93.
13. Iranzo A, Molinuevo JL, Santamaria J, et al. Rapid-eye-movement sleep behaviour disorder as an early marker for a neurodegenerative disorder: a descriptive study. Lancet Neurol 2006;5:572–7.
14. Postuma RB, Gagnon JF, Vendette M, et al. Quantifying the risk of neuro-degenerative disease in idiopathic REM sleep behavior disorder. Neurology 2009;72:1296–300.
15. Claassen DO, Josephs KA, Ahlskog JE, et al. REM sleep behavior disorder may precede other manifestations of synucleinopathies by up to half a century. Neurology 2010;75:494–9.
16. Lai Y-Y, Siegel JM. Physiological and anatomical link between Parkinson-like disease and REM sleep behavior disorder. Mol Neurobiol 2003;27:137–51.
17. Mahowald MW, Schenck CH. REM sleep parasomnias. In: Kryger MH, Roth T, Dement WC, editors. Principles and practice of sleep medicine, 5th edition. Philadelphia: Elsevier Saunders; in press.
18. Schenck CH, Mahowald MW. Long-term, nightly benzodiazepine treatment of injurious parasomnias and other disorders of disrupted nocturnal sleep in 170 adults. Am J Med 1996;100:333–7.
19. Gagnon JF, Postuma RB, Montplaisir J. Update on the pharmacology of REM sleep behavior disorder. Neurology 2006;67:742–7.
20. Gugger JJ, Wagner ML. Rapid eye movement sleep behavior disorder. Ann Pharmacother 2007;41: 1833–41.
21. Schuld A, Kraus T, Haack M, et al. Obstructive sleep apnea syndrome induced by clonazepam in a narcoleptic patient with REM-sleep-behavior disorder. J Sleep Res 1999;8:321–2.
22. Kunz D, Bes F. Melatonin as a therapy in REM sleep behavior disorder patients: an open-labeled pilot study on the possible influence of melatonin on REM-sleep regulation. Mov Disord 1999;14:507–11.
23. Takeuchi N, Uchimura N, Hashizume Y, et al. Melatonin therapy for REM sleep behavior disorder. Psychiatry Clin Neurosci 2001;55:267–9.
24. Boeve BF, Silber MH, Ferman JT. Melatonin for treatment of REM sleep behavior disorder in neurologic disorders: results in 14 patients. Sleep Med 2003;4:281–4.
25. Fantini ML, Gagno J-F, Filipini D, et al. The effects of pramipexole in REM sleep behavior disorder. Neurology 2003;61:1418–20.
26. Schmidt MH, Koshal VB, Schmidt HS. Use of pramipexole in REM sleep behavior disorder. Sleep Med 2006;7:418–23.
27. Kumru H, Iranzo A, Carrasco E, et al. Lack of effects of pramipexole on REM sleep behavior disorder in Parkinson disease. Sleep 2008;31:1418–21.
28. Ringman JM, Simmons JH. Treatment of REM sleep behavior disorder with donepezil: a report of three cases. Neurology 2000;55:870–1.
29. Simmons J. Treatment of REM behavior disorder with acetylcholinesterase inhibitors. Sleep 2009;32:A292.
30. Shneerson JM. Successful treatment of REM sleep behavior disorder with sodium oxybate. Clin Neuropharmacol 2009;32:158–9.
31. Iranzo A, Graus F, Clover L, et al. Rapid eye movement sleep behavior disorder and potassium channel antibody-associated limbic encephalitis. Ann Neurol 2005;59:178–82.
32. Rye DB, Dempsay J, Dihenia B, et al. REM-sleep dyscontrol in Parkinson's disease: case report of effects of elective pallidotomy. Sleep Res 1997;26:591.
33. Hublin C, Kaprio J, Partinen M, et al. Prevalence and genetics of sleepwalking: a population-based twin study. Neurology 1997;48(1):177–81.
34. Ohayon MM, Guilleminault C, Priest RG. Night terrors, sleepwalking, and confusional arousals in the general population: their frequency and relationship to other sleep and mental disorders. J Clin Psychiatry 1999;60(4):268–76.
35. Pressman MR. Disorders of arousal from sleep and violent behavior: the role of physical contact and proximity. Sleep 2007;30(8):1039–47.
36. Harris M, Grunstein RR. Treatments for somnambulism in adults: assessing the evidence. Sleep Med Rev 2009;13(4):295–7.
37. Kavey NB, Whyte J, Resor SR Jr, et al. Somnambulism in adults. Neurology 1990;40(5):749–52.
38. Cooper AJ. Treatment of coexistent night-terrors and somnambulism in adults with imipramine and diazepam. J Clin Psychiatry 1987;48(5):209–10.

39. Lillywhite AR, Wilson SJ, Nutt DJ. Successful treatment of night terrors and somnambulism with paroxetine. Br J Psychiatry 1994;164(4):551–4.

40. Wilson SJ, Lillywhite AR, Potokar JP, et al. Adult night terrors and paroxetine. Lancet 1997;350(9072):185.

41. Hurwitz TD, Mahowald MW, Schenck CH, et al. A retrospective outcome study and review of hypnosis as treatment of adults with sleepwalking and sleep terror. J Nerv Ment Dis 1991;179:228–33.

42. Hauri PJ, Silber MH, Boeve BF. The treatment of parasomnias with hypnosis: a 5-year follow-up study. J Clin Sleep Med 2007;3:369–73.

43. Schenck CH, Arnulf I, Mahowald MW. Sleep and sex: what can go wrong? A review of the literature on sleep related disorders and abnormal sexual behaviors and experiences. Sleep 2007;30:683–702.

44. Rosenfeld DS, Elhajjar AJ. Sleepsex: a variant of sleepwalking. Arch Sex Behav 1998;27:269–78.

45. Guilleminault C, Moscovitch A, Yuen K, et al. Atypical sexual behavior during sleep. Psychosom Med 2002;64:328–36.

46. Shapiro CM, Trajanovic NN, Fedoroff JP. Sexsomnia—a new parasomnia? Can J Psychiatry 2003;48:3110317.

47. Della Marca G, Dittoni S, Frusciante R, et al. Abnormal sexual behavior during sleep. J Sex Med 2009;6:3490–5.

48. Bejot Y, Juenet N, Garrouty R, et al. Sexsomnia: an uncommon variety of parasomnia. Clin Neurol Neurosurg 2010;112:72–5.

49. Krol DGH. Sexsomnia during treatment with a selective serotonin reuptake blocker. J Psychiatry 2008;50(11):735–9.

50. Schenck CH, Mahowald MW. Parasomnias associated with sleep-disordered breathing and its therapy, including sexsomnia as a recently recognized parasomnia. Somnology 2008;12:38–49.

51. Howell MJ, Schenck CH, Crow SJ. A review of nighttime eating disorders. Sleep Med Rev 2009;13:23–34.

52. Winkelman JW, Herzog DB, Fava M. The prevalence of sleep-related eating disorder in psychiatric and non-psychiatric populations. Psychol Med 1999;29:1461–6.

53. Schenck CH, Hurwitz TD, Bundlie SR, et al. Sleep-related eating disorders: polysomnographic correlates of a heterogeneous syndrome distinct from daytime eating disorders. Sleep 1991;14:419–31.

54. Howell MJ, Schenck CH. Treatment of nocturnal eating disorders. Curr Treat Options Neurol 2009;11:333–9.

55. Morgenthaler TI, Silber MH. Amnestic sleep-related eating disorder associated with zolpidem. Sleep Med 2002;3(4):323–7.

56. Sansone RA, Sansone LA. Zolpidem, somnambulism, and nocturnal eating. Gen Hosp Psychiatry 2008;30(1):90–1.

57. Chiang A, Krystal A. Report of two cases where sleep related eating behavior occurred with the extended-release formulation but not the immediate-release formulation of a sedative-hypnotic agent. J Clin Sleep Med 2008;4(2):155–6.

58. Dang A, Garg G, Rataboli PV. Zolpidem induced Nocturnal Sleep-Related Eating Disorder (NSRED) in a male patient. Int J Eat Disord 2009;42:385–6.

59. Tsai MJ, Tsai YH, Huang YB. Compulsive activity and anterograde amnesia after zolpidem use. Clin Toxicol (Phila) 2007;45:179–81.

60. Schenck CH, Mahowald MW. Combined buproprion-levodopa-trazadone therapy of sleep-related eating disorder and sleep disruption in two adults with chemical dependency. Sleep 2000;23:587–8.

61. Schenck CH, Mahowald. Dopaminergic and opiate therapy of nocturnal sleep-related eating disorder associated with sleepwalking or unassociated with another nocturnal disorder. Sleep 2002;25(Suppl):A249–50.

62. Provini F, Albani F, Vetrugno R, et al. A pilot double-blind placebo-controlled trial of low-dose pramipexole in sleep-related eating disorder. Eur J Neurol 2005;12(6):432–6.

63. Winkelman JW. Treatment of nocturnal eating syndrome and sleep-related eating disorder with topiramate. Sleep Med 2003;4(3):243–6.

64. Martinez-Salio A, Soler-Algarra S, Calvo-Garcia I, et al. Nocturnal sleep-related eating disorder that responds to topiramate. Rev Neurol 2007;45(5):276–9.

65. Schenck CH, Mahowald MW. Topiramate therapy of sleep related eating disorder (SRED). Sleep 2006;29:A268.

66. Winkelman JW. Efficacy and tolerability of open-label topiramate in the treatment of sleep-related eating disorder: a retrospective case series. J Clin Psychiatry 2006;67:1729–34.

67. Schenck CH, Hurwitz TD, O'Connor KA, et al. Additional categories of sleep-related eating disorders and the current status of treatment. Sleep 1993;16:457–66.

68. Spaggiari MC, Granella F, Parrino L, et al. Nocturnal eating syndrome in adults. Sleep 1994;17(4):339–44.

69. Miyaoka T, Yasukawa R, Tsubouchi K, et al. Successful treatment of nocturnal eating/drinking syndrome with selective serotonin reuptake inhibitors. Int Clin Psychopharmacol 2003;18(3):175–7.

70. O'Reardon JP, Allison KC, Martino NS, et al. A randomized, placebo-controlled trial of sertraline in the treatment of night eating syndrome. Am J Psychiatry 2006;163:893–8.

71. Sleep runners: the stories behind everyday parasomnias (1 hour DVD documentary film). Slow-Wave Films, LLC 2004 (Deluxe Academic Edition, 2007). Available at: www.sleeprunners.com. Accessed August 11, 2010.

Therapeutics for Circadian Rhythm Sleep Disorders

Ehren R. Dodson, PhD, Phyllis C. Zee, MD, PhD*

KEYWORDS

- Circadian rhythm sleep disorders • Treatment
- Melatonin • Light therapy • Sleep

Circadian rhythm sleep disorders (CRSD) are caused by a misalignment between the timing of the endogenous circadian rhythm and the desired or socially acceptable sleep-wake schedule, or dysfunction of the circadian pacemaker and its afferent/efferent pathways. CRSDs include delayed sleep phase disorder, advanced sleep phase disorder, non−24-hour sleep-wake disorder, irregular sleep-wake rhythm disorder, shift work sleep disorder, and jet lag disorder.

The central circadian pacemaker in mammals is located in the suprachiasmatic nucleus (SCN). The endogenous period of circadian rhythms in humans is typically slightly longer than 24 hours.[1] Therefore, to maintain a stable relationship with the recurring daily changes in the 24-hour physical environment, circadian rhythms are entrained by light, social and physical activity cues, and melatonin. Of these, light is the strongest entraining agent for the circadian clock. Light-dark cycle information is relayed from the retina to the SCN primarily via the retinohypothalamic tract, a neural pathway that is distinct from the visual system.[2] The timing of light exposure is crucial, and determines its ability to effect changes in the timing of circadian rhythms. According to the phase response curve in humans, exposure to bright light in the early morning (after the nadir of the core body temperature rhythm) induces phase advances, whereas light exposure in the evening (before the nadir of the core body temperature rhythm) delays the phase of circadian rhythms (**Fig. 1**).[3]

Although less potent than bright light, melatonin also has circadian phase shifting properties. The timing of melatonin release from the pineal gland is regulated by the SCN and its secretion is suppressed by exposure to bright light.[4] In individuals with a typical sleep-wake schedule, endogenous melatonin levels begin to rise approximately 2 hours before sleep onset,[5] and remain elevated during the habitual sleep hours. Melatonin onset measured in dim light (DLMO) has been shown to be a stable marker of circadian phase,[6,7] and can be used to determine the timing of endogenous circadian rhythms in the research setting as well as in clinical practice. The phase response curve for melatonin is approximately 12 hours out of phase with that for light, but with similar crossover points.[8] Melatonin administration in the early morning (after the nadir of the core body temperature rhythm) cause phase delay shifts, whereas when given in the evening, it elicits phase advance shifts (see **Fig. 1**).[9]

Because the primary synchronizing agents of the circadian system are the light-dark cycle and melatonin, timed exposure to bright light and administration of melatonin have often been used as treatments of CRSD. Although the authors focus here on pharmacologic therapies, it must be borne in mind that timed exposure to bright light is an indication, as either a guideline or option, by the American Academy of Sleep Medicine (AASM) Clinical Practice Parameters for the treatment of most CRSDs.[10] Exogenous melatonin is widely used as a pharmacologic treatment and is

Department of Neurology, Circadian Rhythms and Sleep Center, Northwestern University, 710 North Lake Shore Drive, Suite 520, Abbott Hall, Chicago, IL 60611, USA
* Corresponding author.
E-mail address: p-zee@northwestern.edu

Sleep Med Clin 5 (2010) 701–715
doi:10.1016/j.jsmc.2010.08.001

sleep.theclinics.com

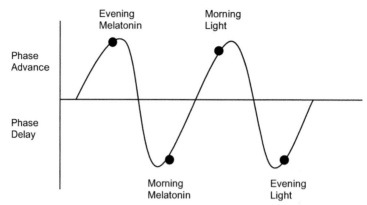

Fig. 1. The human phase response curve (PRC) to melatonin and light. The black circles along the PRC indicate exposure to stimuli (eg, light or melatonin). The position during which the stimulus occurs indicates whether the effect would result in a phase delay or advance of the circadian rhythm. Melatonin administration in the evening induces a phase advance, whereas administration in the morning causes a phase delay. Morning light exposure results in a phase advance, whereas light exposure in the evening elicits a phase delay.

recommended as either a guideline or option by the AASM Clinical Practice Parameters for the treatment of CRSDs. Melatonin is classified as a nutritional supplement and has been approved by the Food and Drug Administration (FDA) as a treatment for sleep disorders.

DELAYED SLEEP PHASE DISORDER

Delayed sleep phase disorder (DSPD) is one of the most common of the CRSD. Limited data suggest that the prevalence rate is about 1.7% in the general population[11] and 7% in those with insomnia complaints.[7] Onset of this disorder typically occurs during adolescence or early adulthood.[12,13]

DSPD often presents as sleep-onset insomnia and/or excessive morning sleepiness associated with the chronic inability to fall asleep and wake up at socially acceptable times as required for work or school.[12] Sleep onset time typically occurs between 2 AM and 6 AM, and wake times delayed into the late morning or early afternoon. When unrestricted by an imposed schedule, sleep latency and duration are normal.[14] Waking in the early morning (ie, 6–8 AM) is very difficult for these patients, often requiring multiple alarms and the assistance of family members. DSPD patients report excessive sleepiness and impaired functioning in the morning, with marked improvement in alertness in the evening/night.

According to the International Classification of Sleep Disorders (ICSD-2) the diagnosis is made by a history of a stable delay of the major sleep period relative to the desired sleep and wake times for at least 1 to 3 months, and is accompanied by clinically significant insomnia and/or

excessive sleepiness.[15] When allowed to sleep at the preferred delayed sleep phase, sleep quality and duration are typically within the normal range for age. In addition, sleep logs or actigraphy monitoring for at least 7 days is recommended to confirm a delayed pattern of the habitual sleep and wake cycle.[15] These diagnostic features and those for other CRSDs are listed with guidelines for assessment and treatment in **Table 1**.

Although the exact etiology of DSPD is unknown, it has been suggested that genetic predisposition, a longer than average endogenous circadian period or alterations in entrainment pathways can result in a delayed circadian phase.[12,13] There is evidence of increased sensitivity to the phase shifting effect of evening light in DSPD patients.[16] Thus, exposure to even moderate levels of light in the evening could delay circadian rhythms, as well as suppress the normal increase in melatonin in the evening, resulting in the delayed onset of the sleep-wake cycle.[16] Furthermore, the typical late rise time of patients with DSPD reduces exposure to morning light in the phase advance zone of the phase response curve, which will perpetuate or exacerbate the already delayed circadian phase. In addition, recent evidence indicates that genetic mechanisms may also play a role. For example, the DSPD phenotype has been associated with polymorphisms of the circadian genes, *Clock*[17] and *Per3*.[18]

Therapeutic Approaches

Patients with DSPD commonly experience repeated unsuccessful attempts at trying to fall asleep earlier, and often resort to the use of

Table 1
Circadian rhythm sleep disorders: essential features, diagnostic assessment, and treatment

Type	Essential Features	Diagnostic Assessment	Treatment
Delayed sleep phase disorder	Delayed sleep onset and wake times in relation to desired sleep schedule Inability to sleep at conventional sleep times Most common onset in childhood or adolescence	Sleep log and/or actigraphy monitoring for a minimum of 7 d	Melatonin administration before desired bedtime Timed bright light exposure in the morning Chronotherapy
Advanced sleep phase disorder	Advanced sleep onset and wake times in relation to desired sleep schedule Inability to sleep at conventional sleep times Rare occurrence, typically in elderly	Sleep log and/or actigraphy monitoring for a minimum of 7 d	Timed bright light exposure in the evening Prescribed sleep schedule Appropriately timed melatonin administration[a]
Free-running disorder	Sleep onset and wake times are progressively delayed 1–2 h each day Complaints of insomnia or excessive sleepiness More common in blind, rare in sighted individuals	Sleep diary and/or actigraphy monitoring for a minimum of 7 d; longer monitoring is best to document drift in sleep pattern Circadian phase markers are also an option for confirming diagnosis	Timed bright light exposure in the morning, prescribed sleep schedule (sighted only) Melatonin administration several hours before desired bedtime
Irregular sleep-wake rhythm	Complaints of insomnia and/or excessive sleepiness Multiple sleep bouts within 24-h period Common in individuals with neurologic impairment	Sleep diary and/or actigraphy monitoring for a minimum of 7 d At least 3 sleep episodes during 24-h period Total sleep time in 24-h period is normal for age	Timed daytime bright light exposure Melatonin administered before desired bedtime (in populations other than elderly demented patients) Multimodal approach combining bright light exposure, physical activity, and behavior modification
Jet lag disorder	Complaints of insomnia and daytime impairment and sleepiness associated with travel across time zones Symptoms occur 1–2 d after travel across at least 2 time zones	Diagnostic assessment usually not indicated	Keep home-based sleep schedule for short trips Melatonin or hypnotic administered before desired bedtime Timed bright light exposure Caffeine
Shift work disorder	Complaints of insomnia or excessive sleepiness associated with work schedule that overlaps usual sleep period Symptoms occur with shift work schedule occurring at least 1 mo	Sleep diary and/or actigraphy monitoring for a minimum of 7 d	Planned napping before shift, minimize morning light exposure Caffeine or modafinil during night shift Melatonin or hypnotic administered before daytime sleep Timed bright light during shift

[a] Theoretical rationale; no reported clinical evidence to support this treatment.
Data from Morgenthaler TI, Lee-Chiong T, Alessi C, et al. Practice parameters for the clinical evaluation and treatment of circadian rhythm sleep disorders. Sleep 2007; 30(11):1445–59; and American Academy of Sleep Medicine. The international classification of sleep disorders: diagnostic & coding manual. 2nd edition. Westchester (IL): American Academy of Sleep Medicine; 2005.

sedating medications and alcohol.[12] Effective treatment requires a multimodal approach aimed to realign circadian rhythms with the desired sleep and wake schedule. Nonpharmacologic approaches including adherence to good sleep hygiene, avoidance of bright light in the evening, and increasing light exposure in the morning are basic in any treatment program for DSPD. Based on the strength of evidence, the AASM practice parameters recommend timed morning light exposure and/or appropriately timed melatonin administration as effective treatments for DSPD.[10]

Numerous studies have demonstrated the ability of appropriately timed bright broad-spectrum light, typically between 2500 and 10,000 lux, to induce phase advancement of circadian rhythms.[19-21] For the treatment of DSPD, exposure to bright light shortly after awakening in the morning (close to but after the nadir of the circadian core body temperature rhythm) will advance the timing of circadian rhythms and improve synchronization with the desired sleep and wake times. For example, bright light (2500 lux) for 2 hours in the morning has shown to successfully phase advance the circadian rhythm of core body temperature in DSPD patients.[19]

There is very limited evidence that methylcobalamin (vitamin B12) when combined with bright light in the morning may be effective for the treatment of DSPD.[22-25] Findings that vitamin B12 injected intravenously (0.5 mg/d) at 12:30 PM for 11 days, followed by oral administration (2 mg 3 times per day) for 7 days increased the phase shift induced with a single morning exposure to bright light led to further examination of its effectiveness in treating CRSDs.[22] In an open-label study, 28% of patients were effectively treated with vitamin B12 either alone or in combination with bright light.[23] Similar success has been reported in several individual cases.[24] However, administration of 1 mg methylcobalamin 3 times per day after each meal for 4 weeks alone did not show improvements compared with placebo, which suggests that its effects may be dependent on its interaction with light.[25] Therefore, there is insufficient evidence to support vitamin B12 as a treatment for DSPD.[10]

Of the pharmacologic approaches for DSPD, exogenous melatonin has been the most studied. The relatively small number of participants and the variability in the dose and timing of melatonin administration have limited most of these studies. Melatonin (5 mg) given 5 hours before sleep onset advanced sleep onset time by about 1.3 hours, wake time by 2 hours[26] and DLMO by 1.5 hours,[27] compared with placebo over a 4- to 6-week treatment period. In one study, patients also reported feeling more refreshed in the morning with melatonin treatment.[27] However, treatment with 5 mg did not change sleep architecture.[28] Timing of melatonin administration can influence the magnitude of the phase shift in patients with DSPD, with earlier times being most effective. Melatonin given 5 to 6.5 hours before the individual DLMO resulted in the largest phase advances of melatonin profiles compared with administration closer (1.5 hours) before the DLMO.[27,29]

Long-term effectiveness of melatonin for the treatment of DSPD has also been evaluated. One year after initiating a 6-week treatment with 5 mg melatonin taken daily at 10 PM, participants were surveyed regarding the efficacy of their treatment.[30,31] Almost 97% of patients reported improvement, 80% of whom noted the change within the first 2 weeks. Side effects were usually minor, with 57% reporting none at all and 34% noting slight morning fatigue. Of those helped by melatonin, 91% relapsed after treatment discontinued, with almost 30% reporting relapse within first 7 days, 15% within the first month, and 42% within 2 to 6 months after treatment had stopped. Patients who relapsed immediately were found to have more severe symptoms of DSPD based on pretreatment actigraphy measures than those with a delayed relapse.[30]

Melatonin has also been investigated for the treatment of DSPD in children with attention-deficit/hyperactivity disorder (ADHD), and has been found to be effective and well tolerated, except for the rare occurrence of new-onset seizures.[31] In an open-label study, daily use of melatonin 3 mg at bedtime for 1 week to 3 months significantly shortened sleep onset latency (median = 135 min) in children with ADHD.[32] In a larger study, children aged 6 to 12 years taking either 3 or 6 mg of melatonin at 7 PM daily for 3 weeks were shown to improve sleep onset and advance DLMO by 44 minutes on average.[33] Improvements of core behavioral problems were also noted. A follow-up study found that approximately 65% of these children were still using melatonin daily and 11% occasionally, with parents reporting its effectiveness in improving sleep onset in 88% of participants.[34] Parents also reported improvements in behavior (71%) and mood (61%) with long-term melatonin treatment.[34] However, recurrence of delayed sleep timing occurred with discontinuation of treatment in most cases,[34] similar to previous studies in adults with DSPD.[26,30]

ADVANCED SLEEP PHASE DISORDER

Advanced sleep phase disorder (ASPD) is characterized by a recurrent pattern of early evening sleepiness and early morning awakening. This earlier than desired sleep propensity (7 PM to 9 PM) can interfere with social and work schedules. When trying to maintain a socially desired schedule, and even if sleep onset is delayed, early morning awakening (eg, before 5 AM) still occurs, and results in shortened sleep duration and excessive daytime sleepiness.

Diagnostic criteria for ASPD includes a stable advance in the timing of the major sleep period relative to the desired sleep time in conjunction with an inability to delay sleep onset and remain asleep until the desired conventional clock time.[15] Given the opportunity to sleep at their preferred sleep schedule, patients also display normal sleep duration and quality. Sleep logs or actigraphy monitoring for at least 7 days are recommended to demonstrate a stable advance in the timing of the sleep period.[15]

ASPD is thought to be less common than DSPD. ASPD is reported more often among older populations.[35] Etiology remains unclear, although patients with ASPD have an earlier timed temperature and melatonin circadian phase, which may be preventing them from sleeping later.[36] Multiple cases of familial advanced sleep phase pattern have been identified in which the ASPD trait segregates with an autosomal dominant mode of inheritance.[37–39] Two gene mutations have been identified, the clock gene *hPer2* in one family with advanced sleep phase,[40] and the *casein kinase 1 delta* gene in another family,[35] suggesting that there is heterogeneity of this disorder. Other underlying mechanisms that may be involved include having a short (less than 24 hours) endogenous circadian period[38] or an attenuated ability to phase delay owing to a dominant phase advance region of the phase response curve (PRC) to light.

Therapeutic Approaches

Treatment approaches for ASPD include chronotherapy, timed light exposure in the evening, and pharmacotherapy with melatonin or hypnotics for sleep maintenance insomnia. However, there is very little evidence of the effectiveness of pharmacologic therapy in ASPD. The AASM Practice Parameters recommend prescribed sleep scheduling and timed bright light exposure as treatments for ASPD.[10] Bright light therapy in the evening (between 7 and 9 PM) is typically used and has been shown to delay the timing of circadian rhythms, and improve sleep and daytime performance in older individuals with advanced circadian phase and sleep maintenance insomnia symptoms,[41,42] although limited compliance may limit its practicality as a long-term treatment.

Based on the PRC to melatonin, early morning administration of melatonin (after the nadir of the core body temperature rhythm) would fall in the curve's advance portion and thus advance the timing of sleep-wake cycle rhythm. However, clinical evidence is lacking regarding its efficacy, and concerns have been raised regarding the safety of taking a potentially sleep promoting agent in the morning.[43,44] Hughes and colleagues[45] evaluated different delivery strategies of melatonin for ASPD in a controlled study. A 2-week administration of immediate release melatonin 0.5 mg, 4 hours after bedtime or controlled-release melatonin 0.5 mg, 30 minutes before bedtime did not improve sleep maintenance, but did result in a nonsignificant phase delay of approximately 27 minutes.[45] Although hypnotics are used in clinical practice to treat the sleep maintenance symptoms of patients with ASPD, their efficacy and safety in this population has not been specifically studied.[46]

FREE-RUNNING DISORDER (NONENTRAINED TYPE)

Individuals with free-running disorder (FRD) typically have a longer than 24-hour circadian rhythm, similar to those living in temporal isolation.[47] Because these patients are unable to entrain to the external 24-hour physical, social, or activity cycles, sleep and wake periods progressively drift later each day.[48] Although there is an overlap between DSPD and FRD, this inability to stably entrain to a 24-hour sleep-wake cycle is what clinically sets FRD from those with DSPD, who are delayed, but stably entrained.[49] Depending on whether the circadian propensity for sleep and wake falls within the day or night, individuals may present with either insomnia symptoms or excessive sleepiness. These periods of insomnia and sleepiness, usually lasting several days to a few weeks, are intermixed with periods of relatively normal sleep and wake times (when the endogenous circadian rhythm is aligned with the conventional clock times).

Diagnosis of FRD includes complaints of insomnia or excessive sleepiness associated with the misalignment between the endogenous circadian rhythm and the light-dark cycle that cannot be explained by other causes.[15] Sleep logs or actigraphy monitoring for at least 7 days is recommended for diagnosis, although a longer duration is preferred to demonstrate the drift in sleep times from one day to the next.[10]

FRD is most common in blind people who lack, or have greatly diminished ability for photic entrainment. It is estimated that approximately 50% of blind persons have nonentrained circadian rhythms.[49] Because light cues are unavailable, sleep disturbances are common.[50] In fact, the degree of visual loss is related to the occurrence of FRD.[51] The insomnia and daytime sleepiness that occur when the circadian pacemaker is out of phase with the desired sleep time have been noted as being second in debilitation next to the blindness itself.[52] However, a good proportion of blind individuals maintain some light perception and/or are able to entrain to recurring social and activity schedules and thus can maintain entrainment.[51] The disorder is thought to be rare among sighted individuals.[53,54] FRD in sighted individuals is more common in men than in women,[55] and onset is typically in adolescence or early adulthood.

Although the etiology of this disorder is unknown, it has been hypothesized that sighted FRD patients may have a blunted response to light or have a limited ability to phase advance, but this has yet to be tested.[53,56] Patients have reported symptoms consistent with DSPD before the onset of FRD, a development that may occur during failed treatment attempts similar in nature to chronotherapy.[56] The development of FRD after traumatic brain injury has also been noted.[57]

Therapeutic Approaches

Both behavioral and pharmacologic options are available for the treatment of FRD, depending on whether the patient is sighted or blind. For sighted patients, the AASM Practice Parameters recommend planned sleep schedules, timed bright light exposure, and melatonin administration as treatment options, and timed melatonin administration for treating FRD in blind individuals.[10] There was insufficient evidence for using vitamin B12 for the therapy of sighted patients with FRD.[10]

Due to the rarity of the disorder in sighted individuals, most published treatments have been case reports. Exposure to bright light during the day and maintaining regular sleep, wake, and work schedules can increase the strength of entrainment, and thus should be the basic approach for all sighted patients. In addition, administration of timed melatonin in the evening has been shown to be beneficial. For example, low-dose exogenous melatonin (0.5 mg) taken at 9 PM entrained a sighted FRD patient's sleep-wake cycle to a 24-hour period.[56] Hayakawa and colleagues[58] described an FRD patient who was able to successfully entrain with light therapy in the morning. However, the patient became noncompliant with light therapy and the sleep-wake cycle began to drift. At this point, administration of melatonin, 1 mg per day at 9 PM successfully

re-entrained his sleep-wake cycle to the 24-hour day. Another FRD patient had long-term success with 3 to 5 mg melatonin taken between 9 PM and 10 PM each night, with continued response to daily treatment at a 15-month follow-up.[59] However, another study using low-dose melatonin (0.3 mg) at 5 hours, 3 hours, and 1 hour before habitual sleep-onset time demonstrated only limited effectiveness.[60]

In blind people with FRD, timed exposure to nonphotic entraining agents such as planned social and physical activities and melatonin are the primary therapies. There is strong evidence for the effectiveness of melatonin for the treatment of FRD in the blind. However, the appropriate timing and dosage of melatonin is especially important for determining its effectiveness and avoidance of side effects, such as daytime sleepiness.[61] For optimal effectiveness, the initial time of melatonin administration should be adjusted so that it occurs a few hours before the predicted endogenous melatonin onset (DLMO).[62] This methodology was used to entrain blind patients using melatonin 10 mg, 1 hour before their preferred bedtime over 3 to 9 weeks.[63,64] Once entrained to the 10-mg dose, patients maintained entrainment for 4 months with daily administration with 0.5 mg. Patients had less wake after sleep onset (WASO) and great sleep efficiency after melatonin than after placebo. However, after just several days to 1 month after discontinuation of this lower dose, there was a recurrence of a free-running rhythm.

Alternatively, treatment may be initiated with lower doses. For example, a patient with an unusually long circadian period (24.6) was unable to entrain with a 10 mg dose of melatonin,[64] but was able to successfully entrain for 161 days with a daily dose of 0.5 mg administered before bedtime.[65] Entrainment to a 24-hour period occurred by day 47 of this low dose. Before trying this lower dosage, investigators attempted a treatment of 20 mg melatonin for 60 days, which also failed to entrain this patient. It has been postulated that the higher dose may spill over into the delay phase of PRC, which would prevent entrainment. Demonstration of successful entrainment with low doses of melatonin has important clinical implications because chronic treatment with low doses may be better tolerated than high doses.[65]

Melatonin treatment of blind patients with FRD typically is considered a long-term therapy because phase drifts typically occur not long after melatonin is discontinued. Because higher doses of melatonin have been associated with sleepiness, determining the lowest effective dose is important. Using a step-down method to find the lowest effective melatonin dose in series of physiologic doses, entrainment to a normal circadian phase occurred on varying doses between 20 and 300 μg.[66] In fact, there appeared to be a linear relationship between the lowest entraining dose and the length of the patients' circadian period (tau) beyond 24 hours (tau minus 24 hours). For example, a patient with tau = 24.15 entrained at the lowest dose of 20 μg, whereas someone with a tau = 24.55 responded best to a dose of 200 μg melatonin.

IRREGULAR SLEEP-WAKE RHYTHM

Irregular sleep-wake rhythm (ISWR) is a circadian rhythm disorder characterized by the absence of a clear sleep-wake pattern. Patients with ISWR present with symptoms of insomnia, excessive daytime sleepiness, fragmented sleep, and frequent napping, depending on the timing of the sleep-wake episode. Total sleep time within a 24-hour period is typically normal, but may consist of several sleep bouts without one primary nocturnal sleep period. ISWR is most common among older adults, especially those in nursing home or care facilities, and is associated with neurologic disorders such as dementia, mental retardation, and brain injury.[67,68]

An ISWR diagnosis requires chronic complaints of insomnia and/or excessive sleepiness, the total time slept in a 24-hour period to be of normal duration for age and for symptoms to be unexplained by another sleep disorder, medication use, or medical condition.[15] Sleep logs or actigraphic monitoring for at least 7 days is recommended to reveal 3 or more irregular sleep bouts during a 24-hour period, although actigraphy may be a useful option in situations when sleep log documentation may be unreliable. Individuals who voluntarily maintain an irregular sleep schedule, perhaps due to rotating work shifts, and engage in poor sleep hygiene may report similar sleep-wake irregularities as those with ISWR, but do not meet criteria for diagnosis.[15]

Multiple factors, from a lack of exposure to structured social and physical activities and bright light[67,69] to degeneration of the central circadian clock regulation, have been proposed to be involved in the development of ISWRs. Compared with age-matched controls, there is evidence of increased loss of SCN neurons in patients with Alzheimer disease (AD).[70,71] Findings that nursing home residents who slept during the day were also found to engage in fewer physical and social activities, less light exposure, more disturbed nighttime sleep, and decreased amplitude of circadian rhythms demonstrate the importance of zeitgebers in regulating the endogenous rhythms and sleep-wake cycle.[67] Although there are no direct findings for a genetic role in ISWR, evidence demonstrates that the variance associated with longitudinal sleep disturbances in patients with AD are related to "trait"-like characteristics more so than "state" components,[72] suggesting that more genetic research is needed to determine a genetic role in the development of ISWR.

Therapeutic Approaches

The overall goals of treatment of ISWR are to increase the duration of consolidated sleep periods during the night and improve daytime function. A multitherapeutic approach combining bright light exposure, physical activity, and other behavioral modifications are indicated as effective treatments for both young and older patients with ISWR.[10] Encouraging good sleep habits and increasing the strength of circadian synchronizers, such as bright light, are basic approaches. Appropriately timed bright light therapy alone has been shown to strengthen circadian rhythms and improve sleep in patients with dementia.[73-75] In addition, behavioral strategies including structured social and physical activities and decreasing nocturnal noise in nursing homes can help improve sleep in institutionalized older adults.

Although melatonin is indicated for children with ISWR or those with psychomotor retardation, it is not recommended for older adults with dementia.[10] The efficacy of melatonin for improving sleep disturbances in patients with AD has yielded inconsistent effects, and thus was not recommend in the recent AASM Practice Parameters.[10] In a randomized multicenter clinical trial, patients with AD were assigned to take either 2.5 mg sustained-release melatonin, 10 mg immediate-release melatonin, or placebo for 8 weeks about 1 hour before habitual bedtime.[76] A nonsignificant trend toward increases in nocturnal sleep duration was found in the melatonin groups compared with placebo. However, another more recent study using either melatonin alone, bright light alone, or combined treatment of bright light (>1000 lux) and melatonin (2.5 mg) in elderly residents of group care facilities for a mean of 15 months showed improvements in sleep efficiency with the combined treatment, decreased sleep latency with melatonin, and increased sleep duration in both individual therapies.[77] Of note, treatment with only melatonin adversely affected mood. These results suggest that in an older population, a combined approach using low-dose melatonin and bright light may be the most efficacious for improving sleep and daytime function.[77]

The use of melatonin to treat circadian rhythm disorders in children with developmental disorders has shown more consistent results than in elderly nursing home patients. However, most of the evidence is derived from case reports or case control studies. Early case reports described the successful treatment of 15 multiply disabled children with melatonin therapy ranging in duration from 3 months to 1 year.[78] Doses of 2.5 to 5 mg melatonin administered at bedtime were found to induce and improve sleep, increase daytime alertness, decrease behavioral problems, and often alleviate other symptoms (eg, seizures) without any adverse effects. The 6:30 PM administration of 3 mg melatonin in children with psychomotor retardation for 4 weeks nightly improved sleep-wake patterns by increasing nocturnal sleep duration and quality while decreasing daytime sleep.[79] Comparisons of fast-release (FR) and controlled-release (CR) forms of melatonin in this population administered at bedtime for 22 days revealed that FR was better at initiating sleep, while CR helped improve sleep maintenance, early morning awakenings, and fragmentation.[80] The most effective average dose for both forms was slightly higher than that required in adults (CR mean = 5.7 mg; FR mean = 7 mg).

JET LAG DISORDER

Travel across multiple time zones can lead to jet lag, which is characterized by symptoms such as sleepiness, insomnia, fatigue, and even gastrointestinal problems.[81] Jet lag is caused by the misalignment of the endogenous circadian rhythm to the destination clock time. For example, if individuals travel from New York to London across 5 time zones, they will need to phase-shift advance about 5 hours to be fully entrained to the destination time. The more time zones crossed, the longer it takes to re-entrain the circadian rhythm.[82] Symptoms typically are transient and improve after several days at the destination location. Diagnosis of jet lag disorder requires a complaint of insomnia or excessive daytime sleepiness, as well as daytime functioning impairment or general illness linked with travel across more than 2 time zones that cannot be attributed to other causes.[15] Due to the circadian period in humans of longer than 24 hours, phase delays are typically easier to achieve[83]; thus adjustments to westward travel occur more rapidly than eastward travel.

Therapeutic Approaches

Treatments for jet lag disorder are focused on adjustment of the endogenous circadian rhythm to the destination time zone, as well as strategies aimed at improving sleep and daytime alertness. Nonpharmaceutical treatments such as good sleep hygiene, adjusting the sleep schedule before travel (when possible), and appropriately timed exposure to light have also been shown to accelerate circadian adjustment and to decrease symptoms of jet lag.[82] Appropriately timed bright light exposure and avoidance of light at the wrong time of the day have been shown to be effective strategies to accelerate entrainment of circadian rhythms. The timing of light exposure depends on the direction of travel and the number of time zones crossed. For example, on an eastward flight from New York to London, when arriving in the early morning one should avoid bright light, but get as much light as possible in the late morning to early afternoon.[84] In summary, strategic exposure to light seems to be a safe and potentially beneficial therapy for air travelers who suffer from jet lag.[85,86]

Pharmacologic approaches include melatonin and hypnotic medications. Data support the use of melatonin to minimize jet lag, although it is not FDA-approved for the treatment of jet lag disorder. The general recommendation is melatonin, 2 to 5 mg be taken before bedtime on arrival, and dosing may be repeated for up to 4 days as needed.[84,87] Potential adverse effects such as headaches, nausea, and exacerbation of cardiovascular disease in patients at risk should be considered. Subjects who took 5 mg melatonin for 3 days preflight at 6 PM and for 4 days at bedtime after eastward travel subjectively rated their jet lag symptoms as less severe than those in the placebo group.[88] Melatonin treatment with 5 mg administered 3 days before departure (between 10:00 AM and noon) and while at the destination time zone (between 10 PM and midnight) on both outbound (eastward) and inbound (westward) flights across 12 time zones decreased jet lag symptoms compared with placebo.[89] A comparison of 0.5 mg FR, 5 mg FR, 2 mg CR melatonin, and placebo administered at bedtime for 4 days after the flight was conducted on individuals traveling eastward across 6 to 8 time zones.[90] The 5-mg FR group had significantly improved sleep quality, shortened sleep latency, and decreased wake during the night by day 2 of the treatment, and continued to increase sleep duration compared with the other groups. All doses of melatonin made it easier to get up in the morning, and patients felt more rested and improved mood versus placebo.[90] Beaumont and colleagues[91] showed that 5 mg melatonin taken at bedtime improved measures of sleep and subjective sleepiness following an eastbound flight across 7 time zones, and 300 mg of slow-release caffeine taken at 8 AM reduced self-rated sleepiness but negatively affected sleep maintenance. These results suggest that slow-release caffeine and melatonin may be of value for alleviating some symptoms of jet lag.

The use of hypnotic medications specifically focused on promoting nocturnal sleep at the new destination has also been studied. Benzodiazepines and newer nonbenzodiazepines, typically used to treat insomnia, were examined to determine their efficacy in the treatment of jet lag. In a simulation study, the short-acting benzodiazepine triazolam was administered 3 hours before bedtime for 5 days after the 8-hour delayed shift (westbound travel across 8 time zones).[92] Administration of 0.5 mg triazolam at bedtime for the first 4 nights significantly improved circadian adaptation compared with placebo, with triazolam inducing an additional shift delay of more than 2 hours by day 3. In contrast, 10 mg of the benzodiazepine temazepam at bedtime for 3 nights after a 5-hour westbound flight revealed no improvements of jet lag symptoms compared with placebo.[93] In an operational setting, 5 mg zopiclone and 2 mg melatonin, single doses taken near bedtime, equally facilitated sleep after an eastbound flight across 5 time zones.[94] Participants had longer sleep duration, shorter sleep latency, less time awake, and reported an overall better quality of sleep after both treatments versus placebo. Zopiclone (7.5 mg) administered at bedtime for 4 nights diminished jet lag—related sleep disturbances following transatlantic westward flights including increased sleep duration, reduced sleep fragmentation, and improved sleep quality compared with placebo.[95] The rest-activity cycle and core body temperature rhythm synchronized and adapted to the destination clock time more rapidly after zopiclone than with placebo, even though jet lag ratings did not differ between groups. Zolpidem (10 mg) taken at bedtime for 3 nights increased sleep duration, decreased nocturnal awakenings, and improved sleep quality compared with placebo during the first 2 nights taken after transatlantic eastward travel (5—9 time zones).[96] Subjective ratings of mood and alertness did not differ between the 2 groups, suggesting that the effects of circadian misalignment involved with jet lag were still apparent, even though sleep itself had improved. A recent study of ramelteon, a melatonin receptor agonist, showed an improvement in the latency to persistent sleep with a 1 mg dose administered before bedtime for 4 nights after eastward travel.[90]

Pycnogenol, an extract from the bark of the French maritime pine, has been shown to help prevent edema associated with long flights.[97]

Recent preliminary results showed that administration of 50 mg oral pycnogenol 3 times daily commencing 2 days before the 7- to 9-hour flight significantly decreased the severity and duration of jet lag symptoms (fatigue, sleep disturbance, and short-term memory).[98] In addition, computed tomography scans performed within 28 hours post flight revealed less brain edema in the pycnogenol group.

Based on the evidence, the AASM Practice Parameters recommend timed melatonin administration to reduce jet lag symptoms.[10] Other treatment options indicated include maintaining home-based sleep hours for brief travel, short-term hypnotic use for insomnia, and caffeine to counteract sleepiness. For eastward travel, the combination of shifting sleep schedule an hour earlier for 3 days before travel and morning light exposure is also suggested to improve symptoms.[10,82]

SHIFT WORK DISORDER

Many American workers have jobs requiring evening, night, or rotation work schedules. Approximately 30% of this population[99] complains for at least 1 month of excessive sleepiness and insomnia in relation to a work schedule falling during the time of habitual sleep, which are the symptoms that characterize shift work disorder (SWD).[15] Sleep logs or actigraphy monitoring for at least 7 days is recommended for diagnosis of SWD, and other sleep disorders and conditions should be ruled out.[15] This disorder has also been associated with poor performance, cardiovascular, gastrointestinal, and reproductive problems, accidents, illness, and depression.[99,100] These issues occur because the endogenous circadian rhythms are not synchronized with the altered sleep-wake cycle because of shift work.

Sleep is curtailed typically by 1 to 4 hours in patients with SWD, with most complaints associated with night and early morning work. These sleep problems may be misinterpreted as either sleep initiation or maintenance issues, as the individual is attempting to sleep at a clock time misaligned with the endogenous rhythm. Also, reports of excessive sleepiness occur during their work shift when they are awake, but sleep propensity is high. Symptoms may persist during days off due to the circadian rhythm disruption, often resulting in reverting back to a normal schedule of sleeping at night when not working.

Therapeutic Approaches

Clinical management of SWD is aimed at realigning circadian rhythms with the sleep and work schedules, as well as improving sleep, alertness, and safety. Although early morning and rotational shifts are commonly associated with SWD, most of the strategies developed for adjustment to shift work have focused on the night-shift worker. Non-pharmacologic treatments are basic to the management of SWD. Family and social factors that disturb sleep can impair adjustment to shift work. Optimizing the sleep environment, adherence to healthy sleep habits, and planned naps, when possible, should be encouraged for all patients.[101]

Similar to jet lag, appropriately timed bright light therapy and avoidance of light at the wrong time of the day can help accelerate and maintain entrainment to the shift schedule. For night workers circadian rhythms need to be delayed, so that the highest sleep propensity occurs during the day rather than at night. Most studies used light intensities between 1200 and 10,000 lux for a period of 3 to 6 hours during the night shift.[102] Intermittent bright light exposure (~20 min/h blocks) has also being shown to accelerate circadian adaptation to night-shift work.[103,104] In addition to its circadian phase resetting effects, light has acute alerting effects that can be useful during the work period.[105] Another complementary strategy is to avoid exposure to morning bright light during the morning commute home.[104,106] Recently in a simulated shift work paradigm, a combination of enforced sleep-wake schedule and intermittent bright light exposure during the night shift was used to achieve a compromised phase position, including on the days off. Under these conditions, there was improvement in performance.[107] A compromise phase position has the potential to improve performance and sleep on work days as well as on days off.

Studies on the effectiveness of melatonin for the treatment of SWD have been mixed,[108–114] and may be limited by use of different doses and formulations. For example, melatonin (6 mg) taken before daytime sleep after 4 to 6 consecutive nights of shift work was ineffective,[108] whereas other studies showed increased alertness during the subsequent night shift after taking 10 mg in the morning before bedtime for 2 to 5 days,[110] and overall improvement in sleep quality when treated with 5 mg in the morning for 6 consecutive days.[111] In addition, the administration of 1.8 mg CR melatonin after 2 consecutive night shifts before daytime sleep increased sleep duration and sleep quality after the first administration, but not after the second.[112] Although it appears that when taken at bedtime after the night shift melatonin can improve daytime sleep, it may have limited effects on alertness at work.[102]

Melatonin is not approved by the FDA for the treatment of SWD, and one should also be aware of potential side effects such as headaches, vivid dreams, nausea, and cardiovascular effects.

Other pharmaceuticals often used for the treatment of sleep disturbance and excessive sleepiness in shift workers include hypnotics for sleep and stimulants for maintaining alertness. However, these approaches do not specifically address the issue of circadian misalignment, and thus should be used in concert with behavioral strategies as already discussed. Several studies have used benzodiazepine receptor agonist hypnotics. For example, treatment with temazepam (20 mg), single dose administered at bedtime, increased daytime sleep duration but did not improve nighttime sleepiness,[115] and zopiclone (7.5 mg), taken 30 minutes before bedtime, increased sleep quality in shift workers without negatively impacting night work performance.[116]

Stimulants such as caffeine can be used to help manage sleepiness. The combination of napping and caffeine alleviated negative symptoms associated with shift work.[117] Naps of 2 to 2.5 hours in the evening before the first 2 of 4 consecutive simulated nights in addition to 4 mg/kg (laboratory study) or 300 mg (field study) caffeine administered 30 minutes before each night shift was more effective at improving alertness and performance than caffeine or naps alone.

Therapy with wake-promoting agents such as modafinil and armodafinil reduced sleepiness associated with night-shift work. Administration of 200 mg of modafinil before commencing a simulated night shift was shown to increase alertness, and maintain levels of vigilance and cognitive function, without disruptions to daytime sleep compared with placebo,[118] and in a multicenter field study modafinil (200 mg) reduced sleepiness and increased alertness in patients with SWD.[119] Recent studies with armodafinil (an isomer of modafinil) 150 mg before the night shift reduced sleepiness into the morning, improved cognitive performance at night, and diminished severity of SWD symptoms.[120] Both modafinil and armodafinil have been approved by the FDA for the treatment of excessive sleepiness associated with SWD.

A combination of optimizing the sleep environment, planned naps, timed bright light exposure at work, avoiding bright light exposure in the early morning (for night-shift workers), and melatonin before bedtime can both facilitate circadian adaptation and improve symptoms of SWSD. However, when excessive sleepiness persists, the use of wake-promoting agents such as modafinil or armodafinil is indicated. Based on the evidence, practice parameters set forth by the AASM indicate planned napping before or during a work shift, timed light exposure, and stimulants such as caffeine of modafinil during the night shift to improve alertness.[10]

SUMMARY AND FUTURE DIRECTIONS

The impact of CRSD is likely greater than estimated in terms of limited recognition, misdiagnoses, and health consequences. This situation may in part be due to a combination of a lack of practical tools to measure circadian rhythms and that most therapies, including light and melatonin, have not been rigorously tested in multicenter randomized clinical trials. Therefore, with the exception of modafinil and armodafinil for the treatment of excessive sleepiness associated with SWD, there are no other FDA-approved therapies for the treatment of CRSDs.

Of the pharmacologic approaches, melatonin has shown the most success for improving the alignment or amplitude of circadian rhythms, including the sleep-wake cycle, especially in patients with DSPD, FRD, children with ISWR, and jet lag disorder. In addition, hypnotic and wake-promoting agents have been used for the symptomatic management of insomnia symptoms and excessive sleepiness associated with various CRSDs, particularly SWD and jet lag. Despite its potential, the pharmacotherapy for CRSD using melatonin has been limited by the inconsistent dose, timing of administration, and differences in formulations used in the various studies. There are also limited data from randomized large scale clinical trials on its effectiveness and long-term safety.

New formulations, including sustained-release and transdermal delivery, have shown clinical potential. Furthermore, recent data demonstrating the ability of selective melatonin receptor agonists such as ramelteon, tasimelteon, and agomelatine to induce phase shifts of the circadian clock has prompted investigation of their usefulness in the treatment of several CRSDs. There is clearly a need for clinically definitive randomized clinical trials in patient populations with CRSDs to determine the efficacy and safety of behavioral and pharmacologic therapies, either alone or in combination.

REFERENCES

1. Wever RA. Light effects on human circadian rhythms: a review of recent Andechs experiments. J Biol Rhythms 1989;4(2):161–85.

2. Sadun AA, Schaechter JD, Smith LE. A retinohypothalamic pathway in man: light mediation of circadian rhythms. Brain Res 1984;302:371–7.

3. Czeisler CA, Richardson GS, Coleman RM, et al. Chronotherapy: resetting the circadian clocks of patients with delayed sleep phase insomnia. Sleep 1981;4(1):1–21.

4. Lewy AJ, Wehr TA, Goodwin FK, et al. Light suppresses melatonin secretion in humans. Science 1980;210:1267–9.

5. Zawilska JB, Skene DJ, Arendt J. Physiology and pharmacology of melatonin in relation to biological rhythms. Pharmacol Rep 2009;61:383–410.

6. Lewy AJ, Sack RL. The dim light melatonin onset as a marker for circadian phase position. Chronobiol Int 1989;6:93–102.

7. Lewy AJ, Cutler NL, Sack RL. The endogenous melatonin profile as a marker for circadian phase position. J Biol Rhythms 1999;14(3):227–36.

8. Lewy AJ, Bauer VK, Ahmed S, et al. The human phase response curve (PRC) to melatonin is about 12 hours out of phase with the PRC to light. Chronobiol Int 1998;15:71–83.

9. Lewy AJ, Ahmed S, Jackson JML, et al. Melatonin shifts circadian rhythms according to a phase-response curve. Chronobiol Int 1992;9:380–92.

10. Morgenthaler TI, Lee-Chiong T, Alessi C, et al. Practice parameters for the clinical evaluation and treatment of circadian rhythm sleep disorders. Sleep 2007;30(11):1445–59.

11. Schrader H, Bovim G, Sand T. The prevalence of delayed and advanced sleep phase syndromes. J Sleep Res 1993;2:51–5.

12. Weitzman ED, Czeisler CA, Coleman RM, et al. Delayed sleep phase syndrome. Arch Gen Psychiatry 1981;38:737–46.

13. Regestein QR, Monk TH. Delayed sleep phase syndrome: a review of its clinical aspects. Am J Psychiatry 1995;152(4):602–8.

14. Chang AM, Reid KJ, Gourineni R, et al. Sleep timing and circadian phase in delayed sleep phase syndrome. J Biol Rhythms 2009;24(4):313–21.

15. American Academy of Sleep Medicine. The international classification of sleep disorders: diagnostic & coding manual. 2nd edition. Westchester (IL): American Academy of Sleep Medicine; 2005.

16. Aoki H, Ozeki Y, Yamada N. Hypersensitivity of melatonin suppression in response to light in patients with delayed sleep phase syndrome. Chronobiol Int 2001;18(2):263–71.

17. Wakatsuki Y, Kudo T, Shibata S. Constant light housing during nursing causes human DSPS (delayed sleep phase syndrome) behaviour in *Clock*-mutant mice. Eur J Neurosci 2007;25:2413–24.

18. Archer SN, Robilliard DL, Skene DJ, et al. A length polymorphism in the circadian clock gene *Per3* is

linked to delayed sleep phase syndrome and extreme diurnal preference. Sleep 2003;26(4): 413–5.

19. Rosenthal NE, Joseph-Vanderpool JR, Levendosky AA, et al. Phase-shifting effects of bright morning light as treatment for delayed sleep phase syndrome. Sleep 1990;13(4):354–61.

20. Cole RJ, Smith JS, Alcala YC, et al. Bright-light mask treatment of delayed sleep phase syndrome. J Biol Rhythms 2002;17:89–101.

21. Boivin DB, Duffy JF, Kronauer RE, et al. Dose-response relationships for resetting of human circadian clock by light. Nature 1996;379:540–2.

22. Hashimoto S, Kohsaka M, Morita N, et al. Vitamin B12 enhances the phase-response of circadian melatonin rhythm to a single bright light exposure in humans. Neurosci Lett 1996;220:129–32.

23. Yamadera H, Takahashi K, Okawa M. A multicenter study of sleep-wake rhythm disorders: therapeutic effects of vitamin B12, bright light therapy, chronotherapy and hypnotics. Psychiatry Clin Neurosci 1996;50:203–9.

24. Okawa M, Uchiyama M, Ozaki S, et al. Circadian rhythm sleep disorders in adolescents: clinical trials of combined treatments based on chronobiology. Psychiatry Clin Neurosci 1998;52(5):483–90.

25. Okawa M, Takahashi K, Egashira K, et al. Viatmin B12 treatment for delayed sleep phase syndrome: a multi-center double-blind study. Psychiatry Clin Neurosci 1997;51:275–9.

26. Dahlitz M, Alvarez B. Delayed sleep phase syndrome response to melatonin. Lancet 1991; 337:1121–4.

27. Nagtegaal JE, Kerkhof GA, Smits MG, et al. Delayed sleep phase syndrome: a placebo-controlled crossover study on the effects of melatonin administered five hours before the individual dim light melatonin onset. J Sleep Res 1998;7:135–43.

28. Kayumov L, Brown G, Jindal R, et al. A randomized, double-blind, placebo-controlled crossover study of the effect of exogenous melatonin on delayed sleep phase syndrome. Psychosom Med 2001;63:40–8.

29. Mundey K, Benloucif S, Harsanyi K, et al. Phase-dependent treatment of delayed sleep phase syndrome with melatonin. Sleep 2005;28(10): 1271–8.

30. Dagan Y, Yovel I, Hallis D, et al. Evaluating the role of melatonin in the long-term treatment of delayed sleep phase syndrome. Chronobiol Int 1998; 15(2):181–90.

31. Smits MG, Nagtegaal EE, van der Heijden J, et al. Melatonin for chronic sleep onset insomnia in children: a randomized placebo-controlled trial. J Child Neurol 2001;16:86–92.

32. Tjon Pian Gi CV, Broeren JPA, Starreveld JS, et al. Melatonin for the treatment of sleeping disorders in children with attention deficit/hyperactivity disorder: a preliminary open label study. Eur J Pediatr 2003;162:554–5.

33. Van der Heijden KB, Smits MG, Van Someren EJW, et al. Effect of melatonin on sleep, behavior, and cognition in ADHD and chronic sleep-onset insomnia. J Am Acad Child Adolesc Psychiatry 2007;46(2):233–41.

34. Hoebert M, van der Heijden KB, van Geijlswijk IM, et al. Long-term follow-up of melatonin treatment in children with ADHA and chronic sleep onset insomnia. J Pineal Res 2009;47:1–7.

35. Ebisawa T. Circadian rhythms in CNS and peripheral clock disorders: human sleep disorders and clock genes. J Pharmacol Sci 2007;103:150–4.

36. Lack LC, Mercer JD, Wright H. Circadian rhythms of early morning awakening insomniacs. J Sleep Res 1996;5:211–9.

37. Satoh K, Mishima K, Inoue Y, et al. Two pedigrees of familial advanced sleep phase syndrome in Japan. Sleep 2003;26(4):416–7.

38. Jones CR, Campbell SS, Zone SE, et al. Familial advanced sleep-phase syndrome: a short-period circadian rhythm variant in humans. Nat Med 1999;5(9):1062–5.

39. Reid KJ, Chang AM, Dubocovich ML, et al. Familial advanced sleep phase syndrome. Arch Neurol 2001;58:1089–94.

40. Toh KL, Jones CR, He Y, et al. An hPer2 phosphorylation site mutation in familial advanced sleep phase syndrome. Science 2001;291:1040–3.

41. Lack L, Wright H. The effect of evening bright light in delaying the circadian rhythms and lengthening the sleep of early morning awakening insomniacs. Sleep 1993;16(5):436–43.

42. Lack L, Wright H, Kemp K, et al. The treatment of early-morning awakening insomnia with 2 evenings of bright light. Sleep 2005;28(5):616–23.

43. Lack LC, Wright HR. Treating chronobiological components of chronic insomnia. Sleep Med 2007;8(6):637–44.

44. Zee PC. Melatonin for the treatment of advanced sleep phase disorder. Sleep 2008;31(7):923.

45. Hughes RJ, Sack RL, Lewy AJ. The role of melatonin and circadian phase in age-related sleep-maintenance insomnia: assessment in a clinical trial of melatonin replacement. Sleep 1998;21(1): 52–68.

46. Taylor SR, Weiss JS. Review of insomnia pharmacotherapy options for the elderly: implications for managed care. Popul Health Manag 2009;12(6): 317–23.

47. Kamgar-Parsi B, Wehr TA, Gillin JC. Successful treatment of human non-24-hour sleep-wake syndrome. Sleep 1983;6(3):257–64.

48. Uchiyam M, Shibui K, Hayakawa T, et al. Larger phase angle between sleep propensity and

melatonin rhythms in sighted humans with non-24-hour sleep-wake syndrome. Sleep 2002;25(1):83–8.

49. Sack RL, Lewy AJ, Blood ML, et al. Circadian rhythm abnormalities in totally blind people: incidence and clinical significance. J Clin Endocrinol Metab 1992;75(1):127–34.

50. Nakagawa H, Sack RL, Lewy AJ. Sleep propensity free-runs with the temperature, melatonin and cortisol rhythms in a totally blind person. Sleep 1992;15(4):330–6.

51. Lockley SW, Skene DJ, Arendt J, et al. Relationship between melatonin rhythms and visual loss in the blind. J Clin Endocrinol Metab 1997;82(11):3763–70.

52. Lewy AJ, Emens JS, Bernert RA, et al. Eventual entrainment of the human circadian pacemaker by melatonin is independent of the circadian phase of treatment initiation: clinical implications. J Biol Rhythms 2004;19:68–75.

53. Hashimoto S, Nakamura K, Honma S, et al. Free-running circadian rhythm of melatonin in a sighted man despite a 24-hour sleep pattern: a non-24-hour circadian syndrome. Psychiatry Clin Neurosci 1997;51:109–14.

54. Hayakawa T, Uchiyama M, Kamei Y, et al. Clinical analyses of sighted patients with non-24-hour sleep-wake syndrome: a study of 57 consecutively diagnosed cases. Sleep 2005;28(8):945–52.

55. Kamei Y, Urata J, Uchiyaya M, et al. Clinical characteristics of circadian rhythm sleep disorders. Psychiatry Clin Neurosci 1998;52:234–5.

56. McArthur AJ, Lewy AJ, Sack RL. Non-24-hour sleep-wake syndrome in a sighted man: circadian rhythm studies and efficacy of melatonin treatment. Sleep 1996;19(7):544–53.

57. Boivin DB, James FO, Santo JB, et al. Non-24-hour sleep-wake syndrome following a car accident. Neurology 2003;60:1841–3.

58. Hayakawa T, Kamei Y, Urata J, et al. Trials of bright light exposure and melatonin administration in a patient with non-24-hour sleep-wake syndrome. Psychiatry Clin Neurosci 1998;52:261–2.

59. Siebler M, Steinmetz H, Freund HJ. Therapeutic entrainment of circadian rhythm disorder by melatonin in a non-blind patient. J Neurol 1998;245:327–8.

60. Kamei Y, Hayakawa T, Urata J, et al. Melatonin treatment for circadian rhythm sleep disorders. Psychiatry Clin Neurosci 2000;5:381–2.

61. Lockley SW, Skene DJ, Tabandeh H, et al. Relationship between napping and melatonin in the blind. J Biol Rhythms 1997;12:16–25.

62. Lockley SW, Skene DJ, James K, et al. Melatonin administration can entrain the free-running circadian system of blind subjects. J Endocrinol 2000;164:R1–6.

63. Lewy AJ, Hasler BP, Emens JS, et al. Pretreatment circadian period in free-running blind people may predict the phase angle of entrainment to melatonin. Neurosci Lett 2001;313:158–60.

64. Sack RL, Brandes RW, Kendall AR, et al. Entrainment of free-running circadian rhythms by melatonin in blind people. N Engl J Med 2000;343:1070–7.

65. Lewy AJ, Emens JS, Sack RL, et al. Low, but not high, doses of melatonin entrained a free-running blind person with a long circadian period. Chronobiol Int 2002;19(3):649–58.

66. Lewy AJ, Emens JS, Lefler BJ, et al. Melatonin entrains free-running blind people according to a physiological dose-response curve. Chronobiol Int 2005;22(6):1093–106.

67. Martin JL, Webber AP, Alan T, et al. Daytime sleeping, sleep disturbance, and circadian rhythms in the nursing home. Am J Geriatr Psychiatry 2006;14(2):121–9.

68. Jacobs D, Ancoli-Israel S, Parker L, et al. Twenty-four-hour sleep-wake patterns in a nursing home population. Psychol Aging 1989;4(3):352–6.

69. Campbell SS, Kripke DF, Gillin JC, et al. Exposure to light in healthy elderly subjects and Alzheimer's patients. Physiol Behav 1988;42(2):141–4.

70. Swaab DF, Fliers E, Partiman TS. The suprachiasmatic nucleus of the human brain in relation to sex, age and senile dementia. Brain Res 1985;342:37–44.

71. Swaab DF. Ageing of the human hypothalamus. Horm Res 1995;43(1–3):8–11.

72. Yesavage JA, Taylor JL, Kraemer H, et al. Sleep/wake cycle disturbance in Alzheimer's disease: how much is due to an inherent trait? Int Psychogeriatr 2002;14(1):73–81.

73. Dowling GA, Mastick J, Hubbard EM, et al. Effect of light treatment for rest-activity disruption in institutionalized patients with Alzheimer's disease. Int J Geriatr Psychiatry 2005;20:738–43.

74. Ancoli-Israel S, Gehrman P, Martin JL, et al. Increased light exposure consolidates sleep and strengthens circadian rhythms in severe Alzheimer's disease patients. Behav Sleep Med 2003;1(1):22–36.

75. Fetveit A, Skjerve A, Bjorvatn B. Bright light treatment improves sleep in institutionalized elderly—an open trial. Int J Geriatr Psychiatry 2003;18:520–6.

76. Singer C, Tractenberg RE, Kaye J, et al. A multi-center, placebo-controlled trial of melatonin for sleep disturbance in Alzheimer's disease. Sleep 2003;26(7):893–901.

77. Riemersma-van der Lek RF, Swaab DF, Twisk J, et al. Effect of bright light and melatonin on cognitive and noncognitive function in elderly residents of group care facilities. JAMA 2008;299(22):2642–55.

78. Jan JE, Espezel H, Appleton RE. The treatment of sleep disorders with melatonin. Dev Med Child Neurol 1994;36:97–107.

79. Pillar G, Shahar E, Peled N, et al. Melatonin improves sleep-wake patterns in psychomotor retarded children. Pediatr Neurol 2000;23:225–8.

80. Jan JE, Hamilton D, Seward N, et al. Clinical trials of controlled-release melatonin in children with sleep-wake cycle disorders. J Pineal Res 2000; 29:34–9.

81. Arendt J, Marks V. Physiological changes underlying jet lag. BMJ 1982;284:144–6.

82. Burgess HJ, Crowley S, Gazda CJ, et al. Preflight adjustment to eastward travel: 3 days of advancing sleep with and without morning bright light. J Biol Rhythms 2003;18(4):318–28.

83. Czeisler CA, Weitzman ED, Moore-Ede MC, et al. Human sleep: its duration and organization depend on its circadian phase. Science 1980; 210:1264–7.

84. Herxheimer A, Waterhouse J. The prevention and treatment of jet lag. BMJ 2003;326(7384):296–7.

85. Boivin DB, James FO. Phase-dependent effect of room light exposure in a 5-h advance of the sleep-wake cycle: implications for jet lag. J Biol Rhythms 2002;17(3):266–76.

86. Boulos Z, Campbell SS, Lewy AJ, et al. Light treatment for sleep disorders: consensus report. VII. Jet lag. J Biol Rhythms 1995;10(2):167–76.

87. Herxheimer A, Petrie KJ. Melatonin for the prevention and treatment of jet lag. Cochrane Database Syst Rev 2002;(2):CD001520.

88. Arendt J, Aldhous M, Marks V. Alleviation of jet lag by melatonin: preliminary results of a controlled double blind trial. BMJ 1986;292:1170.

89. Petrie K, Conaglen JV, Thompson L, et al. Effect of melatonin on jet lag after long haul flights. BMJ 1989;298:705–7.

90. Suhner A, Schlagenhauf P, Johnson R, et al. Comparative study to determine the optimal melatonin dosage form for the alleviation of jet lag. Chronobiol Int 1998;15(6):655–66.

91. Beaumont M, Batejat D, Pierard C, et al. Caffeine or melatonin effects on sleep and sleepiness after rapid eastward transmeridian travel. J Appl Physiol 2004;96:50–8.

92. Buxton OM, Copinschi G, Onderbergen AV, et al. A benzodiazepine hypnotic facilitates adaptation of circadian rhythms and sleep-wake homeostasis to an eight hour delay shift simulating westward jet lag. Sleep 2000;23(7):915–27.

93. Reilly T, Atkinson G, Budgett R. Effect of low-dose temazepam on physiological variables and performance tests following a westerly flight across five time zones. Int J Sports Med 2001;22:166–74.

94. Paul MA, Gray G, Sardana TM, et al. Melatonin and zopiclone as facilitators of early circadian sleep in operational air transport crews. Aviat Space Environ Med 2004;75:439–43.

95. Daurat A, Benoit O, Buguet A. Effects of zopiclone on the rest/activity rhythm after a westward flight across five time zones. Psychopharmacology 2000;149:241–5.

96. Jamieson AO, Zammit GK, Rosenberg RS, et al. Zolpidem reduces the sleep disturbance of jet lag. Sleep Med 2001;2(5):423–30.

97. Cesarone MR, Belcaro G, Rohdewald P, et al. Prevention of edema in long flights with Pycnogenol. Clin Appl Thromb Hemost 2005;11(3):289–94.

98. Belcaro G, Cesarone MR, Steigerwalt RJ, et al. Jet-lag: prevention with Pycnogenol. Preliminary report: evaluation in healthy individuals and in hypertensive patients. Minerva Cardioangiol 2008; 56(Suppl 5):3–9.

99. Drake CL, Roehrs T, Richardson G, et al. Shift work sleep disorder: prevalence and consequences beyond that of symptomatic day workers. Sleep 2004;27(8):1453–62.

100. Knutsson A. Health disorders of shift workers. Occup Med 2003;53:103–8.

101. Purnell MT, Feyer A-M, Herbison GP. The impact of a nap opportunity during the night shift on the performance and alertness of 12-h shift workers. J Sleep Res 2002;11:219–27.

102. Burgess HJ, Sharkey KM, Eastman CI. Bright light, dark and melatonin can promote circadian adaptation in night shift workers. Sleep Med Rev 2002; 6(5):407–20.

103. Crowley SJ, Lee C, Tseng CY, et al. Combinations of bright light, scheduled dark, sunglasses, and melatonin to facilitate circadian entrainment to night shift work. J Biol Rhythms 2003;18(6): 513–23.

104. Boivin DB, James FO. Circadian adaptation to night-shift work by judicious light and darkness exposure. J Biol Rhythms 2002;17(6):556–67.

105. Campbell SS, Dijk DJ, Boulos Z, et al. Light treatment for sleep disorders: consensus report. III. Alerting and activating effects. J Biol Rhythms 1995;10(2):129–32.

106. Eastman CI, Stewart KT, Mahoney MP, et al. Dark goggles and right light improve circadian rhythm adaptation to night-shift work. Sleep 1994;17(6): 535–43.

107. Smith MR, Fogg LF, Eastman CI. Practical interventions to promote circadian adaptation to permanent night shift work: study 4. J Biol Rhythms 2009; 24(2):161–72.

108. James M, Trema MO, Jones JS, et al. Can melatonin improve adaptation to night shift? Am J Emerg Med 1998;16(4):367–70.

109. Sadeghniiat-Haghighi K, Aminian O, Pouryaghoub G, et al. Efficacy and hypnotic effects of melatonin in shift-work nurses:

double-blind, placebo-controlled crossover trial. J Circadian Rhythms 2008;6:10.

110. Jorgensen KM, Witting MD. Does exogenous melatonin improve day sleep or night alertness in emergency physicians working night shifts? Ann Emerg Med 1998;31:699–704.

111. Folkard S, Arendt J, Clark M. Can melatonin improve shift workers' tolerance of the night shift? Some preliminary findings. Chronobiol Int 1993; 10(5):315–20.

112. Sharkey KM, Fogg LF, Eastman CI. Effects of melatonin administration on daytime sleep after simulated night shift work. J Sleep Res 2001;10: 181–92.

113. Rajaratnam SMW, Polymeropoulos MH, Fisher DM, et al. Melatonin agonist tasimelteon (VEC-162) for transient insomnia after sleep-time shift: two randomized controlled multicentre trials. Lancet 2009;373:482–91.

114. Aeschbach D, Lockyer BJ, Dijk DJ, et al. Use of transdermal melatonin delivery to improve sleep maintenance during daytime. Clin Pharmacol Ther 2009;86(4):378–82.

115. Porcu S, Bellatreccia A, Ferrara M, et al. Performance, ability to stay awake, and tendency to fall asleep during the night after a diurnal sleep with temazepam or placebo. Sleep 1997;20(7):535–41.

116. Monchesky TC, Billings BJ, Phillips R, et al. Zopiclone in insomniac shiftworkers. Int Arch Occup Environ Health 1989;61:255–9.

117. Schweitzer PK, Randazzo AC, Stone K, et al. Laboratory and field studies of naps and caffeine as practical countermeasures for sleep-wake problems associated with night work. Sleep 2006; 29(1):39–50.

118. Walsh JK, Randazzo AC, Stone K, et al. Modafinil improves alertness, vigilance, and executive function during simulated night shifts. Sleep 2004; 27(3):434–9.

119. Czeisler CA, Walsh JK, Roth T, et al. Modafinil for excessive sleepiness associated with shift-work sleep disorder. N Engl J Med 2005;353:476–86.

120. Czeisler CA, Walsh JK, Wesnes KA, et al. Armodafinil for treatment of excessive sleepiness associated with shift work sleep disorder: a randomized controlled study. Mayo Clin Proc 2009;84(11):958–72.

Index

Note: Page numbers of article titles are in **boldface** type.

Sleep Med Clin 5 (2010) 717–724
doi:10.1016/S1556-407X(10)00109-8
1556-407X/10/$ – see front matter © 2010 Elsevier Inc. All rights reserved.

sleep.theclinics.com

United States Postal Service

Statement of Ownership, Management, and Circulation
(All Periodicals Publications Except Requestor Publications)

1. Publication Title	2. Publication Number		3. Filing Date
Sleep Medicine Clinics of North America	0 2 5 - 0 5 3		9/15/10

4. Issue Frequency	5. Number of Issues Published Annually	6. Annual Subscription Price
Mar, Jun, Sep, Dec	4	$150.00

7. Complete Mailing Address of Known Office of Publication (*Not printer*) (*Street, city, county, state, and ZIP+4®*)

Elsevier Inc.
360 Park Avenue South
New York, NY 10010-1710

Contact Person
Stephen Bushing

Telephone (*Include area code*)
215-239-3688

8. Complete Mailing Address of Headquarters or General Business Office of Publisher (*Not printer*)

Elsevier Inc., 360 Park Avenue South, New York, NY 10010-1710

9. Full Names and Complete Mailing Addresses of Publisher, Editor, and Managing Editor (*Do not leave blank*)

Publisher (*Name and complete mailing address*)

Kim Murphy, Elsevier, Inc., 1600 John F. Kennedy Blvd. Suite 1800, Philadelphia, PA 19103-2899

Editor (*Name and complete mailing address*)

Sarah Barth, Elsevier, Inc., 1600 John F. Kennedy Blvd. Suite 1800, Philadelphia, PA 19103-2899

Managing Editor (*Name and complete mailing address*)

Catherine Bewick, Elsevier, Inc., 1600 John F. Kennedy Blvd. Suite 1800, Philadelphia, PA 19103-2899

10. Owner (*Do not leave blank. If the publication is owned by a corporation, give the name and address of the corporation immediately followed by the names and addresses of all stockholders owning or holding 1 percent or more of the total amount of stock. If not owned by a corporation, give the names and addresses of the individual owners. If owned by a partnership or other unincorporated firm, give its name and address as well as those of each individual owner. If the publication is published by a nonprofit organization, give its name and address.*)

Full Name	Complete Mailing Address
Wholly owned subsidiary of	4520 East-West Highway
Reed/Elsevier, US holdings	Bethesda, MD 20814

11. Known Bondholders, Mortgagees, and Other Security Holders Owning or Holding 1 Percent or More of Total Amount of Bonds, Mortgages, or Other Securities. If none, check box ☐ None

Full Name	Complete Mailing Address
N/A	

12. Tax Status (*For completion by nonprofit organizations authorized to mail at nonprofit rates*) (*Check one*)
The purpose, function, and nonprofit status of this organization and the exempt status for federal income tax purposes:
☐ Has Not Changed During Preceding 12 Months
☐ Has Changed During Preceding 12 Months (*Publisher must submit explanation of change with this statement*)

PS Form 3526, September 2007 (Page 1 of 3 (Instructions Page 3)) PSN 7530-01-000-9931 PRIVACY NOTICE: See our Privacy policy in www.usps.com

---

13. Publication Title	14. Issue Date for Circulation Data Below
Sleep Medicine Clinics of North America	September 2010

15. Extent and Nature of Circulation			Average No. Copies Each Issue During Preceding 12 Months	No. Copies of Single Issue Published Nearest to Filing Date
a. Total Number of Copies (*Net press run*)			972	961
b. Paid Circulation (By Mail and Outside the Mail)	(1)	Mailed Outside-County Paid Subscriptions Stated on PS Form 3541. (*Include paid distribution above nominal rate, advertiser's proof copies, and exchange copies*)	496	491
	(2)	Mailed In-County Paid Subscriptions Stated on PS Form 3541 (*Include paid distribution above nominal rate, advertiser's proof copies, and exchange copies*)		
	(3)	Paid Distribution Outside the Mails Including Sales Through Dealers and Carriers, Street Vendors, Counter Sales, and Other Paid Distribution Outside USPS®	56	49
	(4)	Paid Distribution by Other Classes Mailed Through the USPS (e.g. First-Class Mail®)		
c. Total Paid Distribution (*Sum of 15b (1), (2), (3), and (4)*)		▶	542	540
d. Free or Nominal Rate Distribution (By Mail and Outside the Mail)	(1)	Free or Nominal Rate Outside-County Copies Included on PS Form 3541	73	62
	(2)	Free or Nominal Rate In-County Copies Included on PS Form 3541		
	(3)	Free or Nominal Rate Copies Mailed at Other Classes Through the USPS (e.g. First-Class Mail)		
	(4)	Free or Nominal Rate Distribution Outside the Mail (Carriers or other means)		
e. Total Free or Nominal Rate Distribution (*Sum of 15d (1), (2), (3) and (4)*)		▶	73	62
f. Total Distribution (*Sum of 15c and 15e*)		▶	615	602
g. Copies not Distributed (*See instructions to publishers #4 (page #3)*)		▶	357	359
h. Total (*Sum of 15f and g*)		▶	972	961
i. Percent Paid (*15c divided by 15f times 100*)			88.13%	89.70%

16. Publication of Statement of Ownership
If the publication is a general publication, publication of this statement is required. Will be printed in the **December 2010** issue of this publication. ☐ Publication not required

17. Signature and Title of Editor, Publisher, Business Manager, or Owner

Stephen R. Bushing

Stephen R. Bushing – Fulfillment/Inventory Specialist   Date September 15, 2010

I certify that all information furnished on this form is true and complete. I understand that anyone who furnishes false or misleading information on this form or who omits material or information requested on the form may be subject to criminal sanctions (including fines and imprisonment) and/or civil sanctions (including civil penalties).

PS Form 3526, September 2007 (Page 2 of 3)

Moving?

Make sure your subscription moves with you!

To notify us of your new address, find your **Clinics Account Number** (located on your mailing label above your name), and contact customer service at:

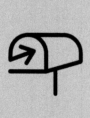

Email: journalscustomerservice-usa@elsevier.com

800-654-2452 (subscribers in the U.S. & Canada)
314-447-8871 (subscribers outside of the U.S. & Canada)

Fax number: 314-447-8029

Elsevier Health Sciences Division
Subscription Customer Service
3251 Riverport Lane
Maryland Heights, MO 63043

ELSEVIER

Printed and bound by CPI Group (UK) Ltd, Croydon, CR0 4YY

03/10/2024

01040357-0012